D0086708

Administrative Topics in Athletic Training

CONCEPTS TO PRACTICE

Administrative Topics in Athletic Training

CONCEPTS TO PRACTICE

Gary L. Harrelson, EdD, ATC

Director, Organizational Development and Education

DCH Health System

Tuscaloosa, Alabama

Greg Gardner, EdD, ATC, LAT

Clinical Associate Professor

Associate Director, School of Nursing

University of Tulsa

Tulsa, Oklahoma

Andrew P. Winterstein, PhD, ATC

Associate Clinical Professor

Program Director—ATEP

Department of Kinesiology

University of Wisconsin–Madison

Madison, Wisconsin

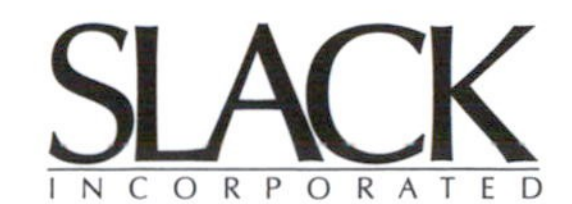

www.slackbooks.com

ISBN: 978-1-55642-739-8

Administrative Topics in Athletic Training: Concepts to Practice Instructor's Manual is also available from SLACK Incorporated. Don't miss this important companion to *Administrative Topics in Athletic Training: Concepts to Practice*. To obtain the *Instructor's Manual*, please visit http://www.efacultylounge.com

SLACK Incorporated uses a review process to evaluate submitted material. Prior to publication, educators or clinicians provide important feedback on the content that we publish. We welcome feedback on this work.

Published by: SLACK Incorporated
6900 Grove Road
Thorofare, NJ 08086 USA
Telephone: 856-848-1000
Fax: 856-853-5991
www.slackbooks.com

Contact SLACK Incorporated for more information about other books in this field or about the availability of our books from distributors outside the United States.

Library of Congress Cataloging-in-Publication Data

Administrative topics in athletic training : concepts to practice / edited by Gary Harrelson, Greg Gardner, and Andrew Winterstein.
p. ; cm.
Includes bibliographical references and index.
ISBN 978-1-55642-739-8 (alk. paper)
1. Physical education and training--Administration. I. Harrelson, Gary L. II. Gardner, Greg, 1960- III. Winterstein, Andrew P., 1962-
[DNLM: 1. Sports Medicine--organization & administration. 2. Allied Health Personnel--organization & administration. 3. Leadership. 4. Professional Role. QT 261 A238 2009]
GV343.5.A365 2009
796.06'9--dc22
2009003393

Last digit is print number: 10 9 8 7 6 5 4 3 2

DEDICATION

Dedicated to Christi, my best friend for life.
There is no one I respect and cherish more than you.
Greg Gardner, EdD, ATC, LAT

To my mentor and friend Jim Gallaspy who taught me that athletic training was not solely about the science but also about how you treat people and build relationships.
I am forever indebted to you for serving as my father away from home for many years.
Also, to Jerry Rhea and the late Roy Don Wilson whom I had the privilege to work under. I still marvel, through my memories, over how you managed the athletes as well as the people around you.
Gary L. Harrelson, EdD, ATC

This text is dedicated to three of my organization and administration mentors:
Donald McCarty, Jacob Stampen, and my "Rabbi" Brad Sherman.
They serve as my standard for professionalism and are, above all, gentlemen.
Of course, Barb.
Andrew P. Winterstein, PhD, ATC

CONTENTS

ABOUT THE AUTHORS

Gary L. Harrelson, EdD, ATC received his bachelor's of science in athletic training, master's of science in exercise physiology, and EdD in administration and teaching all from the University of Southern Mississippi. He is the Director of Organizational Development and Education (ODE) for the DCH Health System in Tuscaloosa, Alabama. In his current role with the DCH Health System, he is responsible for positioning ODE as a strategic partner with many of the system's stakeholders. The Department of ODE has been a catalyst for meaningful organizational development innovations in such areas as employee training and development, large scale change initiatives, performance improvement, and strategic planning processes. Gary is trained as a Gestalt Organizational Systems Development intervener where he contracts with individuals, intact work groups, and cross-functional teams to support them in accomplishing their mission and building relationships. Gary was instrumental in the implementation of Web-based training for the health system as well as being the co-developer and facilitator of a nationally recognized leadership development program by the American Hospital Association in 2002 as a "model program" for leadership development. As a result of his position within the DCH Health System, he either directly or indirectly supports the training and development initiatives across multiple healthcare professions.

Since his certification as an athletic trainer in 1985, Gary has worked as an athletic trainer in multiple settings, including high school, clinic, collegiate, and professional sports. Gary has taught in the athletic training curriculums at the University of Alabama and the University of Southern Mississippi. He was an associate editor for the *Journal of Athletic Training* and *Athletic Therapy Today.* Additionally, he is the coauthor of *Physical Rehabilitation of the Injured Athlete, Third Edition* and *Principles of Pharmacology for Athletic Trainers* as well as a CD-ROM, *Joint Mobilization*, and an 8-video series on evaluation. He has authored numerous articles and made many professional presentations at the state, regional, and national levels as well as internationally.

Gary spends his spare time reading, writing, and bicycling. In 2007, he rode the entire Natchez Trace Parkway (444 miles) on his bicycle in just over 4 days. He has been married to his wife, Lisa, for over 20 years and they have one son, Noah.

Greg Gardner, EdD, ATC, LAT is a Clinical Associate Professor of Athletic Training and Associate Director of the School of Nursing at the University of Tulsa. Dr. Gardner completed his bachelor's degree at the University of Wyoming and holds a master's degree from the University of Arizona. In 1995, Dr. Gardner completed his doctoral work at the University of Southern Mississippi. Dr. Gardner has extensive experience as an athletic trainer and has been a certified athletic trainer for 25 years. His career includes work at the high school, small college, and major college levels. Dr. Gardner served on the JRC-AT and remained with that group as the transition to Commission on Accreditation of Athletic Training Education (CAATE) was completed. In November 2008, Dr. Gardner was elected the first President of the CAATE and began serving in that capacity in 2009.

Andrew P. Winterstein, PhD, ATC is an associate clinical professor in the Department of Kinesiology at the University of Wisconsin–Madison, where he currently serves as the program director of their CAATE accredited undergraduate athletic training education program. He also maintains an affiliate appointment in the Department of Orthopedics and Rehabilitation in the School of Medicine and Public Health. Dr. Winterstein has coordinated the athletic training education efforts since 1999 and has been at the University of Wisconsin since 1986. He provided clinical care as part of the athletic training staff in the Division of Intercollegiate Athletics for 14 years before moving over to direct the AT education program. A 1984 graduate of the University of Arizona with a Bachelor of Science degree in Secondary Education and Biology, Andy has had a variety of athletic training and educational experiences.

Prior to his appointment at the University of Wisconsin–Madison, Andy was a graduate assistant at the University of Oregon in Eugene. At the University of Oregon, he earned a Masters of Science in Applied Physiology and Athletic Training. In 1994, Andy received his Doctorate in Educational Administration with an emphasis in higher education and sports medicine related issues from the University of Wisconsin–Madison. Dr. Winterstein's academic interests include studying emerging technologies and their use in teaching and learning, medical humanities and their application to athletic training education, and the Scholarship of Teaching and Learning (SoTL). His papers and abstracts have appeared in the *Journal of Athletic Training, Athletic Therapy Today,* and *Athletic Training and Sports Health Care.* He has been privileged to make numerous professional presentations at the state, regional, and national level.

A certified member of the National Athletic Trainers' Association since 1985, and certified member of the Wisconsin Athletic Trainers' Association, Dr. Winterstein is active in many aspects of athletic training. He serves as a reviewer for the *Journal of Athletic Training*, is a reviewer and member of the editorial board for the *Journal of Athletic Training Education* and *Athletic Training and Sports Health Care*, and has served on several state, regional, and national committees. Dr. Winterstein has received numerous awards including the 2008 Great Lakes Athletic Training Association Outstanding Educator Award, 2007 Wisconsin Athletic Trainers Association Outstanding Educator Award, and the 2006 UW-Madison School of Education Distinguished Service Award. He and his colleagues are three-time winners of the NATA Educational Multimedia Committee award for educational innovations and have been awarded the MERLOT Classics Award for exemplary on-line learning objects. In addition to this text, he is the author of the *Athletic Training Student Primer: A Foundation for Success* published by SLACK Incorporated.

In his spare time, Andy enjoys fly fishing, fly tying, reading, and writing. He resides in Madison, Wisconsin with his wife, Barb.

CONTRIBUTING AUTHORS

Brian Anderson, ATC (Chapter 9)
President
Collegiate Sports Medicine Foundation
Boca Raton, FL

Gina M. Delmont, MPA, ATC (Chapter 4)
Director of Clinical Operations
Midwest Orthopaedic Institute
Sycamore, IL

Tim McGuine, PhD, ATC (Chapter 7)
Senior Athletic Trainer
Research Coordinator
University of Wisconsin Health Sports Medicine
Madison, WI

Jill H. Murphy, MPT, LAT, ATC, CSCS (Chapter 8)
Affinity Health System
Oshkosh, WI
Department of Kinesiology
University of Wisconsin–Oshkosh
Oshkosh, WI

William A. Pitney, EdD, ATC (Chapter 12)
Associate Professor
Department of Kinesiology and Physical Education
College of Education
Northern Illinois University
DeKalb, IL

Elizabeth Swann, PhD, ATC (Chapter 9)
Director of Athletic Training Education
Nova Southeastern University
Fort Lauderdale, FL

FOREWORD

New practitioner to his or her mentor or supervisor:

"How did I get myself into this situation and what can I do to solve it?"

These words have been spoken by most if not all athletic training students and professionals as they have advanced through their career and need additional managerial skills. This may have been due to having been placed into a role for which they were not prepared or were unaware of the associated responsibilities, ranging from preparing a first time budget or resolving an interpersonal conflict. From a personal perspective, I have been asked this question many times in my roles as a head athletic trainer, clinical supervisor, department chair, academic advisor, or committee chair. While I have been able to refer individuals to portions of other texts, they do not compare to the approach of comprehensive information offered in *Administrative Topics in Athletic Training: Concepts to Practice*.

The authors of *Administrative Topics in Athletic Training: Concepts to Practice* have in essence "been there and done that." Their wealth of experience has culminated in the production of a book that is useful for students, novice practitioners working to establish themselves in a new position within the profession, as well as the current practitioner. The insights provided allow the student or inexperienced practitioner to grasp administrative concepts and implement strategies that allow for administrative maturity. For the seasoned practitioner, the text will serve as a valuable resource when one experiences a change in position or responsibilities that include integration of additional administrative knowledge and skills. Tools such as case studies, sidebars, and realistic examples are provided, allowing for problem solving through critical thinking on the part of the reader. Topics such as hiring and employment practices, medical documentation, risk management, fiscal management, planning, evaluation, socialization, and facility design assist in rounding out a comprehensive text for classroom and individual use.

The 3 authors have collaborated to draw on the strengths of each individual's experience, which is evident to those who have practiced with them clinically or administratively. Their combined service to the profession of athletic training through national association committee seats, scholarly publications, and professional presentations speaks highly of their recognized ability to lead, manage, and mentor. The strength of their experience is further contained with their association and employment in a wide variety of clinical settings ranging from hospitals, clinics, and secondary schools to National Collegiate Athletic Association (NCAA) Division I athletics. As administrators, knowledge is provided from the private health care sector, as program directors in undergraduate and graduate athletic training education programs, head athletic trainers, and within the hierarchy of academia in health sciences. As an outcome, the text relates to the various practice settings for athletic trainers and creates a basis for usability in each of these practice settings.

While the text may not solve the dilemma of how we place ourselves in administrative quandaries we are unprepared for, it will provide the tools to assist us to resolve the situation at hand. I encourage all athletic trainers to add *Administrative Topics in Athletic Training: Concepts to Practice* to their professional library.

Peter Koehneke, MS, ATC
Professor and Director
Athletic Training Education Program
Canisius College
Buffalo, New York

PREFACE

The Organization and Administration National Athletic Trainers' Association (NATA) competency domain provides somewhat of a departure from the other domains, which are clinically oriented. When it comes to how well athletic trainers are prepared for specific aspects of their job, the area of organization and administration often leaves new professionals wishing they had received more instruction. Practicing athletic trainers often cite this domain as a general weakness in their preparation, and it is frequently self-identified as a continuing education need. Athletic training educators who teach in this area have often pulled materials from other sources to supplement the few texts dedicated to this subject. It is an interesting area and one that many new athletic training graduates may not attend to since it may be difficult for them to connect to given that it is a departure from the clinical side of athletic training, which is one of the main reasons a student has chosen the profession to start with, and typically undergraduate students do not have the experience to ground themselves in these concepts, thus connecting with the material may be difficult.

Administrative Topics in Athletic Training: Concepts to Practice bridges this instructional gap by providing a text that is authored by 3 individuals who have a long tenure in athletic training in multiple settings and numerous leadership roles. Where they felt their knowledge base and expertise were not adequate, they sought subject matter experts in those areas to give greater depth to the material. The reader will find a text with numerous examples, case studies, boxes, tables, etc instead of page after page of narrative text. Every chapter has activities and/or case studies at the end to aid the learner in synthesis of the material, make "real world" application, and promote learner-centered higher order thinking. There is also an online instructor's manual that contains test questions, slides, and additional activities that the instructor may want to use as a part of his or her teaching methodology. *Administrative Topics in Athletic Training* addresses the multiple settings in which athletic trainers practice as evidenced by Chapter 6, which addresses issues in educational settings and Chapter 7, which explores issues in clinical settings as well as issues common to outreach services found in the clinical environment. Chapters 3 and 9 relate directly to finances by addressing budgeting and reimbursement. Chapter 2 focuses on risk management and Chapter 5 addresses ethical practice issues. Attention is given to personnel management via chapters on human resources and employment issues (Chapters 4 and 12, respectively). Chapters 10 and 11 cover organizational skills and performance improvement. Chapter 8 presents medical record keeping. Unique to this type of text is Chapter 12, which addresses organizational and professional socialization issues.

While the primary audience for this text is the entry-level athletic training student, students enrolled in graduate athletic training education programs may also find this text beneficial to their study. The text will also serve as a resource for those engaged in the delivery of athletic training services, both novice and experienced, as the basic tenets of sound administrative practice remain unchanged, regardless of the career stage of the practitioner.

LEADERSHIP AND MANAGEMENT

OBJECTIVES

At the end of this chapter, the reader will be able to:

- Compare and contrast the difference between manager and leader
- Identify the qualities/behaviors of an effective leader
- Explain emotional intelligence (EI) and why it is an important characteristic
- Differentiate between power and authority
- Explain how Theory X and Theory Y assumptions about people emerge as a part of a leader's pattern of behavior
- Compare and contrast 3 different leadership models: managerial grid, situational leadership, and exemplary leadership practices
- Explain the leader's role as a change agent
- Recognize and categorize patterns of resistance to change and apply the correct intervention depending on the level of resistance
- Employ Bridges' Transition Model as a framework for a change effort

Leadership is an AWESOME responsibility! Many of the skills and behaviors that make people successful and certainly make leaders great are not generally taught through a formal education process, yet they are core leader competencies. So how are these skills learned? Generally, through the modeling of others. The adage, "Great leaders are born and not made" is not necessarily true. While there are people who have the innate characteristics and behaviors to be a successful leader, the behaviors that have been found to translate to successful leadership can be learned if one is willing to change. Much has been written about leadership and leadership qualities, and it is far beyond the scope of this chapter to explore this in depth. The purpose of this chapter is to give you an overview of leadership and how it differs from management, several leadership models, and how a leader serves as a change agent for him- or herself, others, and organizations.

LEADERSHIP VERSUS MANAGEMENT

There is a difference between being a manager and being a leader. Table 1-1 compares and contrasts the two on several different dimensions in an attempt to differentiate them. Warren Bennis's classic quote, "Leaders are people who do the right thing; managers are people who do things right" seems to serve as a demarcation point between the two. In my own interpretation of the literature and experience, I find management to be more focused on the task or getting the work done (see Figure 1-4) with very little concern for the people doing the work. The leader has the capability of not treating the task and people as an "either/or" choice but rather as an "and." He or she understands that both are important for success and to treat one as more important than the other will result in experiencing the downside of neglecting the other.

Table 1-1

A Contrast Between Managers and Leaders

	Managers	Leaders
Necessary characteristics	Persistence, tough mindedness, intelligence, analytical ability, tolerance, goodwill	Imagination, ability to communicate, creativity, readiness to take risks, willingness to use power to influence the thoughts and actions of others
Attitudes toward goals	Have impersonal goals that arise from organizational necessity, respond to ideas	Have personal active goals; shape ideas; seek to change what people think is desirable, possible, or necessary
Conceptions of work	Formulate strategies; make decisions; manage conflict; negotiate, bargain, compromise, balance; limit choices	Create excitement; develop fresh approaches to problems; open up issues; project ideas into images that excite and then develop choices that give the projected images substance
Relations with others	Prefer working with others, with low level of emotional involvement in these relationships; role oriented; concerned with how to get things done	Intuitive, emphatic, intensive; concerned with what events and decisions mean to people
Creating an agenda	Planning and budgeting—establishing detailed steps and timetables for achieving needed results, and then allocating the resources necessary to make them happen	Establishing direction—developing a vision of the future, often the distant future, and strategies for producing the changes needed to achieve that vision
Developing a human network for achieving the agenda	Organizing and staffing—establishing some structure for accomplishing plan requirements, staffing that structure with individuals, delegating responsibility and authority for carrying out the plan, providing policies and procedures to help guide people, and creating methods or systems to monitor imple mentation	Aligning people—communicating the direction by words and deeds to all those whose cooperation may be needed so as to influence the creation of teams and coalitions that understand the vision and strategies, and accept their validity
Execution	Controlling and problem solving—monitoring results versus plan in some detail, identifying deviations, and then planning and organizing to solve these problems	Motivating and inspiring—energizing people to overcome major political, bureaucratic, and resource barriers to change by satisfying very basic, but often unfulfilled, human needs
Outcomes	Produces a degree of predictability and order and has the potential of consistently producing key results expected by various stake holders (eg, for customers, always being on time; for stockholders, being on budget)	Produces change, often to a dramatic degree, and has the potential of producing extremely useful change (eg, new products that customers want, new approaches to labor relations that help make a firm more competitive)

Both concern for work and concern for people are interdependent to each other, not independent. This relationship is referred to as a polarity.[1] Incidentally, the term *total quality management* (TQM) used in the 1970s and 1980s has nothing to do with defining a manager or his or her qualities. Rather it is a quality philosophy that attempts to reduce defects and can be considered a management tool (see Chapter 11).

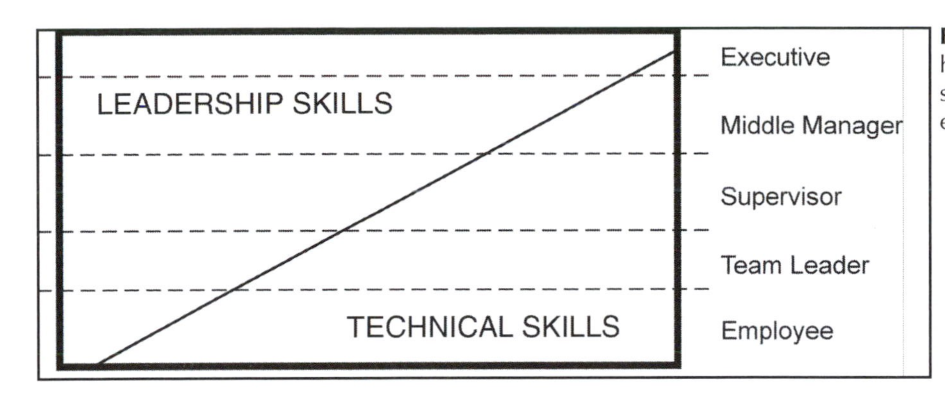

Figure 1-1. As one moves up in the hierarchy of an organization, technical skills become less important and leadership skills become more vital.

What Is a Polarity?

Polarities are a set of opposites that cannot function well independently. The two sides of the polarity are interdependent; you cannot choose one as a "solution" and neglect the other. You do not solve a polarity, you manage it. You cannot choose one pole over the other. It is not an "either/or," but rather an "and." The objective of managing a polarity is to get the best of both opposites while avoiding the limits of each. Other examples of polarities include: reduced cost and improved quality, customer service and financial viability, individual recognition and team recognition, and work and life balance.

There has long been this debate over whether leaders are made or born. While it is true that some people are born with the innate qualities that make them leaders, it is also true that the qualities, skills, and behaviors that make a successful leader can be learned if one is interested in changing his or her behavior.

> *The most dangerous leadership myth is that leaders are born—that there is a genetic factor to leadership. This myth asserts that people simply either have certain charismatic qualities or not. That's nonsense; in fact, the opposite is true. Leaders are made rather than born.*
>
> Warren Bennis

Leadership Qualities

Effective leaders possess qualities and competencies that impact others in a way in which they choose to follow them. The definitions for leadership are as numerous as the scholars that have written about it. John Maxwell[2,3] simply defines leadership as the ability to influence others. In order to have that influence there are behaviors that leaders engage in that cause others to allow themselves to be influenced by them. This does not necessarily come from positional power since we allow ourselves to be influenced by others daily. This section focuses on some of the qualities, characteristics, and behaviors that make a successful leader.

The interesting practice, at least in health care, is that we tend to promote the best clinician and they get promoted into incompetence. Just because someone is an excellent clinician does not mean that he or she will be a successful leader. The reason for this is the skills that made him or her a clinical "super star" are not the same set of skills that will make him or her an effective leader. Figure 1-1 depicts this change in skill sets that must occur in order to be an effective leader. Note that the higher you go in the organizational hierarchy, the fewer clinical/technical skills that are required.

A successful leader must have a heightened awareness about his or her strengths and weaknesses, his or her habitual patterns of behavior, and the impact he or she has on others. There are several ways to heighten awareness, including scanning yourself, scanning others for clues, and seeking feedback from others and/or behavioral instruments/assessments. We all can find ourselves on the competence continuum in Figure 1-2. We all have skills and behaviors that we are good at and aware of (conscious competence). There are also some things we are good at, but we are not aware of our proficiency (unconscious competence). Sometimes these are just things we do naturally (without thinking) such as listening with empathy and encouraging others. Conversely, there are things we are not good at but we do not have a clue that we are not good at them. As a matter of fact, we might believe that we are good at them (unconscious incompetence). An example might be cooking. We believe we are wonderful cooks, yet the recipients of the food believe differently. Then there are those things we are not good at but we are aware of our incompetence (conscious incompetence). The cooking example could also apply here. We know we are not good cooks.

Ideally, our awareness can be heightened around what we are unconsciously incompetent at through

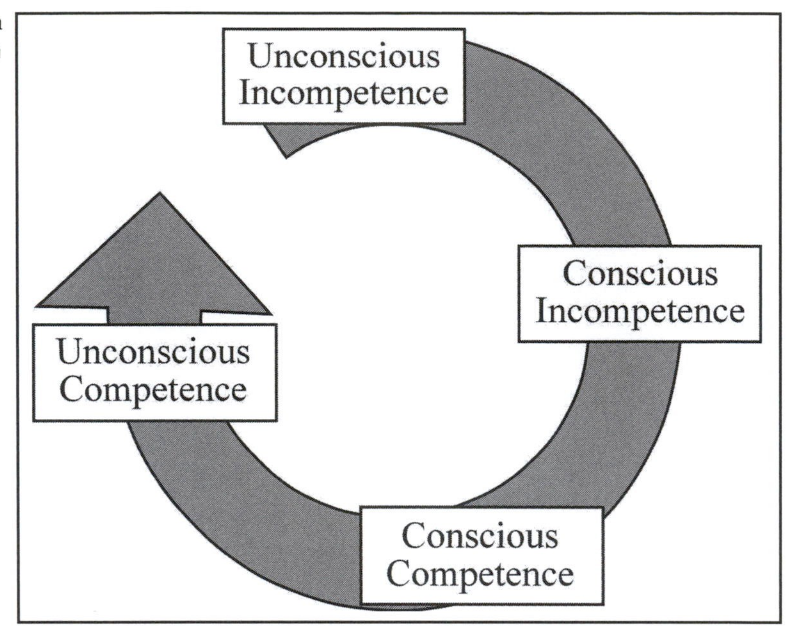

Figure 1-2. When learning a new skill or behavior, a person follows a predictable pattern of moving from unconscious incompetence to unconscious competence.

feedback and since we are now aware of it and believe it, we move to consciously incompetent. Then we can decide if we want to change to become consciously competent and then ultimately, once the skill or behavior becomes a part of us (automated or habitual), we move to unconsciously competent. This model serves as the underpinnings of most leadership development programs and can apply to learning any new skill or behavior. The goal is to heighten people's awareness of their "blind spots" and then help them make conscious choices about what they would like to do with their new awareness.

There are many leadership models and with those models come the qualities, characteristics, and behaviors that successful leaders possess. Table 1-2 gives a sampling of these from 5 authors. While the language to describe characteristics of successful leaders and the segmentation of these characteristics might be different, you will find many of the following words are used: influence, credibility, integrity, trustworthy, thinks in terms of "we" not "I," encourages others, innovative, visionary, catalyst for change, holds people accountable, empathic, respectful, caring, open-minded, and the descriptors can go on.

Maxwell[2] describes 5 levels of leadership (Figure 1-3) that occur in a hierarchical order or progression. Level 1 is labeled as position and this is given to you by your place in the organizational hierarchy and the rights that come with that. This can be also referred to as "positional power." People follow you because they have to. Level 2 is named permission and is related to a leader's ability to connect with people and develop relationships. People will follow you beyond your stated authority. People follow at this level because they want to. Level 3 is termed production. This is where success is sensed by most individuals. Most people like you and what you are doing and they follow because of what you have done for the organization. Level 4 is called people development and people follow because of what you have done for them. This is characterized by a commitment to developing leaders. Personhood is the label associated with Level 5. People follow because of who you are and what you represent. This stage is reserved for leaders who have spent years growing people and organizations. Few make it, but those who do are bigger than life. As this model implies, becoming the leader your subordinates and organization deserve is a lifelong journey.

Emotional Intelligence

While most leaders may be smart people, they also have a developed sense of EI as well. In general, EI implies that smarts are not enough to be successful as a leader or as part of an effective workforce. The term *emotional intelligence* was first coined in 1990 by Salovey and Mayer[4] and became mainstream language with the publication of Daniel Goleman's book, *Emotional Intelligence: Why It Can Matter More Than IQ* in 1995.[5] Trying to define EI can be difficult and attempting to measure one's EI quotient (EQ) is even more complicated. Box 1-1 contains 3 definitions of EI. As a relatively new area of psychological research, the definition of EI is constantly changing.

Skill training for a specific job can be taught, but a positive attitude, acceptable organizational behaviors, interpersonal relationship skills, and EI are much harder to teach and change and in some instances cannot be altered. Some scholars claim that EI is the largest single predictor of success in the workplace.[6,7]

Table 1-2

Overview of Leadership Qualities

Williams[8]	Covey[9]	Kouzes and Posner[10]	Zenger and Folkman[11]	Gebelein et al[12]
Vision Communicating the vision Getting buy-in People skills Be visible and available Listen Delegate Character Honesty Integrity Humility Competence Boldness Servant's heart	**7 Habits** Be proactive Begin with the end in mind Put first things first Think win/win Seek first to understand, then be understood Synergize Sharpen the saw **8th Habit** Find your voice and inspire others to find theirs	Challenge the process Inspire a shared vision Enable others to act Model the way Encourage the heart	Character Interpersonal skills Personal capability Focus on results Leading organizational change	Personal leadership Establish trust Show adaptability Learn continuously Thought leadership Analyze issues Make sound decisions Act strategically Leverage innovation Employ financial acumen Manage globally People leadership Increase cultural competence Manage conflict Establish relationships Write effectively Listen attentively Speak with impact Foster open communication Promote collaboration and teamwork Coach and develop others Build talent Engage and inspire Influence others Results leadership Lead courageously Show drive and initiative Manage change Manage and improve processes Build realistic plans Manage execution Focus on customers

Goleman's[5,6] model views EI as a wide array of competencies and skills that drive performance. He believes that the EI competencies are not innate talents but rather learned capabilities that must be worked on and developed to achieve outstanding performance. He hypothesizes that individuals are born with a general EI that determines their potential for learning emotional competencies. Goleman's[6,13]

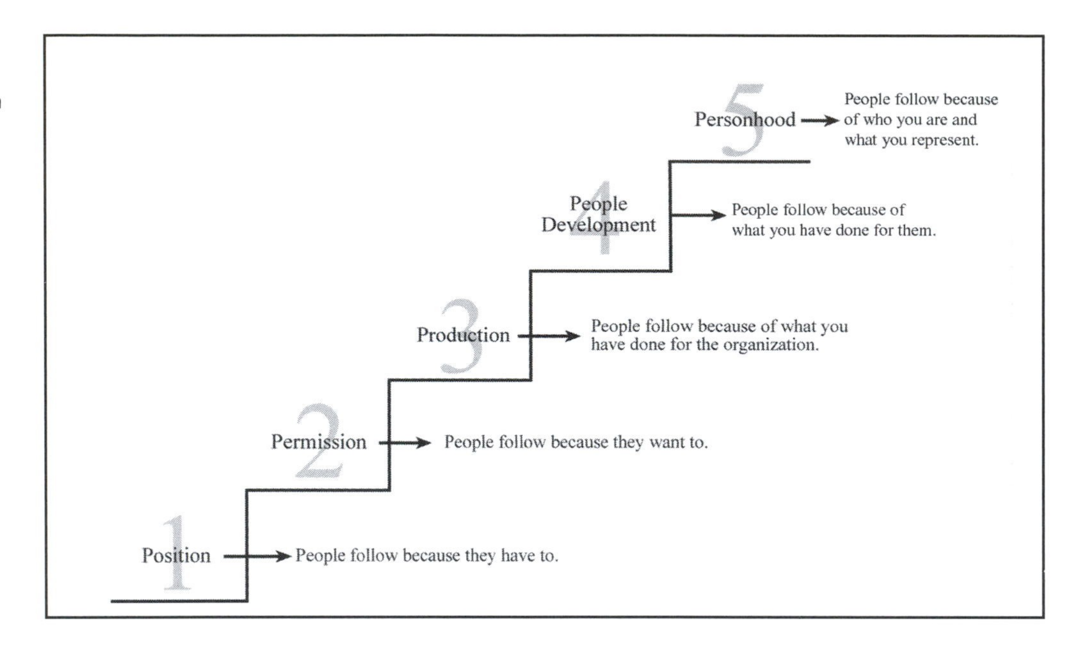

Figure 1-3. Five levels of leadership development based on the work of John Maxwell.

> **Box 1-1**
>
> **Emotional Intelligence Defined**
>
> EI describes an ability, capacity, or skill to perceive, assess, and manage the emotions of one's self, of others, and of groups.[7]
>
> "The ability to perceive emotion, integrate emotion to facilitate thought, understand emotion and to regulate emotions to promote personal growth."[4]
>
> The ability to manage ourselves and our relationships effectively consists of 4 fundamental capabilities: self-awareness, self-management, social awareness, and social skill.[5,6]

EI Competence Framework is summarized in Table 1-3. He segments the Competency Framework into 2 overarching categories: personal competencies that reflect how we manage ourselves, and social competencies that determine how we handle relationships. The competencies lie within each of these 2 categories.

Relative to the leadership qualities discussed above, you should see some overlap with the EI competencies and thus the case that a high EQ is as important, if not more important, than one's intellectual capital in determining one's leadership and workforce capabilities. It is no longer acceptable to be good or even exceptional at the technical components of your job; organizations are demanding that you must also be able to work well with others. EI enables leaders to understand and deal with their own internal responses, feelings, and moods. EI also yields the insight and skills for relating to and with other people. Specifically, EI leaders are self-aware, manage their own and others' emotions, are highly attuned to and skillful in managing the social environment, and have highly developed relationship skills.[14]

Power and Authority

Power is the potential to influence. French and Raven[15] defined 5 bases for power (Table 1-4). All five can be found to be active in all organizations. Legitimate, coercive, reward, and expert come because of the organizational position you hold, referred to as positional power. Referent power on the other hand is based on your personal characteristics and personality attributes, also known as personal power. While formal leaders have positional power, it is their personal power that makes them effective. Athletic trainers have legitimate power because of the position they hold; coercive and reward power over student athletic trainers, and expert power when assessing an athlete's injury and the ability to influence treatment options. Counterpower is the ability to influence the behavior of a superior, such as a coach or in a societal construct a physician, unless the physician holds a formal hierarchical position in the organization. Authority is the aspect of power, granted to either groups or individuals, that legitimizes the right of the group or individual to make decisions on behalf of others. It is how power is applied and without authority positional power would not exist.[16]

Table 1-3

The Emotional Competence Framework

Personal Competence	*Social Competence*
These competencies determine how we manage ourselves	These competencies determine how we handle relationships
Self-Awareness *Knowing one's internal states, preferences, resources, and intuitions* Emotional awareness: Recognizing one's emotions and their effects. Accurate self-assessment: Knowing one's strengths and limits. Self-confidence: A strong sense of one's self-worth and capabilities.	**Social Awareness** *Awareness of others' feelings, needs, and concerns* Empathy: Sensing others' feelings and perspectives, and taking an active interest in their concerns. Service orientation: Anticipating, recognizing, and meeting customers' needs. Developing others: Sensing others' development needs and bolstering their abilities. Leveraging diversity: Cultivating opportunities through different kinds of people. Political awareness: Reading a group's emotional currents and power relationships.
Self-Regulation *Managing one's internal states, impulses, and resources* Self-Control: Keeping disruptive emotions and impulses in check. Trustworthiness: Maintaining standards of honesty and integrity. Conscientiousness: Taking responsibility for personal performance. Adaptability: Flexibility in handling change. Innovation: Being comfortable with novel ideas, approaches, and new information.	**Social Skills** *Adeptness at inducing desirable responses in others* Influence: Wielding effective tactics for persuasion. Communication: Listening openly and sending convincing messages. Conflict management: Negotiating and resolving disagreements. Leadership: Inspiring and guiding individuals and groups. Change catalyst: Initiating or managing change. Building bonds: Nurturing instrumental relationships. Collaboration and cooperation: Working with others toward shared goals. Team capabilities: Creating group synergy in pursuing collective goals.
Self-Motivation *Emotional tendencies that guide or facilitate reaching goals* Achievement drive: Striving to improve or meet a standard of excellence. Commitment: Aligning with the goals of the group or organization. Initiative: Readiness to act on opportunities. Optimism: Persistence in pursuing goals despite obstacles and setbacks.	

Table 1-4

Five Bases for Power

Power	*Description*
Legitimate	Refers to an individual's power based on his or her position in the organization. You can demand compliance of certain people because such authority has been granted to you by the organization. The people over whom you exert legitimate power know that noncompliance would mean certain sanctions (eg, the loss of their jobs). Also referred to as positional power.
Referent	The ability to influence the behavior of another person is based on your personal traits. Can be based on charisma and interpersonal skills of the power holder, where others want to be identified with you.
Coercive	The ability to influence the behavior of someone else is based on fear. This fear can take many forms, such as fear of retribution, fear of punishment, or even the fear of appearing inadequate or incompetent.

(continued)

Table 1-4 (continued)

Five Bases for Power

Power	Description
Reward	The ability to grant rewards influences the behavior of another person. Rewards can be as simple as a smile of approval or as significant as a promotion.
Expert	The ability to influence the behavior of another person based on your expertise in some area. our expertise may be necessary for another person to do his or her job satisfactorily—or superbly; therefore, the person complies with your desires in order to receive your expertise.

Table 1-5

Theory X and Theory Y Assumptions

Theory X Assumptions About People	Theory Y Assumptions About People
Avoid work	Will work toward goal
Avoid responsibility	Will assume responsibility
Need direction	Can self-direct
Cannot make decisions	Can make decisions
Not achievement oriented	Want to achieve
Not dependable	Are dependable
Motivated by money	Motivated by interest or challenges
Not concerned with organization's needs	Are concerned with their organizations
Must be controlled	Want to be supported
Cannot change	Want to develop

LEADERSHIP MODELS

There are many leadership models described in the literature. The 4 models presented here were chosen because of their longevity, practicality, and associated available assessments for 3 of them. I believe that models are important in understanding and explaining some of the phenomena we experience daily, particularly in the behavioral sciences. Many times when we have a model to explain what we are experiencing, we are able to use the model to appreciate the experience and respond in a more productive way.

THEORY X AND THEORY Y

Theory X and Theory Y are based on the work of Douglas McGregor,[17] define 2 sets of assumptions about human nature, and have come to be applied as management styles. The Theories explain how assumptions affect people's attempts to influence the behavior of others—especially how they affect leaders' attitudes toward employees. This model is based on the premise that a leader's effectiveness can be traced to the leader's subtle, frequently subconscious assumptions about people. Table 1-5 lists the assumptions that characterize advocates of Theory X and Theory Y. This is not to say, of course, that all leaders believe entirely in Theory X or Theory Y. Most leaders probably believe that people are a combination of both, with a tendency to behave as one type. The leader's assumption about people impacts his or her style of leadership and has an impact on the environment and people he or she leads.

Theory X

The traditional view of people, which was widely held in the first half of the 20th century, was labeled "X" and based on the following set of assumptions[18]:

- The average human being has an inherent dislike for work and will avoid it if he or she can.
- Because of this human characteristic of dislike for work, most people must be coerced, controlled, directed, or threatened with punishment

to get them to put forth adequate effort toward the achievement of organizational objectives.

- The average human being prefers to be directed, wishes to avoid responsibility, has relatively little ambition, and wants security above all.

These assumptions about people in relationship to their work might seem somewhat antiquated today; however, Theory X assumptions about people are still alive in organizations and "play out" in very subtle and subconscious ways. Robinson[18] provides these examples:

> *...if we examine how organizations are structured and how policies, procedures, and work rules are established, we can see them (Theory X) operating. Job responsibilities are closely spelled out, goals are imposed without individual employee involvement or consideration, reward is contingent on working within the system, and punishment falls on those who deviate from the established rules. These factors all influence how people respond, but the underlying assumptions or reasons for them are seldom tested or even recognized as assumptions. The fact is that most people act as if their beliefs about human nature are correct and require no study or checking.*

Theory Y

Theory Y, which is not necessarily the opposite extreme of Theory X, is characterized by the following set of assumptions about the nature of people, which influences managerial behaviors[18]:

- The expenditure of physical and mental effort in work is as natural as play or rest.
- External control and threat of punishment are not the only means for bringing about effort toward organizational objectives. A person will exercise self-control in the service of objectives to which he or she is committed.
- Commitment to objectives is dependent on rewards associated with their achievement. The most important rewards are those that satisfy needs for self-respect and personal improvement.
- The average human being learns, under proper conditions, not only to accept, but to seek responsibility.
- The capacity to exercise a relatively high degree of imagination, ingenuity, and creativity in the solution of organizational problems is widely, not narrowly, distributed in the population.
- Under the conditions of modern industrial life, the intellectual potential of the average human being is only partially utilized.

This is not a soft approach to managing the human capital within an organization. Rather it can be viewed as a very demanding style; it sets high standards for all and expects people to reach for them.

The focus of a Theory Y manager is on the person as a growing, developing, learning being, while a Theory X manager views the person as static, fully developed, and capable of little change. A Theory X manager sets the parameters of his or her employees' achievements by determining their potential in light of negative assumptions. A Theory Y manager allows his or her people to test the limits of their capabilities and uses errors for learning better ways of operating rather than as clubs for forcing submission to the system. He or she structures work so that an employee can have a sense of accomplishment and personal growth. The motivation comes from the work itself and provides a much more powerful incentive than the external demands or directives imposed in the Theory X assumptions.[18] Theory X and Theory Y assumptions about people are summarized in Table 1-5. These assumptions about people can be detected in the next leadership model, the managerial grid.

Managerial Grid

The managerial grid is based on the work of Blake and Mouton[19] and provides a model for framing leader behavior based on the leader's concern for production and people. Production concerns center around accomplishing an assigned task or attaining desired results and people concerns address the needs, morale, capacities, etc, of the individuals being supervised.[20] By manipulating the concern for people (vertical axis) and concern for production (horizontal axis), the managerial grid provides 5 styles of leading associated with specific behavioral patterns (Figure 1-4). Each of these styles is based on different strategies for dealing with people and production and stems from personal beliefs about what is and what is not possible concerning the two.[20]

These styles are referred to numerically by where they fall on the grid as well as through word labeling. A "1" on either axis indicates a low concern and a "9" denotes a high concern. For example, a 1/9 style implies a low concern for production and a high concern for people. These 5 styles are referred to as follows[19,20]:

1. (9/1) Authoritarian or dictator
2. (1/9) Country club
3. (1/1) Burned out or impoverished
4. (5/5) Politician
5. (9/9) Team manager

The managerial grid is provocative in that it proposes one correct style and that is team manager. Any style other than that misses the mark.

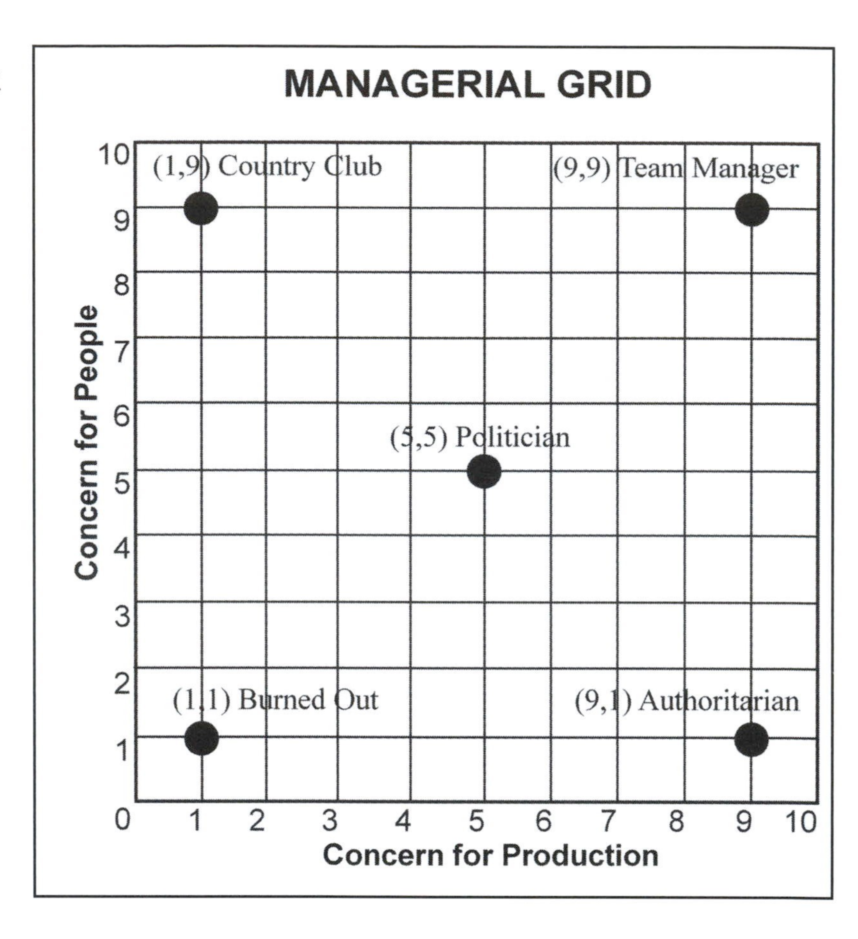

Figure 1-4. Managerial grid. (Adapted from Blake R, Mouton JS. *The New Managerial Grid.* Houston, TX: Gulf Publishing; 1978:11.)

A manager's style is a direct result of that person's particular beliefs about the relationship between people and production and is grounded in McGregor's Theory X and Theory Y assumptions (see previous section).[17,18] Some managers believe that the normal requirements for work and the basic needs of human beings are so different as to be opposed to one another. As a matter of fact, 3 of the 5 managerial styles depicted by the managerial grid stem from managers' personal perceptions that people and work "do not mix."[20]

9/1 Style: Authoritarian or Dictator

The primary concern for this style is output. The 9/1 manager views people only as contributors to production, and they are expected to carry out plans and directions given to them. They are not often required to understand why nor are they expected to contribute original ideas of their own.[20]

1/9 Style: Country Club

This management style is in direct opposition to the 9/1 style. The style focuses on people and their relationships and pays little attention to production need. In many ways, this style is contradictory to the very purposes of organizations but exists nonetheless.[20]

1/1 Style: Burned Out or Impoverished

This pattern of behavior seeks neither to attain any real production nor to establish sound relationships. The major goal is to stay out of trouble by avoiding risk and to meet only minimum requirements for both production and relationships. This style can be adopted by people who have been repeatedly passed over for promotion or realize they will not go any higher in the organization and instead of moving elsewhere they adopt the 1/1 pattern of behavior.[20]

5/5 Style: Politician

The 5/5 manager adopts a "middle of the road" stance, where compromise is his or her way of reconciling the perceived conflict between people and work. This manager still views the concern for people and concern for production as a dilemma that he or she has difficulty reconciling in his or her mind and thus this confusion shows up in his or her behaviors. While he or she believes it is important to be concerned about both people and production, he or she believes a manager cannot realistically hope to get the best from either one.[20]

9/9 Style: Team Manager

The 9/9 manager believes that work is healthy for people, that people have an innate need to work, and

Table 1-6

Characteristics of the Five Managerial Grid Styles

Dictator (9/1)	*Country Club (1/9)*	*Impoverished (1/1)*	*Politician (5/5)*	*Team Manager (9/9)*
Controlling Cuts people off Decides and then tells people what to do Decisions are final Demanding Expects compliance Fault finding Gets into win-lose fights Hard driving Has all the answers Impatient Interrogates Others keep their distance Overpowering Pushy Quick to blame Sees things in black/white terms Stubborn Taskmaster Tells people what to do but not why	Agreeable Appreciative Avoids negatives Cannot say no Deferential Dislikes disagreements Excessively complimentary Overly eager to help Over trusting Remorseful at unintended slights Says nice and thoughtful things Sensitive, easily hurt Supporting and comforting Sympathetic and soft Thrives on harmony Uncontroversial Unlikely to probe Waits to hear what others think before speaking Withholds controversial convictions Yields to gain approval	Apathetic Bystander Defers Disclaims responsibility Feedback does not register Gives up easily Hands-offish Inconspicuous Indifferent Keeps out of the way Lets things run their course Likely to miss new things that need to be done Neglects task responsibilities Neutral Noncommittal Noncontributor Putting in time Resigned Stays out of the line of fire Volunteers few opinions Waits for others to take action Weak follow-through Withdrawn	Accommodates Cautious Compromises Conformist Evasive when challenges Expedient Indirect Likes the tried and true Negotiates Prefers middle ground Prefers to act on precedent Pulls punches Sandwiches bad between good comments Soft-pedals agreements Stays on majority side Straddles issues Swallows convictions in the interest of progress Waffles Waits to see where others stand	Candid and forthright Confident Decisive Determined Enjoys working Fact-finder Focuses on real issues Follows through Gets issues into the open Has a "can do" spirit High standards Identifies underlying causes Innovative Open-minded Positive Priorities are clear Reflective Sets challenging goals Speaks mind Spontaneous Stands ground Stimulates participation Unselfish

that they must achieve some productive issue in order to feel good about themselves. This manager believes that people and production are not in conflict with each other, but that they are interdependent. They view people and production not as an "either/or" choice but as an "and." This is a core characteristic of an exemplary leader; he or she does a magnificent job of managing daily the concern for people and concern for production not as mutually exclusive opposites but interdependent to each other. This type of management style is not only concerned about employee morale but also does not permit unsatisfactory performance.[20]

Table 1-6 provides a summary of characteristics for each of the 5 managerial styles denoted in the managerial grid. The 9/9 style is the preferred or ideal style and those leaders that engage in this type of behavior do not view the concern for people and concern for production as being independent of each other, but rather realize the need to manage both of these dimensions to be successful. You cannot chose one over the other and be an exemplary leader. The Styles of Management Inventory (Telemetrics International, Waco, TX, www.telemetrics.com) is a self-assessment inventory based on the managerial grid concept developed by Blake and Mouton[19] and provides insight

Table 1-7

Summary of Directive and Supportive Behavior

	Directive Behavior	Supportive Behavior
Definition	The extent to which a leader engages in one-way communication, spells out the employee's role; tells the employee what to do, where to do it, when to do it, how to do it; and closely supervises performance.	The extent to which a leader engages in two-way communication, listens and provides support and encouragement, facilitates interaction, and involves the employee in decision making.
Actions	When using directive behavior, the leader: Sets goals or objectives Plans and organizes work in advance Identifies job priorities Clarifies the leader's and employee's roles Establishes time lines Determines methods of evaluation and checks work Teaches an employee how to do a specific task Supervises progress	When using supportive behavior, the leader: Encourages, reassures, and praises Listens Asks for suggestions or input Explains why Encourages self-reliant problem solving Makes information about the organization accessible Discloses information about self
Key words	When using directive behavior, you would: Structure Organize Teach Supervise	When using supportive behavior, you would: Encourage Listen Ask Explain

into your primary and secondary management styles based on the managerial grid model.

Situational Leadership

The situational leadership (SL) model described here is based on the work of Ken Blanchard[3] and is referred to as SLII and serves as a guide to choosing the leadership style(s) that will have the greatest probability of success for the specific person in a particular skill/task. The underpinnings of the SLII model are based on flexibility, diagnosis, and partnering for performance.[21]

Flexibility

Flexibility in this model refers to the leader's ability to manipulate the amount of and use appropriately 2 core behavioral sets: directive behavior and supportive behavior. Table 1-7 contrasts the difference between directive and supportive behavior. Based on altering the amount of directive behavior (low to high) and the amount of supportive behavior (low to high), 4 leadership styles are created that fall into 4 quadrants (Figure 1-5).

Directing (S1)

This behavior is known as "telling" because the behavior is highly directive with low support. The leader gives specific instructions about the skill/task and then closely observes as the employee perform it. This is best used when the person is a novice at the skill/task. It is basically telling and showing the employee how to do the skill/task with the person having little to no input on how it should be done. Decision making lies with the leader.

Coaching (S2)

This behavior is high both in directive and supportive behavior. The leader uses praise to reinforce those things the employee does correctly or almost correctly in the skill/task and may solicit suggestions from the employee but is still highly directive in telling the person how the task should be performed and why. The final decision rests with the leader.

Supporting (S3)

Supportive behavior is characterized by low directive and high supportive behavior. Here the leader's

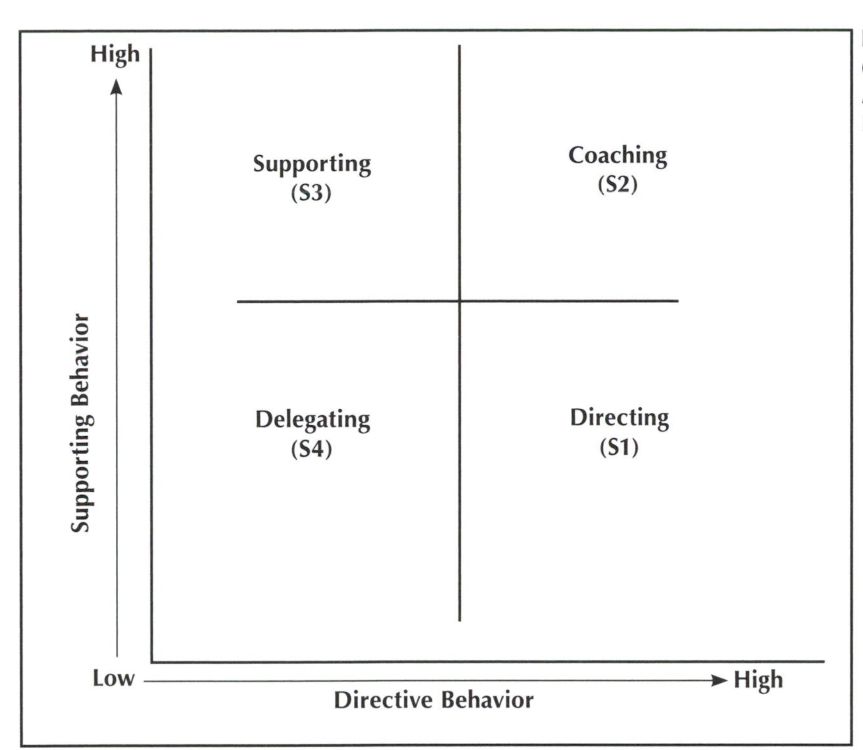

Figure 1-5. Situational leadership model. (Adapted from Blanchard K. *Situational Leadership II: The Article*. Escondido, CA: Ken Blanchard Co; 1994:4.)

behavior is more facilitative in nature and the employee is more involved in decision making and problem solving. Instead of telling the employee what he or she did correctly or incorrectly and how to fix it, the leader might pose questions such as, "What do you believe you did well?" "What do you believe you could improve upon next time?" and "How might you do it differently next time?" Decision making begins to shift from the leader to the employee.

Delegating (S4)

This behavior is low both in supportive and directive behavior. It is at this point that the employee has become proficient at the skill/task and should be able to perform it independently. Decision making is the responsibility of the employee with little if any input from the leader.

Table 1-8 summarizes the 4 leadership styles. While these leadership styles are generally grounded in the context of helping a person grow from a novice to expert on a given skill or task, this same philosophy (styles) can be used to help mold or change a person's behavior(s) in order to help assimilate him or her into an organization's culture. For this reason, although referred to as a leadership model at its core, it is a teaching model, and has been written about as such.[22]

Diagnosis

The SL model not only takes into account the leader's style but also the developmental level of the employee and consists of 4 developmental levels that correspond with the 4 leadership styles. The 4 development levels are determined by the amount (high or low) of competence and commitment the employee has for the task or skill to be learned. Competence is defined as the knowledge and skills a person brings to a skill/task. It can be developed over time with appropriate direction and support during the learning process. Commitment is a combination of an employee's motivation and confidence to learn a new skill/task. Motivation is the level of interest and enthusiasm the employee has for learning a particular skill. Conversely, confidence is characterized by an employee's self-assuredness, which translates into the extent to which an employee trusts his or her own ability to perform the skill/task.[21]

Developmental levels are labeled as D1, D2, D3, and D4 and are characterized by combinations of varying amounts of competence and commitment (Table 1-9). The goal is to progress a learner from D1 (a novice) to D4 (self-reliant person that can make decisions on his or her own). Low competence and high commitment characterize a D1 level. Although the person's confidence may be somewhat waning, he or she is eager to learn and is referred to as the enthusiastic beginner by Blanchard.[21]

The D2 level is referred to as the disillusioned learner[21] and is characterized by both low to some competence and low commitment. This occurs when the employee discovers that the skill/task is more difficult then he or she thought and he or she experiences frustration in trying to learn it, resulting in a decrease in his or her commitment.

Table 1-8

Overview of Situational Leadership II Leadership Styles

Style	Description	Behavior	Definition
Directing (S1)	Leader is in charge	High directive Low supportive	Leader provides specific instructions about roles and goals and closely supervises the employee's performance. Most decisions are made by the leader.
Coaching (S2)	The employee is more involved in decision making, but when push comes to shove, the leader decides	High directive High supportive	Leader explains decisions, solicits suggestions, praises behaviors that are approximately right, and continues to direct task accomplishment. Input is considered, although final decisions are made by the leader.
Supporting (S3)	The employee's role is to decide how the task is to be accomplished. The leader's role is to listen and provide assurance, support, resources, and ideas if requested.	High supportive Low directive	The leader and employee make decisions together. The role of the leader is to facilitate, listen, draw the associate out, encourage, and support.
Delegating (S4)	The employee decides how, when, where, and with whom the goal is to be accomplished.	Low supportive Low directive	Leader turns over responsibility for task accomplishment to the employee; the employee provides his or her own direction and support.

Table 1-9

Developmental Levels

Developmental Level	Competence	Commitment (Motivation and Confidence)
D4	High	High
D3	Moderate to high	Variable
D2	Low to some	Low
D1	Low	High

Adapted from Gardner G, Harrelson GL. Situational teaching: meeting the needs of the evolving learner. *Athletic Therapy Today.* 2002;7(5):18-22.

The D3 level is the self-doubt stage. The employee has moderate to high competence but variable commitment due to his or her lack of confidence. He or she has acquired the necessary knowledge and skill to perform the task but questions if he or she can perform it correctly on his or her own.

Finally, level D4 is characterized by both high competence and high commitment and is labeled by Blanchard[21] as the self-reliant achiever. The employee is capable of correctly performing a given skill/task independently of the leader.

Development level is skill specific, therefore allowing the employee to be at different developmental levels for different skills/tasks. It is generally beneficial to have someone guide the learning process as we learn new or different skills, tasks, or behaviors and we are all at many developmental levels for any given skill, task, or behavior.

Table 1-10

Matching Leader's Behavior With Developmental Level

If developmental level is...	Then use leadership style...
D1	Directing (S1)
D2	Coaching (S2)
D3	Supporting (S3)
D4	Delegating (S4)

Adapted from Gardner G, Harrelson GL. Situational teaching: meeting the needs of the evolving learner. *Athletic Therapy Today.* 2002;7(5):18-22.

Matching Leadership Style to Developmental Level

By knowing the employee's development level, a leader can match it to the appropriate amount of directive and supportive behavior (Table 1-10). For example, a leader who assesses an employee to be at a D1 level would use a directing leadership style (S1), and a D2-level assessment would get a coaching style (S2).

A directing style is used for employees at a D1 level because of the employee's lack of knowledge and skill. There is less need for support at this level because the person is eager to learn. Employees at a D2 level need the continued high directive behavior to help them develop competence and also high supportive behavior to offset the decrease in commitment they might experience as they struggle with the new skill/task or behavior.

As a learner becomes competent, the leader needs to reduce the amount of directive behavior because the employee should have acquired the knowledge and skills necessary to perform the skill/task but needs his or her confidence and self-esteem reinforced and maintained (D3 level).

The employee at the D4 level is both proficient and committed to the new skill, task, or behavior; thus, low directive and supportive behavior are needed from the leader. The person at a D4 level should be able to effectively perform the skill independently.

Partnering for Improvement

SLII is not something done to an employee by the leader, but rather something done *with* him or her. Teaching this model to employees can help improve communication between the leader and employee. Since determining the developmental level is not an exact science (but determined through observed performance), this dialogue is necessary to help the leader "hit the mark" with his or her leadership behavior.

Under- and over supervision occurs when the leader does not match his or her leadership style with the development level of the employee. Under supervision occurs when the leader is not as directive as he or she needs to be. An example would be when an employee who is at a D1 level is engaged by the leader with a supportive leadership style. Over supervision happens when the leader is too directive and should be more supportive. An example of this is when the leader uses a directing leadership style with an employee who is at a D4 level. Both examples result in "missing the mark" and lessen the chance for success. SLII is a developmental model to help people grow professionally and personally. Matching the leadership style and developmental level is critical to having the highest probability for success. A self-assessment inventory (Leader Behavior Analysis II) is available to help assess your primary and secondary leadership style and your developing leadership style(s) (The Ken Blanchard Companies, San Diego, CA, www.kenblanchard.com). Observer assessments are also available for this leadership model in which one can receive feedback from his or her leader, peers, and/or direct reports. These instruments are required to be administered by a facilitator that has been certified by The Ken Blanchard companies.

This model requires the leader to broaden his or her repertoire of leadership behaviors he or she uses to support the employee's growth. The leader must alter the amount of supporting and directive behavior based on the specific skill/task that is being acquired or behavior modified.

Give a man a fish and you feed him for a day.
Teach a man to fish and you feed him for a lifetime.
Chinese Proverb

Exemplary Leadership Practices

The exemplary leadership practices model is based on the work of James Kouzes and Barry Posner and described in their book *The Leadership Challenge*.[10] Their research, which included interviewing thousands of leaders in regards to their personal best leadership experiences, revealed 5 patterns of behavior that were seen in successful leaders who get extraordinary things done in an organization. They found leadership is not about personality, but about practice. These 5 practices of exemplary leaders include the following:

1. Model the way
2. Inspire a shared vision
3. Challenge the process
4. Enable others to act
5. Encourage the heart

These 5 practices are not just available to a select few, but they are available to anyone in any organization or situation who wants to make a difference in the lives of people and organizations and achieve extraordinary results. Table 1-11 summarizes the 5 practices and each practice is examined further below.

Model the Way

Exemplary leaders know that if they want to gain commitment and achieve the highest standards, they must be models of the behavior they expect of others.[10] In order to model the way, you must open up to others and let them know what you are thinking, what you believe in, and what values guide you and then give voice to these beliefs and values. Words will only take you so far; your actions and deeds must be congruent with your spoken beliefs and values. Modeling the way is essentially about earning the right and the respect to lead through direct individual involvement and action.[10]

You must be the change you wish to see in the world.
Mohandas K. Gandhi

Inspire a Shared Vision

Exemplary leaders have a vision of what the future can be and the ability to communicate that vision to others as well as the confidence in their abilities to make something happen, to change the way things are, and to create something that no one else has ever created before. People move toward the pictures they create in their mind. Leaders must have and communicate a compelling picture and then enlist people to move toward it. In order to enlist support, leaders must have intimate knowledge of people's dreams, hopes, aspirations, visions, and values. Leaders breathe life into the hopes and dreams of others and enable them to see the exciting possibilities that the future holds.[10]

In the absence of a great dream pettiness prevails.
Peter Senge

It is always important to have something yet to do in life.
Victor Frankel

Challenge the Process

Leaders are pioneers who are willing to step out into the unknown and take risks. They challenge the status quo, searching for opportunities to innovate, grow, and improve. Many times the innovations come not from themselves, but from listening to others and recognizing good ideas; supporting those ideas; and challenging the system to move, change, and adopt these ideas. In order to challenge the process, leaders must be willing to experiment and know that failure is a possibility and realize that learning can be gleaned from failed experiments. Leaders are learners and learn from their failures as well as their successes.[10]

Experience is simply the name we give our mistakes.
Oscar Wilde

I have not failed. I've just found 10,000 ways it won't work. (in reference to the light bulb)
Thomas Edison

Enable Others to Act

Leaders know that achieving a vision does not come through the actions of one person but rather through the efforts and commitment of others. Exemplary leaders foster collaboration and trust. They create an environment that allows others to do good work and feel empowered by making people feel strong and capable, to achieve more than they thought they were capable of. When leadership is founded on trust and confidence, people take risks, make changes, and keep organizations and movement alive. Through that relationship, leaders turn their workforce into leaders themselves.[10]

To help others become something that they could never on their own become, is putting value into that other person.
Unknown

Table 1-11

Overview of Exemplary Leadership Practices

Practice	Characteristics	Commitments Required
Model the way	A leader who models the way: Is clear about his or her values and beliefs Keeps people and projects on course by consistently behaving according to these values Models the behaviors that he or she expects from others Plans thoroughly and divides projects into achievable steps, thus creating opportunities for small wins Focuses on key priorities, which makes it easier for others to achieve goals	A leader who models the way must be committed to: Setting an example Planning small wins
Inspire a shared vision	A leader who inspires a shared vision: Looks toward and beyond the horizon Envisions the future with a positive and hopeful outlook Is expressive; his or her genuine nature attracts followers Shows others how mutual interests can be met through commitment to a common purpose	A leader who inspires a shared vision must be committed to: Envisioning the future Enlisting the support of others
Challenge the process	A leader who challenges the process: Is a pioneer Seeks out new opportunities and is willing to change the status quo Is innovative, experimental, and explores ways to improve his or her organization Views mistakes as learning experiences and is prepared to meet any challenge that confronts him or he	A leader who challenges the process must be committed to: Searching for opportunities Experimenting and taking risks
Enable others to act	A leader who enables others to act: Instills followers with spirit-nurturing relationships based on mutual trust Stresses collaborative goals Actively involves others in planning and permits others to make their own decisions Makes sure followers feel strong and capable	A leader who enables others to act must be committed to: Fostering collaboration
Encourage the heart	A leader who encourages the heart: Recognizes accomplishments and contributes to the organization's vision Lets others know that their efforts are appreciated Expresses pride in his or her team's accomplishments Finds ways to celebrate accomplishments Nurtures team spirit, which enables people to sustain continued efforts	A leader who encourages the heart must be committed to: Recognizing contributions Celebrating accomplishments

There is no more noble occupation in the world than to assist another human being to succeed.
Alan McGinnis

Encourage the Heart

Exemplary leaders encourage others to dream, to act, and to take risks; moreover, they encourage people when things get tough. They create a culture that fosters appreciation through recognition and celebration, linking rewards to performance. Leaders that encourage the heart are capable of not only correcting poor performance, but also looking for what is right and encouraging others to achieve more. Leaders know that celebrations and rituals, when done with authenticity and from the heart, build a strong sense of collective identity and community spirit that can carry a group through tough times.[10,23]

Catch someone doing something right.
Ken Blanchard and Spencer Johnson

People who produce good results feel good about themselves.
Ken Blanchard

From the work of Kouzes and Posner[10] we learn that leadership is an identifiable set of skills and practices that are available to all of us, not just a few charismatic men and women. Leadership skills can be learned if we choose to change. We also find that leadership is not determined by one's status within an organization, rather leaders are all around us. Finally, leadership is about desiring, creating, and nurturing relationships with others. Extraordinary things get done in organizations not because people are told to do something but because they choose to follow someone else. Leadership is a relationship between those who aspire to lead and those who choose to follow. Leadership success is grounded in the relationships forged between leaders and their subordinates. This success is dependent upon the capacity to build and sustain those human relationships that enable people to get extraordinary things done on a regular basis.[10]

The Leadership Practices Inventory (LPI)[24] (Pfeiffer, San Francisco, CA, www.pfeiffer.com) is a self-assessment inventory that can provide insight into how one perceives him- or herself in regards to the 5 exemplary leadership practices. There is also an observer version of the LPI that can be given to bosses, peers, and direct reports to assess how others see you in the light of these 5 practices.

360-Degree Feedback Assessment

Instruments that allow for 360-degree feedback are commonly used in organizations to provide feedback to leaders on their leadership behaviors. The assessments can be a combination of quantitative and qualitative data collection and are generally not recommended to be tied to a performance evaluation, rather they should be used for personal growth and development. The reason they are referred to as 360-degree feedback is that the leader receives feedback from multiple levels of the organization and includes feedback at a minimum from his or her boss, peers, or colleagues and direct reports, thus providing the leader with a 360-degree view of how others perceive him or her. This is generally compared to a self-assessment of themselves as well. There are numerous instruments that can provide this information. Both Situational Leadership and the Leadership Practices Inventory mentioned in this chapter can provide this information based on that particular leadership/management model. There are others instruments that are much more robust in the feedback they provide to the leader. Two such examples can be found from Personnel Decisions International (Minneapolis, MN, www.personneldecisions.com) and The Center for Creative Leadership (Greensboro, NC, www.ccl.org).

LEADER AS CHANGE AGENT

Successful leaders must be a catalyst for change (ie, challenge the process) and as a proponent of change they must manage the transition of change and the resistance associated with it. Figure 1-6 represents the "Formula for Change" where "D" signifies the dissatisfaction with how things are now, "V" equals vision for what is possible, and "F" stands for first concrete steps toward the vision. If the product of these 3 factors is greater than the resistance (R), then change is possible. Because of the multiplication of D, V, and F, if any one is absent or low, then the product will be low and therefore not capable of overcoming the resistance.[25] For instance, if I am satisfied with the current state, then change is unlikely and I will resist that change in whatever way I can. In order for change to be successful, stakeholders impacted by the change must believe a change is needed and it is the leader's job to make a case for the change.[26]

All 5 exemplary leadership practices identified from Kouzes and Posners'[10] research are required to

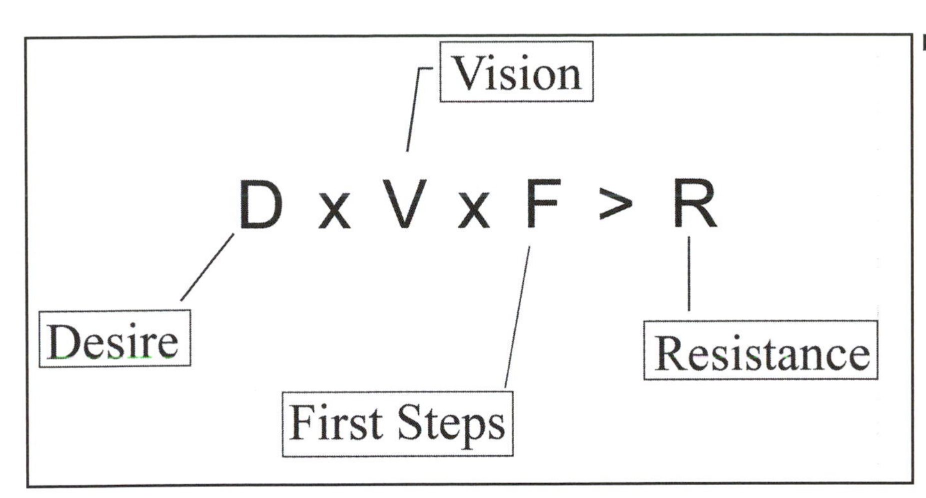

Figure 1-6. Formula for change.

manage successful change. The change itself is about challenging the process through an inspired and compelling vision of the future, modeling the way through the change, and encouraging others during the difficult and successful times as the leader enables others to act by having input and involvement into the change.

An interesting observation in my experience with organizations is the surprise many leaders have when there is resistance to change. Many times leaders want employees to meet them where they are and fail to meet the employees where they are. Often the leader has been aware of a change event for days, weeks, or months before it occurs and has had time to prepare for it and make meaning of the change for him- or herself. The same time should be afforded to others who are affected by the change and to expect someone to "swallow change whole" is just not realistic. Resistance is a natural response to change and if there is no overt resistance to change, then that should be of concern itself. Leaders use their skills to help people work through their resistance to change. Box 1-2 lists 5 pitfalls that need to be avoided when making the case for change.[26]

Resistance

The reason for the resistance to change can be explained through the metaphor of an ocean wave (Figure 1-7). There is a current that carries that wave onto shore and underneath that wave is a countercurrent. In any change event, there is the desire to change (current) and the desire for sameness (countercurrent). It is this desire for sameness that results in resistance. Obviously, when the desire for change is greater than the desire for sameness, change will occur (see Figure 1-6). Making a case that something needs to change is the first step toward overcoming this resistance.

Box 1-2

Pitfalls in Managing the Change Process

Pitfall 1: How Before Why

People need to know *why* something is important before they are interested or even willing to entertain *how* you want them to do it. Too often the "why" something is important is not addressed before launching into "how" it should get done.

Pitfall 2: Rushing From Change Event to Change Event

We rush from one change to the next, never building sufficient support. This invites resistance when we do not take time to make a case for the change.

Pitfall 3: All We Need To Do Is Tell Them

Explaining things is important but it does not address the emotional concerns and fears, nor the trust and respect for those delivering the message.

Pitfall 4: We Can Force Them to Do It

You cannot force people to change; they will come up with very creative ways to stop you.

Pitfall 5: Taking Time Will Waste Time

Regardless of how quickly change must occur, not taking time up-front to make your case will only result in increased resistance and more energy used to keep the change on track, with a high possibility of the change effort failing in the end.

Adapted from Maurer R. *Making a Compelling Case for Change.* Fairfax, VA: Maurer & Associates; 2004.

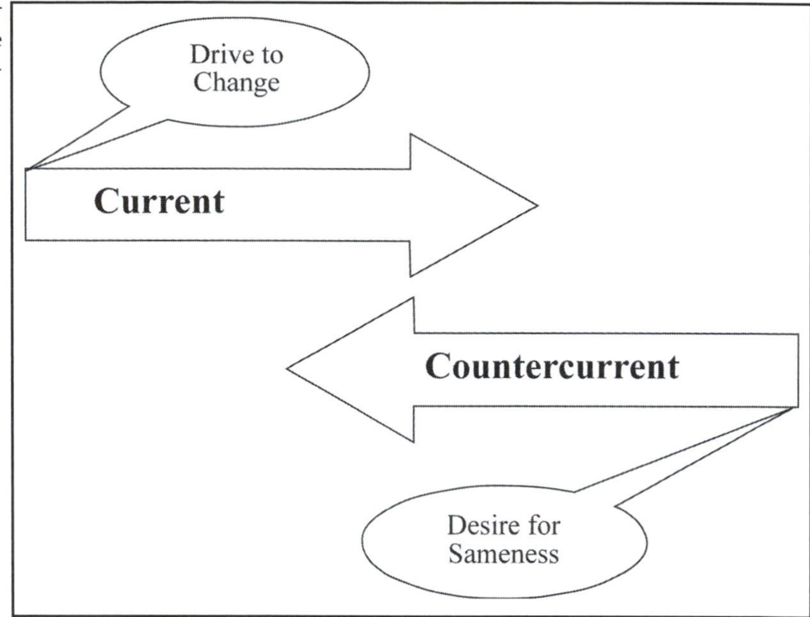

Figure 1-7. Illustrates the desire one has for change (current) and at the same time one's desire for sameness (countercurrent). This countercurrent is referred to as resistance.

Maurer[26,27] provides a way to frame resistance in 3 levels:

- Level 1: They do not get it.
- Level 2: They do not like it.
- Level 3: They do not like you.

Level 1 resistance is about information. People need to intellectually understand why change needs to occur and this is accomplished by sharing information. Level 2 reactions to change center around emotional responses based on fear that can be attached to loss of job or job security, loss of money, reduction in quality, etc. While organizations may address Level 1 issues, the emotional reactions associated with Level 2 are rarely attended to. If not addressed, these reactions do not easily go away and may crop up months or even years later. Level 3 addresses the need for those impacted by change to trust and have confidence in leadership, otherwise people will be skeptical of anything leadership has to say and will undermine the change effort. If resistance is Level 3, then the reason(s) for the lack of trust must be attended to in order for change to be successful. Remember, Level 3 resistance is about you as the leader or the group of leadership you represent. These 3 levels are summarized in Table 1-12.

Even when leaders want to take resistance seriously and deal with it responsibly, most strategies are Level 1. There is a belief that if leaders give people just a little more information, then they will certainly come around. Newsletters, video, and PowerPoint presentations are all Level 1 approaches. There is nothing wrong with presentations if people are confused or need more facts, but Level 1 tactics do not work at Levels 2 and 3. To make a compelling case for change, the change plan needs to address all aspects of the 3 levels of resistance and minimize the pitfalls listed in Box 1-2. Additional tips for managing resistance are found in Box 1-3.

Box 1-3

Tips for Managing Resistance

- Find "common ground" (ie, where you agree and disagree)
- Build strong working relationships
- Embrace resistance
- Explain the 3 levels of resistance to the individual or group
- Match your intervention to the level of resistance. If people have Level 2 concerns, address with Level 2 interventions
- Level 2 and 3 resistance will probably require having a "difficult conversation(s)" (see Chapter 10)

Given that resistance has been framed in 3 levels, it may now be clear how resistance is a natural human response to new ideas or change. Maurer[27] explains the relationship of resistance to the 3 levels in the following way:

> *People resist us, change and/or new ideas for good reasons. Take something as simple as Level 1 understanding. If they do not understand the idea or why change is needed, it makes sense that they will not get behind it. Why should they? And if the*

Table 1-12

Overview of Resistance Levels

Level of Resistance	Description	Examples
1	This resistance is based on information: Level 1 may come from: Facts Figures Ideas Many make the mistake of treating all resistance as if it were Level 1	Level 1 may come from: Lack of information Disagreement with idea itself Lack of exposure Confusion
2	This is a physiological and emotional reaction to change. This resistance is based on fear; people fear they will lose face, friends, and even their jobs. It is physiological and uncontrollable; can be triggered without conscious awareness.	Level 2 may come from fear over a perceived: Loss of power or control Loss of status Loss of face or respect Made to seem incompetent Fear of isolation or abandonment Worn out (too much change)
3	This is deeply entrenched beliefs, experiences, and biases. It is bigger than the ideas at hand. People are not resisting the idea—in fact they may love the idea itself—they are resisting you. History tells them to be wary—it is a trust issue. Level 3 is also the domain of cultural, religious, and racial differences. In other words, people may be resisting who you represent.	Level 3 may come from: Personal history of mistrust Cultural, ethnic, racial, gender differences Significant disagreement over values Transference. The person being resisted represents someone else such as a mother or father.

idea or change threatens them (Level 2), there is absolutely no reason why they should support us. And if they believe we represent all that is bad and wrong in the organization (Level 3), they would be foolish to jump on our bandwagon. People resist due to lack of understanding, negative reaction to the new idea or change effort, or lack of trust for the leadership. (p. 46)

The appropriate level of resistance needs to be addressed in its own specific way (Table 1-13). Additionally, to navigate the murky waters of change we should continually ask 3 questions[27]:

1. Do they understand?
2. Are they reacting positively or negatively to the idea or change effort?
3. Is there sufficient trust between us for them to support me in the idea or change effort?

Transition

Bridges[28] provides a model that can be useful for managing transition during the change process (Figure 1-8). Bridges[28] views change as situational (eg, move to a new site, retirement of a leader, new or revised of a policy or procedure, the reorganization of the roles on the team, the revisions to the pension plan). Transition on the other hand is psychological; it is a 3-phase process that people go through as they internalize and come to terms with the details of the new situation that the change brings about. The 3 phases are as follows[28]:

1. Ending, losing, letting go
2. The neutral zone
3. The new beginning

Transition is a way in which people unplug from an old world and plug into a new world. Getting people through the transition is essential if the change is actually to work as planned. In my experience, the interesting thing is that executives/administrators generally do not put nearly as much thought into managing the change after it occurs as they do in orchestrating the change itself. Bridges' Transitional Model can explain some of the phenomenology people experience during change and can give a leader a "road map" to navigating change.

Table 1-13

Actions to the Three Levels of Resistance

If resistance is...	*Then...*
Level 1	Explain the idea using language and examples that the other person or group will understand.
Level 2	You must engage in conversation—not presentation. Only by finding the true resistance can you hope to transform it into support for your idea.
Level 3	Begin by repairing burned bridges and building relationships.

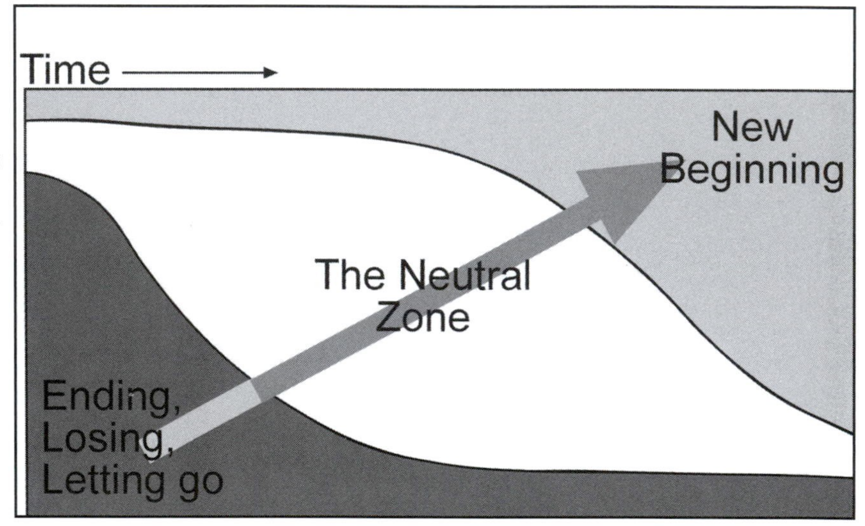

Figure 1-8. Bridges' transition model. Note from the illustration that even in the early changes of transition there is a new beginning (ie, a new leader) and even in the later stages of the transition, there is still ending, losing, and letting go. (Adapted from Bridges W. *Managing Transitions: Making the Most of Change.* 2nd ed. Cambridge, MA: Perseus Book Group; 2003:5.)

I do not care how much you know until I know how much you care.
Unknown

Ending

Transition starts with an ending and begins with letting go of something. This first phase of transition is an ending and a time leaders need to help people deal with their losses. This can involve letting go of old ways and old identities people had. The starting point for transition is not the outcome of change (or the change itself) but rather the ending that you will have to make to leave the old situation behind. It is important for employees to think about what is ending and what is going to remain the same for them personally and for the organization as a whole.

Neutral Zone

The neutral zone lies in between the time when the old is gone but the new is not fully operational. It is both dangerous and an opportune place to capitalize on the change; it is the very core of the transition process and can be a difficult time. People wonder during this time how the change will impact them and their livelihood. If you do not understand and expect it, you are more likely to try and rush through the neutral zone or even bypass it. The confusion and chaos you experience may be mistaken as a sign that something is wrong. However, this is the area of opportunity for the individual's and organization's best chance to be creative, to develop into what they need to become, and to renew themselves. It is the chaos into which the old form dissolves and from which the new form emerges. Employees need to have some sense of where the organization is going and how they are going to get there. Communication is key. Informing people about what is changing, what activities have to continue, and what activities can wait helps them understand what is required of them during the transition. This will also send a message that the organization cares about its employees and wants them to manage the transition successfully.

New Beginning

The third phase is referred to as a new beginning. This is when people develop the new identity, experience the new energy, and discover the new sense of purpose that makes the change begin to work. Employees need to know what in fact changed and what has remained the same. They must also understand the new vision and goals to see how they fit into the new reality and to be clear on what is now expected of them.

These phases do not happen separately; they often occur at the same time. They serve to reorient and renew people when things are changing all around them. Unfortunately, most organizations pay little attention to endings, do not acknowledge the neutral zone (and try to avoid it), and do nothing to help people make a fresh, new beginning even as they trumpet the changes. Living in the past and consistently referring to events where they believe they were wronged that occurred many years ago can be indicators that transition with a change event has not been completed by the individual and is referred to as "unfinished business."

People respond differently to change and it is not change they fear, but rather the fear of the unknown that change can produce. Putting as much effort into planning the transition of change as is put into orchestrating the change will go a long way toward minimizing the resistance to the change and increase the likelihood of a successful change effort. Know that when new ideas are proposed and/or change is inevitable, people will resist until their levels of resistance are overcome. Leaders should not only embrace change, but more importantly the fears and emotions associated with it.

SUMMARY

- Compare and contrast the difference between manager and leadership.

  A multitude of characteristics are listed to help differentiate manager behaviors from leadership behaviors. In the end, these differences can be summarized by how well a person balances getting the work done (task) with the people doing the work and their needs and wants. A manager's behaviors can be thought of as relating to getting the task or work done with little concern for the people, while a leader is concerned about getting the work done and is also equally as concerned about the people doing the work.

- Identify the qualities/behaviors of an effective leader.

  There are many qualities/characteristics/behaviors of effective leaders, some of which include the ability to influence others, visionary, encourage others, trustworthy, innovative, listen attentively, servant's heart, integrity, humility, exceptional communicator and foster open communication, results oriented, change agent, embrace conflict, and promote collaboration and teamwork just to name a few.

- Explain EI and why it is an important characteristic trait.

  It is key to be able to build a relationship in the workforce. It is no longer acceptable to just have a high IQ, but you must also be able to work well with others. *Emotional intelligence* is the term coined for this new set of behaviors that employers are requiring of employees. An effective leader has a high EI quotient. EI can be defined as the ability, capacity, or skill to perceive, assess, and manage the emotion of one's self, of others, and of groups.[7]

- Differentiate between power and authority.

  Power is basically the potential to influence, and 5 types of power have been defined: legitimate, referent, coercive, reward, and expert. Most leaders are effective in an organization not because of their positional power but rather because of their personal power, which is based on the relationship they develop and the loyalty they create. Authority on the other hand is the aspect of power granted to either groups or individuals that legitimizes the right of the group or individual to make decisions on behalf of others.

- Explain how Theory X and Theory Y assumptions about people emerge as part of a leader's pattern of behavior.

  Theory X and Theory Y can be considered the underpinnings of an individual's leadership philosophy and is based on the assumptions one holds regarding people. Theory X basically believes that people want to avoid work, are lazy, and must be driven and controlled in order for the work to occur. Theory Y philosophy believes people will work toward goals and assume responsibility, they want to achieve, and are motivated by interest and challenges. While a leader's behaviors generally cannot be categorized as solely either Theory X or Theory Y, he or she will generally have a little of both characteristics with a pattern of behavior toward one or the other.

- Compare and contrast 3 different leadership models: managerial grid, situational leadership, and exemplary leadership practices.

  These 3 models serve as a way to frame leadership behaviors and for a person to identify his or her primary pattern of behavior. The managerial grid is based on a leader's concern for production and people. These 2 variables create a horizontal and vertical axis, respectively, resulting in 5 categories of behaviors. The managerial grid is provocative because it promotes that a 9/9 team manager is the ideal style and the rest of the styles miss the mark.

The SL model on the other hand endorses that the leader's style should change based on the development level of the employee. There is not an ideal leadership style, but a leader needs to be able to use several styles given the developmental level of the employee. A leader's style is characterized by the amount of directive behavior and supportive behavior (low to high) demonstrated by the leader given a person's development level on that particular skill, task, or behavior.

The exemplary leadership practices model is based on research that asked thousands of individuals to identify characteristics of exemplary leaders. This research model produced the following 5 practices seen in exemplary leaders: challenge the process, inspire a shared vision, enable others to act, model the way, and encourage the heart.

- Explain the leader's role as a change agent.

  Successful leaders must be a catalyst for change and as a proponent of change they must manage the transition of change and the resistance associated with it. In order for change to be successful, stakeholders impacted by the change must believe a change is needed and it is the leader's job to make a case for the change.[26]

- Recognize and categorize patterns of resistance to change and apply the correct intervention depending on the level of resistance.

  People resist change for 3 reasons: 1) They do not get it, 2) they do not like it, or 3) they do not like you or who you represent. Each of these categories can be thought of as a level. Level 1 resistance is about information—they simply do not understand. Level 2 reactions to change center around emotional responses based on fear that can be attached to the change effort. Level 3 resistance is around trusting those in charge of the change effort. The problem is that all resistance is treated as Level 1 resistance by providing more information and having more meetings to communicate more. Of course these interventions fail when the resistance is Level 2 or 3.

- Employ Bridges' Transition Model as a framework for a change effort.

  The Bridges transition model provides a map for "framing" a change effort and dissecting it into 3 stages: 1) ending, losing, letting go; 2) the neutral zone; and 3) the new beginning. No matter if it is an individual, group, or organization going through a change, people will experience the pain, uncertainty, and at times chaos created by a change effort. This model helps to explain what people are experiencing and gives hope for the future as well as a "road map" for the leader to track the change effort. The problem arises in that organizations typically do not manage the transition of change nor deal with the resistance associated with the change. While the model indicates clear demarcation points between the stages, it is not that "clean." People may still be experiencing a prior stage as they are in a current stage or moving toward the next one.

ACTIVITIES

The following activities are designed to reinforce material presented in the chapter and to allow for discussion among students and instructors.

Situational Leadership

- Think for a moment of a skill or task you would like to teach someone. This should be a skill or task at which the other person would be a beginner. Using the SL model described in this chapter, what would you say and do to progress this person from a D1 developmental level to a D4 on this particular skill or task?

Exemplary Leadership Practices

- Think for a moment of the best leader you have ever been around. Then list all of the characteristics and behaviors that made this person an ideal leader for you.
- Take these characteristics and behaviors and place them in one of the five exemplary practices: challenge the process, inspire a shared vision, enable others to act, model the way, and encourage the heart.

This is not unlike the Kouzes and Posner's leadership model which gives you some specific characteristics and behaviors to associate with each of the 5 practices. If you want to work on improving one of the practices, just look as that specific characteristic or behavior and begin doing that one.

REFERENCES

1. Johnson B. *Polarity Management: Identifying and Managing Unsolvable Problems.* Amherst, MA: HRD Press, Inc; 1996.

2. Maxwell J. *Developing the Leader Within You.* Nashville, TN: Thomas Nelson; 1992.
3. Maxwell J. *The 21 Irrefutable Laws of Leadership.* 2nd ed. Nashville, TN: Thomas Nelson; 2007.
4. Salovey P, Mayer JD. Emotional intelligence. *Imagination, Cognition and Personality.* 1990;9:185-211.
5. Goleman D. *Emotional Intelligence: Why It Can Matter More Than IQ.* New York, NY: Bantam Books; 1995.
6. Goleman D. *Working With Emotional Intelligence.* New York, NY: Bantam Books; 1998.
7. Bradberry T, Greaves J. *The Emotional Intelligence Quick Book.* New York, NY: Simon and Schuster; 2005.
8. Williams P. *The Warrior Within.* Ventura, CA: Regal Books; 2006.
9. Covey S. *The 7 Habits of Highly Effective People.* New York, NY: Simon & Schuster; 1989.
10. Kouzes J, Posner B. *The Leadership Challenge.* 3rd ed. San Francisco, CA: Jossey-Bass; 2002.
11. Zenger J, Folkman J. *The Extraordinary Leader: Turning Good Managers Into Great Leaders.* New York, NY: McGraw-Hill; 2002.
12. Gebelein S, Nelson-Neuhaus KJ, Skube CJ, et al. *Successful Manager's Handbook.* 7th ed. Minneapolis, MN: Personnel Decisions International; 2004.
13. Goleman D. The emotional competence framework. The Consortium for Research on Emotional Intelligence in Organizations. Available at http://www.eiconsortium.org/reports/emotional_competence_framework.htm. Accessed January 27, 2009.
14. McKee A, Frances J. The impact and opportunity of emotion in organizations. In: Jones B, Brazzel M, ed. *The NTL Handbook of Organizational Development and Change: Principles, Practices and Perspectives.* San Francisco, CA: Pfeiffer; 407-423.
15. French J, Raven B. The bases of social power. In: Cartwright D, ed. *Studies in Social Power.* Ann Arbor, MI: Institute for Social Research, University of Michigan; 1959:150-167.
16. Ray R. *Management Strategies in Athletic Training.* Champaign, IL: Human Kinetics; 2005.
17. McGregor D. *The Human Side of Enterprise.* New York, NY: McGraw-Hill; 1961.
18. Robinson A. *McGregor's Theory X-Theory Y Model.* The Pfeiffer Library. Vol 20. San Francisco, CA: Pfeiffer; 2003.
19. Blake R, Mouton, JS. *The New Managerial Grid.* Houston, TX: Gulf Publishing Co; 1978.
20. Hall J, Harvey J, Williams M. *Styles of Management Inventory.* Waco, TX: Teleometrics International; 2000.
21. Blanchard K. *Situational Leadership II: The Article.* Escondido, CA: Ken Blanchard Co; 1994.
22. Gardner G, Harrelson GL. Situational teaching: meeting the needs of the evolving learner. *Athletic Therapy Today.* 2002; 7(5):18-22.
23. Kouzes J, Posner B. *Encouraging the Heart.* San Francisco, CA: Jossey-Bass; 2003.
24. Kouzes J, Posner B. *Leadership Practices Inventory: Facilitators Guide.* 3rd ed. San Francisco, CA: Pfeiffer; 2003.
25. Beckhard R. *Organization Development: Strategies and Models.* Reading, MA: Addison-Wesley; 1969.
26. Maurer R. *Making a Compelling Case for Change.* Fairfax, VA: Maurer & Associates; 2004.
27. Maurer R. *Why Don't You Want What I Want?* Atlanta, GA: Bard Press; 2002.
28. Bridges W. *Managing Transitions: Making the Most of Change.* 2nd ed. Cambridge, MA: Perseus Book Group; 2003.

Chapter

RISK MANAGEMENT IN ATHLETIC TRAINING

OBJECTIVES

At the end of this chapter, the reader will be able to:

- Identify the 4 elements of negligence
- Articulate common defenses against negligence and incorporate appropriate risk management strategies such as policy and procedure
- Explain standard of care and apply current practice standards published by professional agencies and societies
- Develop policies and procedures to aid in risk management, including emergency action plans and standard operating procedures
- Identify key legal issues encountered in a drug-testing program
- Differentiate between licensure and certification and explain the implications of each
- Recognize common legal and ethical issues facing the team physician

If the risk of injury was not associated with participation in physical activity or athletics, there would be little need for athletic trainers or even the profession of athletic training. However, the risk of injury is undeniable. While it is not possible to eliminate all risks associated with participation in athletic or physical activity, every effort must be made to minimize or control those risks. Failure to do so can jeopardize the health and safety of the athlete/client/patient with whom you are working as well as placing your career, possibly even your well being, at risk.

This chapter presents the basic concept of risk management and introduces elementary legal concepts that are fundamental to the understanding of risk management. Unfortunately, the concept of risk management is much too complex to address with a simple adage such as "be careful" or "always use good judgment." One must first understand a few basic legal concepts in order to appreciate risk management. Legal concepts such as liability, negligence, and standard of care are central to developing a greater awareness of risks. Perhaps more importantly, these and other concepts that will be discussed in this chapter act as the basis for identifying risk management strategies that will help protect the athlete or patient with whom you are working, the institution or entity for which you are working, and yourself in your role as health care provider.

LIABILITY AND NEGLIGENCE

Athletic trainers and other health care professionals have a legal responsibility to the patients or athletes with whom they work. *Black's Law Dictionary* defines liability as a "quality or state of being legally obligated or accountable; legal responsibility to another or to society."[1] Without question, a certified athletic trainer has a legal responsibility to provide care for the patient or athlete with whom they are working. Taking this concept a step further, the certified athletic trainer has a legal responsibility to provide a certain standard, or quality, of care. Negligence exists when an individual fails to provide the standard of care that a reasonably prudent person would have provided in a similar situation, but perhaps more importantly, negligence exists when an athletic trainer's actions fall below the legal standard established to protect others against unreasonable risk of harm.

Negligence is a relatively complex legal concept that is composed of 4 basic elements. Initially, a duty must exist between the person whose actions are being called into question and the individual or individuals who have been injured or harmed by those actions. Secondly, the duty that has been established must have been breached. The third element of negligence is cause. The actions or failure to act must have caused damage or harm. The fourth element is the actual damage or harm that resulted. In order for negligence to exist, there must be some breach of duty that causes damage or harm. These 4 elements are better understood if they are placed in context or actual cases. Identifying one party as the plaintiff, whose actions or inactions are being called into question, and one party as the defendant or the individual that has suffered injury or damage will facilitate the discussion of the 4 elements.

Duty

At first glance, duty would appear to be the most straightforward of the 4 elements, but there is actually more to the duty relationship than many immediately realize. If an individual has been hired to provide athletic training services for a certain group of individuals such as student-athletes at a junior college or patients in a sports medicine clinic, the duty is clearly established. Other situations may not be so well defined.

Whether or not a school had a duty to provide on-site medical coverage to a lacrosse team in the off-season was the focal point of a case involving the sudden death of a student-athlete.[2] In this particular case, the school did not have a sufficient number of certified athletic trainers employed to provide on-site medical coverage to off-season sports. When the player collapsed in cardiac arrest during an off-season practice, the athletic trainer was summoned but because he was at a different location on campus, several minutes elapsed before the athletic trainer arrived on the scene. Tragically, the student-athlete died as a result of the incident. When the parents of the deceased athlete brought suit against the school, it was due in part to the school's failure to provide adequate medical coverage for student-athletes. The court agreed that such a duty did indeed exist and the case was ruled in favor of the deceased student's parents.

Breach

Complicating the issue is the fact that negligence can be either an act of commission or an act of omission. In other words, a negligent act can be something the athletic trainer did that was performed improperly. Another example of an act of commission would be simply doing the wrong thing. An act of omission differs in that it is simply a failure to act.

A case in Texas[3] in which a coach failed to render medical treatment to an athlete suffering from heat exhaustion is an example of an act of omission. Unfortunately, this failure to act resulted in heat exhaustion escalating into heat stroke. By the time the athlete received proper medical treatment, it was too late. Failure to provide proper care or recognize an ever-worsening heat illness resulted in the tragic death of a high school athlete. An example of an act of commission can be found in the case involving a college football player who was struck in the head during practice.[4] The athlete walked to the side of the field and collapsed, where he was unconscious for close to 10 minutes. Proper care was exercised when an ambulance was summoned to transport the athlete to the emergency room of the nearest hospital. Unfortunately, the athletic training staff failed to communicate the extent of the injury to the emergency room staff and the severity of the injury was grossly underestimated. No magnetic resonance image (MRI) or computed tomography (CT) scan was performed and the athlete was cleared to return to practice in 1 week. The student-athlete was again struck in the head approximately 1 month later during a game. The athlete collapsed, unconscious on the sideline and was subsequently transported to a hospital where he underwent emergency surgery for treatment of a subdural hematoma. During the procedure, physicians found a hematoma that had developed approximately 3 weeks prior to the surgery. As a result of the second injury, the athlete suffered permanent neurological damage, including seizures and significant cognitive impairment. The court ruled in favor of the injured athlete, citing the rendering of improper care in the initial handling of the injury as a causative factor in the resultant permanent damage.

Cause

The third element of negligence is cause. There must be a duty relationship between the plaintiff and the defendant in order for negligence to exist. This duty must have been breached and that breach must be the cause of the resultant damage. The actions of the plaintiff must be the direct cause of the damage. The causal element of negligence is further developed within the concept of proximate cause. Proximate cause is a legal term that identifies an event or action that directly causes another event to occur. The addition of proximate actually clarifies the concept as it implies a close or more direct relationship. The basic test to determine if the actions in question are the proximate cause of an injury or damage is to remove those actions from the fact pattern or sequence of events and then see if the injury or damage would still be present. If removing the actions in question does not alter the damage or injury, those actions were not the proximate cause of the damage or injury.

In the fall of 1991, the rugby team at a state college held the first practice of the season.[5] The team was not an actual varsity sport, but it did receive formal recognition as a club sport and also received funding from the student association of the university. During the practice, the team was divided into 2 groups in order to form 2 scrums so they could practice a specific aspect of the game known as a "scrummage" or "scrum." During this process, one of the players in the front of the scrum was placed in a position that caused a severe injury to the cervical spine. The injured player alleged that the injury occurred because, at the time of the accident, the 2 scrums were on uneven ground. The injured player believed the condition of the playing field caused the injury and brought suit against the college for negligence.

What Is a Scrummage?

A scrummage involves 8 members of one team binding together and facing an equal number of the opposing team. The object is to capture possession of a ball placed on the ground between the 2 scrums.

The court ruled in favor of the college as numerous expert witnesses testified that the injury would have happened in the same situation even if the scrummage had taken place on level ground, therefore raising the issue of proximate cause. To fully appreciate proximate cause, the concept of "fact pattern" must first be understood. The fact pattern of a case is the chain of events that actually transpire when the initial event occurred. If a legal case were a theatrical play, the fact pattern would be the script. That being said, if the actions of the defendant, the school in this particular case, were taken out of the fact pattern, the injury would still result. If the university had provided a level field, the injury would still have happened. Therefore, the actions of the university were not the proximate cause of the injury.

Harm

The fourth element of negligence is harm. Actual harm or damage has to have happened or negligence simply does not exist. A good illustration of the harm element can be seen in a case involving a retiring National Football League (NFL) player and the team with whom he had spent his entire 15-year career.[6] Earlier in his career, the player suffered a torn medial collateral ligament that was surgically repaired. This was common practice at the time and the repair was relatively successful. It was determined during the surgery that the player had also torn his anterior cruciate ligament. However, the player was not informed of the additional damage to the anterior cruciate ligament.

As the seasons went by, the player had several episodes or problems with his knee. Specifically, there was persistent pain and swelling that resulted in the knee being drained repeatedly. Initially, the knee was drained followed by an injection of procaine hydrochloride and cortisone. This procedure was somewhat effective in relieving the symptoms and it was subsequently repeated. The number of injections the athlete received was not exactly determined during the proceedings, but it was estimated that the athlete received between 14 and 20 per year over a 9-year period. Upon retirement, the athlete sought treatment for persistent knee pain and underwent an attempt to surgically repair the damage. By this time the knee had degenerated substantially and the operation did little, if anything, to reduce the pain and discomfort he was experiencing.

Initially, a lower court ruled in favor of the team, citing the tenacity of the player as one of the factors in his continued play. It was believed that even if he had been informed of the potential consequences of continuing to inject his knee, he would have chosen to take the injections in order to continue his career. On appeal, the court ruled in favor of the player, citing the actions of the team and team physician in creating a chronic and debilitating condition of the plaintiff's knee. It was felt that the harm or damage present was the result of the actions of the defendant NFL team.

STANDARD OF CARE

A certified athletic trainer has a duty to provide a certain level of care. Failure to do so can result in charges of negligence. As such, the level of care merits careful consideration. This level, or standard of care, is influenced by many different factors. A prime example of such an influence would be position statements. A position statement is a publicized statement regarding a specific situation or issue from a learned society or group. The most readily identifiable learned society or expert group for athletic trainers is the National Athletic Trainers' Association (NATA). The

Case Study 2-1

Case. You have been employed for the past 4 years by America State Small College as the head athletic trainer. Your primary sport coverage for the spring semester is with the track team. This is one of the more enjoyable aspects of your job as the team is especially good this year. The relay team has recorded times that place it among the top 5 relay teams in the country. During the season, the athlete that typically runs the anchor leg for the relay team begins to complain of pain and swelling in the area of his Achilles' tendon. After evaluation of the injury, you begin a regimen of treatment for tendonitis. As the season progresses, the athlete continues to practice and compete but the injury is really no better than it was during the initial evaluation. In fact, the injury has become worse, and there is now visible deformity of the area and remarkable crepitation with palpation. You realize this athlete has reached a point where he should stop practice and competition until the symptoms can be brought under control. However, the big qualifying meet is this coming weekend and everyone associated with the team, including the athlete, the coach, and yourself, wants to see the team do as well as possible. Although you are concerned about the risk, you allow the athlete to compete. At the track meet the relay team is running well and everything indicates that this performance will result in their best time of the season. However, during the last leg of the relay, the runner you had been treating for Achilles' tendonitis stumbles and falls to the ground, clutching his leg in obvious pain. A quick evaluation confirms your worst fears: the athlete has suffered a complete rupture of the Achilles' tendon.

Debriefing Question

- Can you identify each of the 4 elements of negligence in this case study? As a reminder, the 4 elements you are looking for are duty, breach, cause, and harm.

NATA has published position statements on several issues, including heat illnesses, lightning exposure, and inclement weather.[7-11] Several groups, including the American Academy of Neurology, the Colorado Medical Society, and the Brain Injury Association,[12-15] have published standards for treating athletes who have suffered a head injury. It must be recognized that these guidelines for treatment and management of injuries act as the standard by which the behavior or actions of an athletic trainer will be judged in the event that charges of negligence arise.

The Kleinecht[2] case questioned the extent of athletic training services provided for student-athletes attending a university and playing on the lacrosse team. More specifically, the quantity of athletic training services provided became an issue. The event in question happened during off-season lacrosse practice. Because the university employed only 2 certified athletic trainers, many sports often had to remain "uncovered" during the off-season. Tragically, on the day in question, one of the team members suffered a fatal cardiac arrhythmia. The parents of the deceased athlete brought suit against the college for failing to provide a sufficient standard of care for their son.

Several facts emerge from this case that can serve as key points in developing appropriate policies and procedures. It would have been much better if the university had employed enough certified athletic trainers to provide coverage for all teams, regardless of whether they were in-season or off-season. Short of that, the university should have taken steps to ensure that all coaches were trained in first aid and cardiopulmonary resuscitation (CPR). Neither of the coaches on the scene that day had been trained to handle an emergency in the absence of the certified athletic trainer. There was no plan of action in the event that a medical emergency occurred on that particular field. While it is impossible to determine if the student-athlete would have died if things had been different, the court determined that the university did indeed have a duty "to have measures in place... to provide prompt treatment in the event he or any other member of the lacrosse team suffered a life-threatening injury."[2] The court ruled that the school failed to provide a sufficient level of care for the student-athlete.

RECOGNITION OF APPROPRIATE STANDARDS

Fortunately, athletic trainers and other health care providers do not act without guidance when making decisions that have direct bearing on the health and safety of the athletes or patients for whom they are responsible. As previously mentioned, many sets of guidelines and standards exist. The NATA has sponsored the development of several such guidelines or position statements. Guidelines or position statements exist to help athletic trainers manage heat illnesses, head injuries, and asthma.[8,10,13] Athletic trainers also gain insight from position statements into dealing with situations involving practices or games conducted in inclement weather, including lightning.

One area that unequivocally demands adherence to established guidelines and position statements is cardiac-related illnesses. A classic case involving a player at Northwestern University[16] serves as a clear example of effective risk management and good decision making relative to cardiac problems and the existing guidelines for handling those problems. Nicolas Knapp was recruited by the university to play basketball and had verbally agreed to play for Northwestern. During Knapp's senior year, he collapsed during a pick-up game and had to be resuscitated. Ultimately, the player was diagnosed with mild asymmetric left ventricular hypertrophy. In essence, the left ventricle of his heart was enlarged and had caused a cardiac arrhythmia, resulting in his collapse. An internal defibrillator was implanted to administer an electrical shock to restore normal cardiac rhythm in the event of another episode of cardiac arrhythmia. Team physicians with Northwestern University refused to allow Knapp to compete in intercollegiate basketball. In making the decision, the physicians cited the medical history and relied heavily on guidelines published as proceedings of a conference of the American College of Cardiology. Members of the American College of Cardiology established guidelines for management of cardiac conditions during the meeting, which is now commonly identified simply as the Bethesda Conference. The guidelines established during the conference clearly supported the disqualification of Knapp from participation in intercollegiate basketball.

Knapp brought suit against the university[17] in an attempt to regain the opportunity to participate on the team. It must be noted that Northwestern fully intended to honor the scholarship awarded to Knapp and was perfectly willing to pay for him to attend school at the university. When the case had made its way through the court system, the final decision was in favor of Northwestern University. In this case, the physicians followed definitive guidelines and made decisions based on those guidelines and their actions were supported by a court of law.

DEFENSES AGAINST NEGLIGENCE

There are several commonly used defenses against charges of negligence. Obviously, the best defense against negligence is to act, at all times, in a professional, competent manner and refrain from any action that might put the athlete or patient at risk. However, an examination of some of the more common defenses of negligent actions (see below) can lead to a better understanding of the concept of negligence and how to avoid potentially litigious situations.

ASSUMPTION OF RISK

One of the most common defenses is to claim the athlete/client/patient knew of the dangers involved and voluntarily assumed some level of risk by participating. This is commonly referred to as the doctrine of assumption of risk. Simply stated, if an individual is aware of the risks involved in participating in an activity but still chooses to participate, then he or she is assuming at least part of the responsibility in the event of accident or injury.

There are several significant concepts that factor into the doctrine of assumption of risk. Prior to assuming any risk, the individual in question must be made fully aware of all of the risks associated with the activity. If the idea of warning an athlete about risks associated with participating in a violent, collision sport seems unnecessary, consider the following scenario that occurred in Seattle.[18] A high school sophomore playing football suffered a cervical fracture that resulted in quadriplegia. The family sued the school system, claiming the student would not have participated in the sport had he known the possibility of such catastrophic injury existed. The court ruled in favor of the family because there was no evidence to indicate that the school warned the student of the potential risks.

The failure to warn doctrine plays a vital role in assumption of risk. It must be recognized that no one assumes the responsibility if he or she does not know about the risk. Schools and athletic programs must warn student-athletes about the potential risks involved in participating in athletic activities.

Failure to warn can be taken further to mean an athletic trainer must fully inform an athlete or patient of the risks involved in a course of treatment or rehabilitation plan. The doctrine of informed consent originates from medical malpractice cases[19] and is applicable to all health care professionals. No patient consents to a treatment regime about which he or she was not fully informed. No patient assumes a risk he or she was unaware of. Failure to fully warn or inform an athlete or patient of any potential risks associated with a given medical treatment or procedure is neither ethical nor responsible behavior on the part of the athletic trainer.

Contributory and Comparative Negligence

Historically, the concept of negligence appeared in the American legal system in the early 19th century.[20] The concept of contributory negligence originated in England and appeared as a defense in the American legal system shortly after negligence itself appeared. Contributory negligence exists when the actions of the plaintiff contributed to the injury or harm he or she suffered. If used successfully as a defense, the plaintiff is not allowed to recover any monetary award for his or her injury. This defense was quite common until the 1970s. Most courts have since found contributory negligence to be unduly harsh in light of potentially astronomical medical costs incurred by a plaintiff. Thus, contributory negligence, as a defense, is seen less and less.

Comparative negligence has, for the most part, replaced contributory negligence. Within the doctrine of comparative negligence the plaintiff is still allowed to recover damages but the amount will be reduced based on the extent to which he or she was responsible for his or her injuries. As an example, if a plaintiff was seeking $1 million in damages and a court or jury believed he or she was 30% responsible for his or her injuries, the award would be reduced accordingly. The total award would now be $700,000. While this may not seem like much of a defense at all, it does take into account some level of responsibility for the actions of the plaintiff. Comparative negligence has variations and may differ slightly from state to state or jurisdiction to jurisdiction, and an in-depth discussion of the topic is beyond the scope of this text.

Governmental Immunity

If a plaintiff is protected by governmental immunity, he or she is beyond the reach of an ordinary negligence claim if he or she is acting on behalf of the state government. In essence, an athletic trainer employed by a public school or university is ultimately paid by the state and may be considered a state employee in some circumstances. Using the judicial system, also an agent of the state, to bring suit against another agent of the state is counterproductive. Therein lies the basis of governmental immunity. When it originated in England, the doctrine of governmental immunity simply prohibited suing the king. The government was protected against suits arising from the actions of state agents or officers. The United States government solidified governmental immunity in the federal Tort Claims Act in 1946. Within the Tort Claims Act, an agent of the state was largely protected from legal responsibility for his or her actions provided there was no intentional negligence involved. However, recent cases have seriously eroded the viability of sovereign immunity as a defense against negligence. Most jurisdictions now challenge, if not deny, sovereign immunity as a defense.[21]

A classic representation of governmental immunity involved a college football player who ultimately died because of heat stroke.[22] The athlete in question was taken to the student health center on campus while in the early stages of heat exhaustion. Due to a lack of communication, the athlete was ultimately left unattended for several hours. By the time health care providers grasped the situation, the athlete was beyond help. At first glance, this case seems to be a clear case for negligence; however, neither the university nor the physicians involved in the case were held accountable because they were protected by governmental immunity.

PRACTICING RISK MANAGEMENT

Without question, the best way to deal with a risk is to avoid the risk. As simple as that seems, avoidance is actually one of the best strategies in risk management! Policies and procedures can be developed and implemented that will help you avoid many of the risks associated with the practice of athletic training. If the tactic of risk avoidance is taken to an extreme, you would simply report to the athletic training room or clinic each day and promptly barricade yourself in your office, avoiding all contact with athletes or patients, in an effort to eliminate all risks. Obviously, the strategy of avoiding contact with people will not work. However, there are some areas where proactive steps can be taken to greatly decrease the risk in the situation or avoid the situation altogether.

Emergency Action Plan

A perfect example of planning to avoid a risk is planning what to do in the event of a severe or life-threatening injury. An emergency action plan is a pre-established set of procedures that will be followed when an athlete or client is injured seriously enough to merit activation of the emergency medical system. The NATA, in a published position statement relative to emergency planning, indicates that each institution or entity that sponsors or conducts an athletic event must have a formal, written plan for emergency situations.[23] The NATA is not alone on this issue. The National Collegiate Athletic Association and the National Federation of State High School Associations both support the need for an emergency action plan.

Development of the emergency action plan requires communication with the individuals that will ultimately be charged with carrying out the plan. Certified athletic trainers should play a lead role in working with team physicians, local emergency medical service personnel, and representatives of the school or institution to develop a plan that identifies specific personnel and how they will be contacted. The plan must also specify the location of vital emergency equipment that will be utilized if the plan is enacted. Additionally, emergency action plans should include detailed information about the specific venue or location where the event is taking place, the medical facility to which the injured person will be transported, and procedures for documenting when and how the plan is to be activated. Again, it must be stressed that no emergency plan will be effective if it is not developed with the input and cooperation of all health care providers that will called upon to carry out the plan.[24] The minimal components of an emergency action plan are outlined in Box 2-1.

Box 2-1

Emergency Action Plan

An emergency action plan must minimally address the following considerations:

- Personnel—Which personnel are involved in the plan and what is the specific duty of each individual?
- What emergency care equipment (stretcher, backboards, splints, automated external defibrillator [AEDs], etc) are available and how is this equipment accessed? Is the equipment appropriate for the personnel, activity, and venue involved?
- Communications—What communication channels do on-site personnel use to activate the emergency medical services? Are emergency numbers posted in a readily accessible area?
- Transportation—What methods of emergency transport are available? If an ambulance is not on-site, what is the best route into the specific venue?
- Venue and location—Is there a specific access plan for various locations and venues?
- Emergency care facilities—Which medical facilities will be utilized in the event of an emergency?
- Documentation—Is the overall plan clearly documented? Does the response team document regular rehearsal of plan activation? Is there documentation of personnel training? Is the maintenance of equipment documented?

Athletic training staffs should practice activating the emergency action plan to ensure each person is familiar with his or her role in the event of an emergency. The NATA position statement recommends practicing activation of the plan on at least an annual basis. It would be wise to take that recommendation a step further and practice enacting the plan more often while focusing on different venues.[24] The consequences of not having an emergency action plan in place are too grave to consider operating without one. The position statement from the NATA not only identifies developing the emergency action plan as a professional responsibility of athletic trainers but goes further in stating that doing so is a legal responsibility.

One of the best examples of emergency planning can be seen in the emergency action plan utilized at the University of Maryland,[25] where the use of global positioning system (GPS) data is incorporated in the event that a student-athlete is injured severely enough to merit being transported by air ambulance. The emergency action plan in place at the University of Maryland is a wonderful example of how to plan ahead.[26]

Policies and Procedures

Another critical practice of risk management is developing a policy and procedure document. In the same vein as the emergency action plan, policies and procedures should exist to direct your actions. However, unlike the emergency action plan, a policy and procedure manual focuses more on nonemergency situations. Policies and procedures guide and direct many everyday actions and in doing so will help decrease the risk of finding yourself in a situation where your actions are being questioned in a court of law. While operating "by the book" may seem unimaginative, the benefits of making safe behaviors a matter of routine is a wise plan indeed. Conversely, while policy and procedures are intended to mitigate risk, not following a policy and procedure that is in place can increase your risk of litigation.

Some policies and procedures are naturally better suited for specific clinical settings. As an example, a policy requiring a written release or return to play clearance from a physician after an athlete has been seen by that physician may be more useful in a high school setting. While this policy may function well when working with younger athletes, it may be less useful in a collegiate setting where a physician employed by the university sees the athlete in an on-campus clinic. Conversely, some policies and procedures are critical, regardless of the setting. For instance, a policy requiring inspection of therapeutic modalities and calibration, where appropriate, on an annual basis is vital to the safe operation of an

Case Study 2-2

Case. While you are in the athletic training room at Upstream High School, the assistant swimming coach runs in and breathlessly tells you there has been an accident in the indoor swimming pool. As you hurry to the pool, you ascertain from the assistant coach that one of the divers hit her head on the board and was knocked unconscious. When you arrive at the pool, the head coach and 2 members of the swim team have removed the student athlete from the water and she is lying on the pool deck. A quick primary survey tells you the girl is not breathing. You immediately tell the coach to call an ambulance and then begin rescue breathing. You continue your efforts for well over 15 minutes until the ambulance crew arrives. The paramedics tell you they were delayed because they did not know where the swimming pool was located on campus. When they did locate the pool, they had to try several doors before they found one that was open. The injured girl is transported to the hospital and her parents are contacted. As you talk to the medical team that is handling the case that evening, they share with you that it is too early to tell how much residual damage is present but they are certain of one thing: the delay in getting the airway open and initiating rescue breathing was long enough to be a substantial factor.

Debriefing Questions

- How would an emergency action plan have helped in this situation?
- Which elements of an emergency action plan come immediately to mind as being especially beneficial?

athletic training room or therapy clinic regardless of the clientele.

One resource available for assistance in developing policies and procedures is the Collegiate Sports Medicine Foundation (www.csmfoundation.org).[6] The Collegiate Sports Medicine Foundation exists to provide support to athletic trainers in developing policy and administrative procedures. The Foundation's Web site acts as a repository of policies and procedures that have been submitted by collegiate athletic trainers from around the country. The site includes policies related to a variety of areas, including emergency action plans, pre-participation physical examinations, environmental conditions, catastrophic injuries, drug testing, nutritional supplements, and blood-borne pathogens among others. While the Collegiate Sports Medicine Foundation is not a definitive legal authority, it does provide a substantial resource for policy development based on the experience of other institutions.

Case Study 2-3

Case. During a soccer practice at Upstream High School, one of the best players is injured. She has a lower back strain that you feel should be evaluated by a physician. You explain this to her parents and they agree to try to get her an appointment with her primary care physician. The student athlete is absent from practice the rest of the day but returns a day later and tells you she is cleared to play. You are a little suspicious of this as she gave every appearance of having a rather severe muscle strain of the lower back. You try to question the player but she is evasive and she is somewhat less than cooperative when you try to re-evaluate her injury. Your better judgment tells you she is not being entirely truthful with you and you make the decision that she should not practice. When you convey this information to the coach, a confrontation quickly develops. The coach cannot understand why you are making this decision. The coach sees no reason to doubt the player and questions your judgment. The situation continues to become worse and finally the coach agrees to hold the player from practice but demands the two of you meet with the athletic director tomorrow to get this straightened out.

Debriefing Question

- What policies and procedures should have been in place to prevent this situation?

LEGAL ISSUES AND THE PRACTICE OF ATHLETIC TRAINING

DRUG TESTING

Drug testing for competitive athletes is certainly not a new issue.[27] In fact, recent attention on drug testing in major league baseball is evidence that drug testing and athletics have, unfortunately, become inseparable. Because drug testing is a practice issue that has given no indication of going away, it is worthwhile to develop a clear understanding of the basic legal issues associated with drug testing.

Freedom from unreasonable search and seizure is a right guaranteed by the fourth amendment of the United States Constitution. The fourth amendment of the United States Constitution was enacted in an effort to protect citizens from unwarranted searches conducted by the government or agents of the government. During the Revolutionary War, blanket search warrants were issued that allowed the military to search entire towns in an attempt to find untaxed goods or subversive literature. Clearly, this was in the mind of those who authored the fourth amendment. Specifically, the fourth amendment states that citizens have a right to remain free of unreasonable search and seizure without probable cause. The connection between a search or seizure of property and drug testing may not be readily apparent at first glance. However, the connection becomes obvious if one equates drug testing with a search. This is indeed the case in the eyes of the law.[28] Searching student-athletes without a warrant, the fundamental problem arising from the fourth amendment, has played a role in several court cases.[22,28,29] However, courts have consistently pointed to the fact that athletes shower and dress in a communal environment and their expectations of privacy are subsequently diminished.

A second sticking point for drug testing comes from the 14th amendment of the United States Constitution. The 14th amendment guarantees that people shall not be denied life, liberty, or the pursuit of happiness without due process of the law, nor shall any individual be denied equal protection of the law. The 14th amendment makes it quite clear that the rights of citizens cannot be taken away without due process of the law. Many cases contesting drug testing have used the 14th amendment as a basis. The basic premise of these cases has been that the drug testing program in question deprived the athlete of the opportunity to participate on an athletic team, or perhaps another extracurricular activity, without due process of the law. However, most courts have made the distinction between rights that are protected by the Constitution and the privilege of participating in interscholastic or intercollegiate athletics. It is commonly held that individual's rights enjoy the protection of the Constitution but that same protection is not extended to such privileges as participation on an athletic team. Within that light, the issues of due process and equal protection have little impact on a drug-testing program.

Case law does more than merely establish the legality of drug testing. Careful examination of the structure of the drug-testing programs that have survived legal challenge yields a substantial degree of guidance in developing or refining a drug-testing program. An excellent example is the case that occurred in the Vernonia School District in Oregon.[29] The drug-testing program in that particular case was taken all the way to the US Supreme Court and as such, the decision reached in the case can be applied to any jurisdiction in the country. This successful program was based on the fact that a positive drug test resulted, eventually, in a loss of athletic eligibility, not expulsion from school. The right to a free public education is a protected right that would require due process and equal protection. The focus of the program in the Vernonia school system was not to expel students, and in doing so deny them a protected right, but rather to withhold a privilege in an effort to protect the athlete and the competitive environment. It is critical to remember that the focus of a drug-testing program should be to protect the athlete and the athletic environment as opposed to becoming a police action that is bent on punishing wrongdoers.

Other elements of the Vernonia program[29] included the incorporation of an automatic re-test of a positive test result. In doing so, the school was giving the athlete the benefit of the doubt. The athlete was also given the opportunity to disclose any medications he or she was taking that might have an effect on test results. A positive result was treated with a great deal of discretion. The number of people who actually knew of a positive result was kept to a minimum. The program depicted in the Vernonia case was exemplary on all fronts.

Many athletic programs are seeking outside help in managing drug-testing programs. Several outside agencies offer such services, one of which is the National Center for Drug Free Sport (www.drugfreesport.com). The National Center for Drug Free Sport has the ability to offer administrative services associated with drug testing by which the actual testing protocol and random subject selection is managed. The agency also offers collection services and will ensure all specimens are collected in a consistent and reliable manner. Of course the actual test of the specimen can be done by the agency as well. The National

Center for Drug Free Sport even offers educational sessions for student-athletes and in doing so provides the last ingredient in a comprehensive substance abuse management program. Given the potentially litigious nature of athletics in general and drug testing in particular, the concept of turning over the testing process to an outside agency is especially appealing.

Licensure and Certification

Licensure and certification are 2 related areas that factor into the safe and legal practice of any allied health care profession. Both are mechanisms that exist to protect the public by regulating the individuals that practice a given profession. While the 2 are closely related, they are not synonymous and each merits further investigation.

Certification simply means that an individual has met a certain minimum standard or level of competence. Meeting the minimum standards is usually demonstrated, at least in part, by passing an examination. In the case of athletic training, the examination is the Board of Certification, Inc certification examination. The candidate must have completed an accredited athletic training education program in order to be eligible to sit for the examination. The Board of Certification (BOC) examination has evolved through the years and has kept pace with the practice of athletic training by closely following the role delineation study for the development of examination content. The Role Delineation Study is basically a descriptor of the practice of athletic training that reflects the content knowledge and skills an entry-level athletic trainer should possess. In holding up a standard for minimal competency, certification ensures all individuals bearing the certification have met that minimum standard.

Licensure also governs or regulates a profession but it does so in a different manner than certification. While certification ensures that all individuals holding a certification are minimally competent, licensure is potentially much more restrictive. Licensure exists when some government agency, typically a state board of health or medical licensure and supervision, agrees to police or regulate the practice of a profession within a given geographic region, again, typically a state. In order to practice the profession within the state, the individual must possess a license to do so. Simply because a physician has completed all the necessary training does not mean he or she can practice medicine. The physician has to be licensed by the state in which he or she is practicing. In awarding the license, the state regulatory agency is agreeing to oversee that individual and provide him or her certain guidelines to follow in his or her practice. Certification and licensure is not unique to athletic training, rather other health care providers have certification and/or licensure, such as nursing, physical therapy, physicians, respiratory therapist, etc.

Going a step further, there are 2 basic types of licensure laws: practice act and title act. The practice act (or practice law) regulates the actual practice of the profession and establishes guidelines to direct practice. A title act is different in that it simply regulates who may carry a title or hold him- or herself out as a health care professional. If an individual has completed the BOC certification examination and has accepted a job as an athletic trainer in a high school in a state where there is a title act, he or she must obtain a state license in order to comply with the law. As soon as the individual is paid as an athletic trainer, he or she is in effect holding him- or herself out as an athletic trainer. Likewise, if that same individual is in a different state that has a practice act, he or she must obtain a state license and follow all guidelines and protocols that regulate the practice of athletic training in that state. The practice act is the more restrictive of the 2 types of licensure laws.

As previously stated, certification and licensure are designed to protect the public. Practicing without certification and licensure, where applicable, is simply unacceptable. It is beyond unacceptable if licensure laws exist within the state in question. Practicing without a license is illegal and the consequences can be disastrous.[30] Beyond the fact that the individual is breaking state law, there are other potential consequences. If the individual in question becomes involved in any sort of litigation, the fact that he or she is practicing without a license will compound the situation. It is most unlikely that any professional liability insurance will help protect the individual in this case. Most liability policies are automatically void if the actions being questioned are illegal.

Team Physician

Certified athletic trainers work closely with team physicians and in many cases fall under the direct supervision of the physician in keeping with state licensure laws. The relationship between the physician and the athletic trainer should be collegial and professional, with each being well versed in his or her role and responsibilities relative to the delivery of athletic health care. Although the team physician faces several legal issues the athletic trainer does not, such as conflict of interests between the team and patient or issues related to the handling of prescription medications (which are well beyond the scope of this text), one should still be very familiar with the issues because many of them directly affect the athletic trainer as a member of the athletic health care team.

In some cases, an athletic trainer may be placed in a position to solicit the services of a team physician. In such cases, it is important to remember that there are guidelines for team physicians to follow. The following description of the team physician's qualifications and role is taken directly from the American Academy of Family Physicians[31]:

> *The team physician must have an unrestricted medical license and be an M.D. or D.O. who is responsible for treating and coordinating the medical care of athletic team members. The principal responsibility of the team physician is to provide for the well-being of individual athletes—enabling each to realize his/her full potential. The team physician should possess special proficiency in the care of musculoskeletal injuries and medical conditions encountered in sports. The team physician also must actively integrate medical expertise with other health care providers, including medical specialists, athletic trainers, and allied health professionals. The team physician must ultimately assume responsibility within the team structure for making medical decisions that affect the athlete's safe participation.*

The standard of care for any physician corresponds to his or her level of training and in particular, the level of specialty training he or she possesses. Courts have failed in the past[32] to recognize sports medicine as a national board certification but that may be changing[33] as the practice of sports medicine becomes more widely recognized. Regardless, the team physician should be selected on the basis of his or her training, interests, and commitment.

In working with a physician, there are a certain areas of practice where the diligent efforts of the physician and the athletic trainer can be especially productive in terms of risk management. One of the most obvious areas is the pre-participation physical exam. In many cases, conducting the pre-participation physical exam will be directed by exam form or documentation required by an athletic-associated or similar governing agency. It must be noted, however, that the pre-participation physical examination, even under the best circumstances, is not a comprehensive health care examination and as such has certain limitations. The majority of abnormal findings from the pre-participation come from the musculoskeletal evaluation[34] as opposed to general medical-related issues. It is important that the physician and athletic trainer work together to maximize the effectiveness of the pre-participation physical exam, be cognizant of the limitations of the exam, and remain aware of the most current trends and position statements. As an example, the team physician could use the standards developed at the 36th Bethesda Conference of the American College of Cardiology to assist in refining personal and family medical history elements of the exam.[35]

Prescription drugs are a potential problem area for both the team physician and the athletic trainer. Athletic trainers must stay within their scope of practice and refrain from handling prescription medications. Athletic trainers are not trained as pharmacists and have very limited legal freedom when dealing with prescription medications. Physicians have lost their license to practice or worse[27,36,37] as a result of improper management of prescription medications that pass through the athletic training room.

A FINAL WORD ABOUT RISK MANAGEMENT

No steps can be taken to completely remove the risk of participating in vigorous physical activity or athletic activities. However, many of those risks can be anticipated and controlled. One way of controlling such risks is the provision of athletic accident insurance. Athletic accident insurance can be equated with risk transfer.[38] Oddly enough, courts have been fairly consistent in the position that a school is under no legal obligation to provide such insurance coverage.[39-41] While there is no legal requirement to provide such insurance, it is certainly in the best interest of the school to do so. It is especially important to consider the purchase of a catastrophic injury policy. Catastrophic injury policies pay those medical costs associated with severe, life-changing injuries such as a neck injury that results in permanent disability. In most cases, the policy is guided simply by the accrual of medical bills. Many lawsuits are initiated only when the family of the injured individual is faced with insurmountable medical costs. They may feel they have no place to turn for help. It is quite likely that adequate insurance coverage has prevented many lawsuits by virtue of the provision of funds for medical bills.

SUMMARY

- Identify the 4 elements of negligence.

  The 4 basic elements of negligence include duty, breach, cause, and harm. Each of these elements must be clearly established if a negligence claim is to be successful. The defendant must have had an identifiable duty to the plaintiff and said duty must have been breached or otherwise compromised. Additionally, the breach of duty must have resulted in harm to the plaintiff.
- Articulate common defenses against negligence and incorporate appropriate risk management strategies such as policy and procedure.

Traditional defenses of negligence include governmental immunity, Act of God, and comparative or contributory negligence. None of these traditional defenses are as simple and reliable as they appear. The best defense against a negligence claim is the initiation of carefully thought out policies and procedures that minimize risk.

- Explain standard of care and apply current practice standards published by professional agencies and societies.

  The NATA has published numerous position statements that act to guide the action of a certified athletic trainer. Position statements published by the NATA can reasonably be considered practice standards and as such, serve as a benchmark to judge the actions of certified athletic trainers.

- Develop policies and procedures to aid in risk management, including emergency action plans and standard operating procedures.

  Emergency action plans enable certified athletic trainers to better deal with athletic injuries that are emergency situations. Additionally, failing to develop and follow emergency action plans is failure to provide an acceptable standard of care.

- Identify key legal issues encountered in a drug-testing program.

  The key issues in drug testing revolve around the fact that a drug test is a legal search. Freedom from unwarranted search is provided by the fourth amendment of the United States Constitution. Because of this fact, drug-testing programs must be carefully designed and managed with every consideration being given to protecting the rights of the student-athlete.

- Differentiate between licensure and certification and explain the implications of each.

  Certification represents a minimal standard of competency. An individual typically has to pass an examination in order to attain certification. Licensure is more restrictive that certification. Licensure is a legal status granted to those that meet minimal standards and agree to practice within an established set of guidelines. Licensure also includes a guarantee that a state agency is agreeing to police the profession in question.

- Recognize common legal and ethical issues facing the team physician.

  Team physicians must remain current on all practice standards and advances in their respective field. On occasion, a team physician may feel pressure as he or she balances the well being of the patient with the needs of the team. This is more likely to occur in a professional sport setting.

REFERENCES

1. Garner BA. *Black's Law Dictionary*. 8th ed. Eagen, MN: Thomson West; 2004.
2. *Kleinecht v. Gettysburg College*, 989 F. 2d 1360 (3rd circuit 1993).
3. *Roventini v. Pasadena Independent School District*, 981 Federal Supplement 1016 (U.S. District Court 1997).
4. *Pinson v. State of Tennessee*, 1995 WL 739820 (Tenn. Ct. App 1995).
5. *Regan v. State of New York*, 654 NYS 488 (New York Supreme Court 1997).
6. *Krueger v. San Francisco Forty Niners*, 234 Cal 579 (1987).
7. Andersen J, Courson R, Kleiner D, McLoda T. National Athletic Trainers' Association position statement: emergency planning in athletics. *Journal of Athletic Training*. 2002;37(1):99-104.
8. Binkley HM, Casa D, Kleiner D, Plummer P. National Athletic Trainers' Association position statement: exertional heat illness. *Journal of Athletic Training*. 2002;37(3):329-343.
9. Walsh K, Cooper M, Holle R, Kithil R, Lopez R. National Athletic Trainers' Association position statement: lightning safety for athletics and recreation. *Journal of Athletic Training*. 2000;35(4):471-477.
10. Miller M, Baker R, Collins J, DAlonzo G. National Athletic Trainers' Association position statement: management of asthma in athletes. *Journal of Athletic Training*. 2005;40(3):224-245.
11. Heck J, Peterson T, Torg J, Weis M. National Athletic Trainers' Association position statement: head-down contact and spearing in tackle football. *Journal of Athletic Training*. 2004;39(1):101-111.
12. Maroon J. Cerebral concussion in athletes: evaluation and neuropsychological testing. *Neurosurgery*. 2000;47(3):659-669.
13. Guskiewicz K, Cantu R, Ferrara M, et al. National Athletic Trainers' Association position statement: management of sport-related concussion. *Journal of Athletic Training*. 2004;39(3):280-297.
14. Cantu R. Return to play guidelines after a head injury. *Clinics in Sports Medicine*. 1998;17(1):45-60.
15. Kelly J. The development of guidelines for the management of concussion in sports. *J Head Trauma Rehabil*. 1998;13(2):53-65.
16. Maron J, Quandt E, Zipes D. Competitive athletes with cardiovascular disease: the case of Nicholas Knapp. *N Engl J Med*. 1998;339(22):1632-1635.
17. *Knapp v. Northwestern University*, 117 S.Ct 2454 (Supreme Court 1997).
18. Jackson K. School districts fear suits over athletic injuries. *The Los Angeles Daily Journal*. May 30, 1984:1, 18.
19. *Zebarth v. Swedish Hospital*, 449 Pacific 2d 1.
20. Abraham KS. *The Forms and Function of Tort Law*. 2nd ed. Eagan, MN: Thomson West; 2002.
21. An overview of state sovereign immunity in the federal system. *Utah Bar Journal*. 2004;17(7):22-29.
22. *Bally v. Northeastern University*, 532 N.E. 2d 49.
23. Anderson J, Kleiner D, McLoda T. National Athletic Trainers' Association position statement: emergency planning in athletics. *Journal of Athletic Training*. 2002;37(1):99.

24. Rehberg RS. *Sports Emergency Care: A Team Approach.* Thorofare, NJ: SLACK Incorporated; 2007.
25. University of Maryland Sports Medicine Department. Maryland State Police/Shock Trauma Helicopter Preferred Landing Zones. Available at http://www.csmfoundation.org/Preferred_Landing_Zones.pdf. Accessed February 23, 2009.
26. Collegiate Sports Medicine Foundation, Policies and Procedures. Available at http://www.csmfoundation.org/Policyandprocedures.html. Accessed February 23, 2009.
27. Houglum J, Harrelson, G, Lever-Dunn D. *Principles of Pharmacology for Athletic Trainers.* Thorofare, NJ: SLACK Incorporated; 2005.
28. *O'Halloran v. University of Washington*, 856 F. 2d 1375.
29. *Vernonia School District 47J v. Acton*, 115 S.Ct 2386 (Supreme Court).
30. *Michigan v. Rogers*, 642 N.W. 595.
31. American Academy of Family Physicians. Team physician consensus statement. Available at http://www.aafp.org/online/en/home/clinical/publichealth/sportsmed/teamphys.html. Accessed January 27, 2009.
32. *Fleischmann v. Hanover Insurance Company*, 470 So 2d 216.
33. Mitten M. Emerging issues in sports medicine: a synthesis, summary, and analysis. *St. Johns Law Review.* 2002;76(1):101-182.
34. Wingfield G, Meeuwisse W. Preparticipation evaluation: an evidence based review. *Clin J Sport Med.* 2004;14(3):109-122.
35. Barry J, Maron D. Eligibility recommendations for competitive athletes with cardiovascular abnormalities—general considerations. *J Am Coll Cardiol.* 2005;45(8):1318-1321.
36. *Wallace v. Broyles*, 961 SW 2d 712.
37. *Curry v. State*, 496 NW 2d 512.
38. Appenzeller H, ed. *Risk Management in Sport.* Durham, NC: Carolina Press; 1998.

Chapter 3

BUDGET AND FINANCE

OBJECTIVES

At the end of this chapter, the reader will be able to:

- Describe the 7 steps to the budgeting process
- Define the components of a common athletic training budget
- Differentiate the various budget systems
- Identify common challenges associated with budget administration
- Describe the purchasing process
- Understand the specifics of the competitive bid process
- Explain the role of inventory control in cost containment

Athletic trainers can be found in a range of employment settings providing quality care in the recognition, treatment, and management of injuries and illnesses. The role of the certified athletic trainer is growing in the health care industry. Athletic trainers working as physician extenders, providing care in educational settings, caring for military personnel in the armed services, and providing physical medicine services in rehabilitation clinics all do so under a common theme: provide cost effective quality health care. To the athletic trainer responsible for planning, coordinating, administering, and appraising budgets, the phrase *cost effective* will take on many forms and athletic trainers must understand the role of fiscal stewardship in effective management. The purpose of this chapter is to explain the budget process, explore the relationship between program planning and budget development, describe various budget systems, and shed light on the role of purchasing and inventory.

BUDGET PROCESS

Budget—Defined

- An estimate, often itemized, of expected income and expenses for a given period in the future.
- A plan of operations based on such an estimate.
- An itemized allotment of funds, time, etc, for a given period.
- The total sum of money set aside or needed for a purpose.

Adjective:

- Reasonably or cheaply priced: a budget watch.

Verb:

- To plan the allotment of (funds, time, etc).
- To deal with (specific funds) in a budget.

Adapted from Dictionary.com. Available at http://dictionary.reference.com/browse/budget. Accessed January 29, 2009.

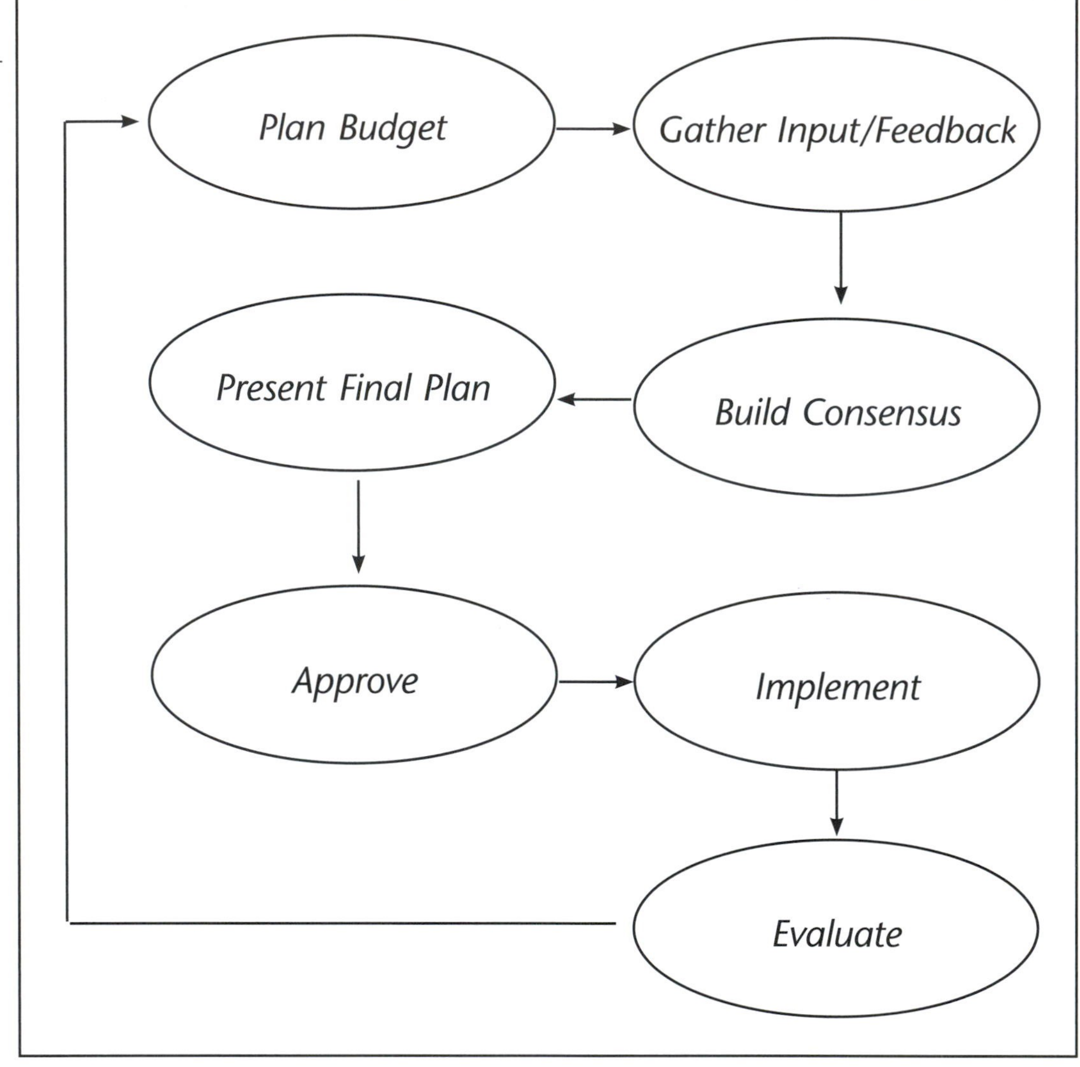

Figure 3-1. The 7 steps of the budgeting process represent an ongoing continuous process that begins with planning and culminates with evaluation. This feedback loop system is similar to other planning and evaluation tools found in Chapter 11. (Adapted from Langley TD, Hawkins JD. *Administration for Exercise-Related Professions*. 2nd ed. Belmont, CA: Thomson-Wadsworth; 2004.)

The development and implementation of a budget may seem like a once a year event for any athletic training heath care organization; simply acquire needed funds and decide how to spend them. In reality, the acquisition and expenditure of funds for the purpose of fulfilling organizational goals and objectives requires an ongoing process with planning and evaluation as key elements. Figure 3-1 outlines a 7-step budget process. These 7 steps include planning, gathering data, analyzing feedback, presenting a final plan, getting approval, implementing the plan, and evaluating the plan.[1] In this form, the budget process forms a feedback loop that allows for continuous monitoring and improvement (see Chapter 11 for a greater discussion of feedback loop systems and organizational effectiveness). While some steps may overlap and could be combined in a smaller organization, the overall themes make up the essential components to the budget planning, implementation, and evaluation process.

Ready or Not...

Be prepared. Athletic trainers must exhibit high levels of preparedness in multiple areas on any given day when they carry out their duties. Developing an emergency plan, carrying out immediate care and treatment protocols, and having a clear cut inclement weather policy are just a few examples that come to mind when we think of the athletic trainer being prepared. However, when it comes to how well athletic trainers are prepared for specific aspects of their job, the area of organization and administration often leaves new professionals wishing they had more instruction. Studies[2,3] show that athletic trainers cite the domain of organization and administration as a general weakness in their preparation. In a study of athletic trainers in Wisconsin, McGuine[2] found that organization and administration was the highest self-identified continuing education need. Within the organization and administration domain, management of human and fiscal resources ranked second only to establishing policies and procedures as the area of greatest continuing education need. These results are in stark contrast to the areas of prevention of injuries and illnesses, recognition and evaluation of injuries and illnesses, and first aid and immediate care. Athletic trainers clearly feel more prepared in these areas.

Understanding the Numbers

Inspection of the organization and administration domain shows several items that directly deal with budget and finance[4]:

- Knowledge of:
    - Institutional budgeting and procurement process
    - Allocation of resources
    - Planning and goal setting
    - Revenue generation strategies
    - Storage and inventory operation
- Skill in:
    - Planning
    - Budgeting
    - Resource allocation
    - Revenue generation

If these facts alone do not encourage prospective certified athletic trainers to dig deeper into this domain, they should consider the following: approximately 16% of the questions on the multiple choice knowledge section of the BOC examination are drawn from the organization and administration domain.[4]

Students and instructors must be sure to give this domain and the specific tasks proper attention. Beyond waiting to "learn on the job," students should participate in authentic learning opportunities that require planning, budgeting, mock purchasing, and evaluation. Students should be proactive and ask questions of clinical instructors about the administrative aspects of their position.

Planning

The planning process is an essential starting point. How a program budget is planned is dependent upon a given program's status. For instance, the director of sports medicine for an intercollegiate athletic training setting with an ongoing program has different planning needs than an athletic training outreach director trying to get a new community program off the ground. Existing programs have a history, and many budget decisions will be based on that history. New programs have no history, and planning for them requires an understanding of similar programs. Budget planners must ask tough questions to insure that the resulting budget is well aligned with organizational needs and mission driven goals and objectives. This idea of budget alignment with goals and objectives is a recurring theme. Budget planning is driven by the following questions:

- What has it cost to provide this program in the past?
- If past budgets serve as a starting point, what needs to change in order to meet changing needs?

- Are there existing programs that can serve as comparisons for our new program?
- Can current staffing needs meet the stated mission?

How the program addresses these questions can vary. Surveying stakeholders and studying previous budgets can glean useful information. More information available to the program will give a clearer understanding of the organizational budget environment.

Gathering Data and Analyzing Feedback

The second step in the budget process is an extension of the initial planning phase. Gathering suggestions and "budget wishes" from staff and other participants is essential. Knowing the wants and needs of the athletic training staff allows for greater ownership in the budget process. While managers cannot make promises beyond the limits of available funding, this step can allow for wider participation in developing the budget and allow the health care administrator an opportunity to educate staff on budget limitations. This is an excellent opportunity for staff to provide justification for budget requests. The process of justifying requests for funds is an important part to some budget systems (see zero base budgeting on p. 48) and, once again, provides another opportunity to align requests with program goals and objectives.

It is unlikely that a head athletic trainer in an intercollegiate setting or program supervisor in a clinical environment will have the final say on his or her overall budget—most will have to present and justify their program budget requests to an administrator, clinic manager, or budget committee. After gathering information and obtaining justifications for budget requests, they will be forced to make decisions on the final budget they wish to present on behalf of the program they manage. It is important at this stage to build consensus for the budget being put forth. Rarely is there enough money to go around and requests tend to outpace funding. When final decisions are made, there is bound to be disagreement. When budget disagreements arise, managers should encourage staff to suggest possible alternatives to budget decisions. This allows staff to better understand the complexity and difficulty in budget decisions and will ultimately lead to greater ownership in the final process.

Presenting the Budget and Getting Approval

The completed budget must be presented in a clear and concise manner to the appropriate administrators. At this point, the budget requests should be finalized and contain no hidden expenditures. Graphs and diagrams may be useful to illustrate aspects of the budget, but they should not detract from the overall presentation. If written justifications have been requested, they should be provided in the final document. Organizations and institutions will have a variety of approval processes. However, upper level administrators will make budget decisions in all cases. To do so, they will rely heavily on the hard work of program managers and staff in the budget process. If the process has been thoughtful and constructive, upper management should be able to see how the budget requests fit with broader program goals. Table 3-1 outlines a 6-month budget development process for an athletic training outreach program that is part of a large hospital-based multidisciplinary sports medicine clinic.

Implementing the Budget

The implementation of the budget requires the program manager to ensure the judicious spending of allocated funds as outlined by the budget. Carrying out the budget requires that proper purchasing and inventory processes are in place. It is also essential that the program manager avoid spending beyond the allocated budget. Clear and open communication with supervising administrators is essential to share information concerning unexpected expenses. Spending beyond the budget limits in one area may require cost containment in other program areas. In some settings it may be required that the budget variance be explained monthly should the expenditures be under or over budget by a threshold set by the organization. The well-prepared athletic training health care administrator should have some contingency plans in mind should the budget require adjustment in mid cycle.

Evaluating the Budget

Evaluating the budget is part of the ongoing budget process. Evaluation closes the feedback loop of the budget cycle and takes the process back to the planning stage (see Figure 3-1). Adhering to the budget requires the diligence of all members of the athletic training organization. It is in the group's interest to take an active role in ensuring that the budget is meeting the desired goals. Observation of daily program services, judicious use of supplies, reasonable purchasing requests, and cautious use of equipment are areas where athletic trainers can make an impact on the budget process. It is essential that rank and file staff have the opportunity to provide feedback on what is and is not working in the budget process. Organizations can provide more structured feedback through monthly accounting summaries for a given

Table 3-1

Sample Budget Calendar for Operational Budget Development Within a Hospital-Based Clinic

Steps to Prepare Next Year's Budget

Month	Steps
January	Ongoing: Release of pertinent data to program areas (eg, patient days, admissions, surgical cases, clinic visits) Budget databases available to all departments for input of operational budget data for upcoming fiscal year Training available to departments on use of hospital budget software
February	Mid month: Deadline for nonrevenue-producing and auxiliary revenue departments to complete operational budgets Ongoing: Hospital administrative budget meetings between departments and hospital budget team End of the month: Deadline for revenue-producing units to complete operational budgets
March	First of the month: Initial review of income statements and FTE (full time equivalency) position counts from hospital budget advisor (first of the month) Ongoing: Additional hospital administrative budget meetings between departments and hospital budget team if needed—final opportunities for adjustments End of the month: Release of preliminary financial statement for upcoming year's budget
April	Mid month: Preparation of formal budget document
May	First of the month: Final budget approval from Hospital Board and Finance Authority
June	Ongoing: Programs are advised of rate increases for services for the upcoming fiscal year
July	First of the month: Implementation of new fiscal year operational budget

Adapted with permission from UW Health Sports Medicine Clinic 2007.

program area. Understanding what is and is not working in the budget process provides information to the next budget cycle.

BUDGETING CYCLES AND BUDGET TYPES

A budget cycle, also known as a budgeting period, is the period of time during the calendar year when the budget is made.[1] The budget cycle should not be confused with the fiscal year. The fiscal year represents the period of time that a specific budget is implemented. July 1 to June 30 is a common fiscal year period. Most organizations will operate on a designated fiscal year. Both short-term and long-term budgets may need to be developed. A short-term budget is most often an annual budget and usually lasts for a period of 1 year. Short-term budgets cover the day-to-day costs of operating a given program. There are 2 types of short-term budgets: operational and equipment/supply. The operational budget includes items like salaries, administrative costs, and office operations (eg, office supplies, phone, and telecommunications). Some organizations may or may not include travel in the operational budget. Operational costs are those that include items needed for the day-to-day operations of the facility or program. The equipment/supplies and services budget will include the expendable and nonexpendable supplies, equipment, and services needed on an annual basis. Expendable items are those that cannot be reused (eg, tape, first aid supplies, over-the-counter medications). Nonexpendable items (eg, orthopedic appliances, elastic wraps, hand weights) are reusable but still have a predetermined minimum lifespan for replacement. Included in the short-term budget would be annual costs associated with maintenance and calibration of equipment and other annual service. Expenses to purchase supplies, equipment, or services that have a known cost are called fixed expenses. By comparison, a variable expense is one that varies throughout the budget and may require an estimate to cover the cost; some maintenance costs are variable depending upon the actual needs (eg, parts, service, repair). Additionally, in some clinical settings, fixed expenses are also determined by the charge per patient treatment. The previous year's average charge per patient treatment is determined by dividing the number of patients treated into the total charges. This number is then used for budgeting in the next fiscal year.

Other short-term budgets may be less than 12 months; they may be related to specific unexpected events. An intercollegiate football team that makes a trip to a bowl game may have additional expenses not covered on the annual budget, but these expenses only would be incurred for a short period of time. A separate operational budget specific to that event may be developed.

A long-term budget involves budget items that exceed the annual budget. These items may be related to long-term projects (building) or equipment purchases of a sufficient expense that they are beyond the limits of the annual budget. Such purchases are called capital expenses or capital outlays. In an athletic training setting, a capital expense may include modalities, ice machines, expensive rehabilitation equipment, and facility remodeling. Capital expenditures may require a separate budget request, additional fund raising, and detailed justification.

BUDGET CLASSIFICATIONS

There are a variety of budget classifications used in both private and public sector athletic training settings. A limited budget is commonly used in educational settings. In this type of budget, the monies are managed throughout the year. If there is money remaining in the budget toward the end of the fiscal year, it is then taken back and can be used in other parts of the organization. A common practice in this model is to spend in order to not lose the budgeted monies, regardless of need. A rollover budget is one that rolls monies not spent in one fiscal year over to the next. Organizations may use one budget system (eg, line item) within a broader classification (eg, limited budget).

The budget systems that follow are part accounting procedure, part program philosophy, and part organizational tool. The budget type will vary by organization type. The budget type may be dictated by the larger organization at the program level. The outreach program in the sports medicine clinic will likely be required to use the budget system put forth by the broader clinic. An athletic training program within an intercollegiate athletic department will be required to use the budgeting process put forth by the department and likely the university as a whole.

LINE ITEM BUDGET

Line item budgeting is a common system used in multiple settings. The budget is separated into various categories or objects on a line (therefore, "line items"). Line items are often assigned numbers to allow for accounting in large organizations.[1] Line items can be plotted over the course of the fiscal year, allowing a view of resource expenditures over time. Such analysis can be helpful in identifying spending trends. However, the use of broad categories in the line item system may limit the ability to analyze specific items. This may reduce the user's ability to monitor how efficiently funds are being used. Fortunately, many purchasing and accounting systems allow for coded line items to be broken down in monthly reports to see spending details for each category.

Although there is freedom to allocate funds toward various items within each budget line, transferring funds from one line to another may or may not be permitted. Programs may be limited if over-spending occurs in one category, even if another line is under budget. Line item budgets that are not program specific may not be very helpful. For instance, if salaries and operational costs for the entire organization are lumped into one budget, meaningful budget analysis is not possible. Individual programs within an organization should have oversight of their own program areas to better understand spending patterns and to influence future budget planning. If individual programs cannot influence the budget planning, administrators may be forced to use line item budgets without having a full understanding of program needs. Figure 3-2 shows some common line items that may be found in a typical intercollegiate-based athletic health care setting.

PROGRAM BUDGETS

Program budgeting is similar to line item budgeting; however, the program budget allows for specific subdivisions of an overall system to have separate accountability. For example, instead of allocating a

Common Line Items for Intercollegiate Athletic Health Care Setting

Account: 0240 **Monthly Summary: October**

Fund Source: Intercollegiate Athletics **Program: Sports Medicine**

Object:	Description:	Year to Date Budget:	Monthly Expenditures:	Year to Date Actual:	Available Balance
2110	Travel/Continuing Ed	$ 10,000.00	$ 0	$ 3,750.00	$ 6,250.00
2140	Interviewing/ Relocation	$ 1,000.00	$ 0	$ 0	$ 1,000.00
3040	Maintenance/Repair	$ 5,000.00	$ 750.00	$ 1,250.00	$ 3,750.00
3060	Memberships	$ 3,000.00	$ 0	$ 0	$ 3,000.00
3100	Postage	$ 3,500.00	$ 598.00	$ 2,621.00	$ 879.00
3110	Printing	$ 6,500.00	$ 1,750.00	$ 2,750.00	$ 3,750.00
3130	Equip. Rental	$ 3,000.00	$ 250.00	$ 1,000.00	$ 2,000.00
3170	Professional Services	$ 35,000.00	$ 6,750.00	$ 16,750.00	$ 18,250.00
3190	Subscriptions	$ 2,700.00	$ 0	$ 600.00	$ 2,100.00
3200	Misc. Equipment	$ 2,000.00	$ 600.00	$ 2,100.00	- $ 100.00
3210	Medical Supplies	$135,000.00	$ 28,250.00	$ 56,350.00	$ 78,650.00
3230	Office Supplies	$ 10,000.00	$ 1,250.00	$ 3,250.00	$ 6,750.00
3240	*Telecommunications	$ 12,000.00	$ 0	$ 0	$ 12,000.00
Totals		$228,700.00	$ 40,198.00	$ 90,421.00	$138,279.00

*Note: Telecommunications will be billed to each department quarterly.

Figure 3-2. The above items are common line items found in a very large intercollegiate athletic health care setting.

general amount of money toward the line item labeled "equipment," the program budget would fraction the equipment category into the specific sub-areas in which the equipment is used (ie, orthopedic goods, rehabilitation equipment, modalities). One major advantage to the program budget is that this option allows for greater prioritizing of items in the budget-planning process. This process can also tie program budget areas directly to goals and objectives by better defining specific budget items. Program budgeting is still just line item budgeting with more categories so some of the same disadvantages exist. A successful program budget places a premium on developing adequate program categories to account for all program needs and allow for cost-benefit analysis.

Incremental Budgets

The incremental budget is based on the line item budget system described above. The incremental budget uses an existing budget and either adds or subtracts a specific percentage based on available funds. Specific line items can be increased or decreased accordingly. If the athletic health care budget were provided a 10% increase, this would allow each budget line item to be increased by 10%. However, shrewd managers will want to analyze budget trends to see if this is logical. It may make more sense to increase one line item by 20% and decrease another by 10% to distribute the incremental increase. This opportunity to make adjustments within each line item is particularly true in times of budget retraction. The freedom to cut from specific lines can help preserve key program functions at the optimal level.

Incremental budget systems treat all areas the same and rely on specific budget management to adjust accordingly. In some organizational structures, like most educational institutions, this is not an issue. However, in certain organizations, like a private sector clinic or a multidisciplinary sports medicine center, multiple areas may have varied levels of performance and still be treated the same with "across the board" budget actions. Such treatment may cause animosity among groups when one area is performing well and increasing revenue and another is performing below par yet both must accept the same budget adjustment.

Such cases rely on effective program leadership (see Chapter 1) and the ability of managers to align goals with budget actions.

Zero-Based Budgets

The zero-based budget (ZBB) approach was designed to help provide a comprehensive, frugal method of financial monitoring. Zero-based budgeting requires that all budget items be fully justified to be included in the annual budget. The development of ZBB grew from the private sector to help control costs.[5] ZBB correctly assumes that many budgets have excess "fat" built in; therefore, the inflated budget becomes the basis for operations. The zero-base assumes you start with nothing and justify everything, therefore no fat. The process gained popularity in government circles in the late 1970s during the Carter administration as a way for government agencies to eliminate wasteful spending. While ZBB received significant press coverage, it does not seem to have had great success.[5] Organizations rarely break out of traditional funding models to shift resources based on a "start from scratch" model annually.

One genuine disadvantage with this mode of budgeting is the enormous time commitment involved during the preparation. The time and money spent on the preparation of the budget justifications can often be spent on other more fruitful ventures. In addition, if ZBB reveals program areas that cannot be justified, who is in a decision-making position to make substantive changes based on the findings of ZBB justifications?[5] ZBB also requires ranking of budget areas to establish funding priorities; in health care this can be particularly challenging. One likely use for ZBB is in the initial start-up of new programs. However, once a budget base is established, it is nearly impossible to create a true "zero" and start over again.

Planning Programming Budget System

Planning programming budget system (PPBS), as the name implies, relies heavily on planning and linking expenditures to specific objectives. PPBS was designed for large institutions and large government organizations like the military.[1] It was popularized in the 1960s and gained widespread use. It was adopted by the US military in the early 1960s after the Rand Corporation developed the system (using new found computer power and prevailing economic theories) to help evaluate budget choices based on comparing alternatives from the point of view of desired objectives and selecting the best alternative.[5] This was logically embraced as a method to insure public funds were spent accordingly. What could be better? Compare all alternatives and move forward.

As expected, it did not prove that easy. Actual examples of successful use of PBSS are challenging to find.[5] While linking budget expenditures and budget desires to program objectives is easily done, adopting budget choices after painstakingly analyzing all alternatives proves time consuming. In addition, budgets tend to exist in a political atmosphere. Assuming all political influence, even within a small organization, can be objectively eliminated by the system is unrealistic. The time and expense of implementing PPBS may outweigh the advantage. The real success may be found in the fact that it rightfully links planning and budgeting together (see Chapter 11). In higher education, PPBS is credited for changing the way management problems could be examined. Beyond its role as a formal budget decision-making tool, PPBS allowed institutions and organizations to think more about goals and objectives and gave legitimacy to planning processes and using greater quantitative analysis.[5]

Fixed and Variable Budgets

A fixed budget system is one that relies on a set budget amount for a given period of time; often a monthly or quarterly basis. This system relies on fixed estimates of available cash for that period to cover expenses. It is adjusted, as needed, at the end of the designated fixed period. The fixed budget system may be used for larger, more established businesses that have good estimates of revenues. A variable budget is also known as a flexible budget. This type of budget system allows for adjustments to monthly expenses based on monthly revenues. Such adjustments are made to insure that expenditures do not surpass the available revenue. Flexible systems are rarely used in institutions or large organizations since monies are usually not distributed on a monthly basis. They may be useful in smaller environments where revenue flows have not been clearly determined. A new private practice sports medicine clinic would need to operate under a variable budget until it was well established. It is worth noting that the fixed and variable budgets are distinctly different from the fixed and variable expenditures described earlier in the chapter.

BUDGET CONSIDERATIONS

The athletic training profession has expanded to many settings in the past 2 decades. Athletic training health care managers find themselves working in a wide range of public and private sector environments. Budget processes, planning, purchasing, and inventory guidelines may vary by setting but the core principle (the cost effective use of available revenues in the interest of program objectives) will remain the same. The majority of certified athletic trainers employed today are found in schools, colleges, universities, and a variety of sports medicine clinics (see Figure 7-1). Many hold jobs that combine clinic duties with outreach to secondary schools. While it is beyond the scope of this text to delineate budget issues for each available employment setting, it is reasonable to explore some issues specific to educational settings and sports medicine clinic settings.

Educational Institutions

The college and university system across the United States encompasses a broad range of institutions with equally varied intercollegiate athletic programs. Community colleges, small liberal arts institutions, and huge comprehensive research institutions all employ athletic trainers to provide care to student-athletes. The financial resources available to athletic trainers at these institutions will vary as well. The ability to use appropriate planning and budget strategies is an essential skill no matter the institution's size. Athletic trainers seeking employment for positions that require controlling resources should clearly understand the financial resources available to them before accepting a specific position. Athletic training health care managers in these settings will be required to learn requisition and purchasing processes specific to their institution in order to maximize available resources.

The interscholastic system may be more challenging given that most school districts are strapped financially for basic instructional resources. Athletic training services, while essential to proper care of student-athletes, are often viewed as a luxury in these settings. In this setting, the financial resources are often controlled at a district level rather than a specific school or program level. Athletic trainers in these settings may need to pool resources to improve purchasing power, work closely with affiliated clinics, and institute strict inventory control plans to get the most out of shrinking resources (see p. 50). Many high school athletic training budgets are a fraction of the budgets found at a major NCAA Bowl Division institution and yet these athletic trainers provide excellent care. How can this be? The creative and judicious use of available resources coupled with caring and compassionate application of clinical skills will result in good care.

Clinical Settings

Athletic training programming in the clinical setting will sit alongside other program areas that contribute to the mission of the sports medicine clinic. Each area, from a budget standpoint, is thought of as either a revenue or cost center. A revenue center is a unit within an organization that is responsible for generating revenues. These are sometimes called profit centers since almost all will incur some costs. Private sector venues are designed to gain profit. Most public sector programs are designed to break even or not go over an established budget. When actual revenue exceeds costs, you have a profit. A cost center is part of an organization that does not produce direct profit and adds to the cost of running the organization. Box 3-1 describes cost and revenue centers

Case Study 3-1

Who Controls Your Budget?

Case. You are the head athletic trainer at a small university with a competitive sports program. You take great pride in the caring and equitable program you have created for all your teams and feel you have made good use of your limited resources. One morning in the hall the volleyball coach shows up with a sales representative from an ankle brace company. She insists that these are the best ankle braces for her volleyball team and implores you to purchase 30 of them for her team. You remind her of your philosophy of bracing athletes who have a specific history of injury and the preventive balance programming you have instituted based on a local study that showed a decrease in ankle injuries with this program. In addition, you inform her that this would not be a wise investment of your budget resources at this time. The coach insists and leaves to seek out her administrator. Later that month on your budget summary you notice a charge for the 30 ankle braces from your sports medicine budget. You are upset and disappointed that this purchase showed up on your budget without your authorization.

Debriefing Questions

- What would you do?
- Do you have all the facts you need?
- How would you approach the coach or administrator?
- What possible solution would you offer?
- Who should be allowed to spend your resources?

Remember, keeping control of your budget is essential. If others can spend your monies in a way that is inconsistent with your program philosophy, you lose your ability to align budget with goals and objectives.

commonly found in a multidisciplinary sports medicine clinic.

Box 3-1

Common Cost/Revenue Centers in a Multidisciplinary Sports Medicine Clinic

- Athletic training outreach program
- Radiology
- Performance and fitness
- Rehabilitation services (physical therapy/athletic training)
- Exercise science lab
- Aquatics program
- Educational classes and community programming
- Physician clinic services
- Pediatric fitness clinic

Just because an area of the organization does not produce a profit does not mean it is not essential. Mission critical programs like marketing, research and development, and community outreach are not revenue centers, but they may be identified as key functions based on organizational goals and objectives. Many athletic training outreach programs run by sports medicine clinics are thought of as cost centers in that the clinic does not make a direct profit from them. However, the presence of the athletic training outreach program can have a direct influence on revenue centers within the clinic (eg, rehabilitation services, physician clinics). Athletic trainers work in and contribute to the revenue generated in many clinic-based revenue centers. Athletic trainers billing for services are generating revenue as are athletic trainers working as physician extenders. As reimbursement for athletic training services becomes more commonplace, a growing number of revenue-generating models are becoming available (see Chapter 9). There are many available models that allow the athletic training programs to contribute to the overall clinic profit (see Chapter 9).

BUDGET ALIGNMENT AND SHRINKING RESOURCES

The concept of aligning the budget with the stated goals and mission of the organization is an essential theme in budget planning and, ultimately, the judicious use of available funds. During times of budget shortfalls, a common occurrence in many institutions, it is necessary to ask hard questions to establish budget priorities. The list of questions below is designed to engage staff members (eg, clinical, academic, private practice) in discussions to identify cost reduction strategies.[6] The order of the questions is deliberate to help insure decisions are made that protect and advance priorities and quality.

Prior to adopting this type of budget discussion strategy, it is important to clarify who will make final decisions regarding budget. Will one leader be taking information in and making a decision or will the group be allowed to advance recommendations? It is helpful to the process to have a clear sense of what level of input the group will have in order to have the most fruitful discussion possible.

Note: The examples in bold below are taken from the perspective of an athletic training outreach program in a multidisciplinary sports medicine clinic. These same questions can be of use in many settings.

Questions to Consider for Shrinking Resources[6]

- Identify principles that will guide the budget deliberations (eg, sustain quality, ensure ability to invest in priorities, etc).
  - **What does the athletic training outreach program hope to accomplish? Can we sustain our previous levels of quality under the current fiscal constraints?**
- List the functions, programs, services, or units most essential to protect.
  - To what extent is the function, program, service or unit a priority in larger strategic planning? (See Chapter 11).
  - **In previous strategic planning exercises, what goals were put forth for the athletic training outreach program?**
- How critical is the function, program, service, or unit to the overall mission or purpose? Why?
  - **How do the athletic training outreach program's goals "fit" into the broader mission of the sports medicine clinic? What would happen if this program no longer existed?**
- What do we know about the quality of the function, program, service, or unit as measured by those served?
  - **What type of feedback has the program received about the quality of the services provided? How recent is that feedback? Does the feedback strengthen the program's case as a critical function to the overall clinic?**

- To what extent does the function, program, service, or unit generate resources?
    - **Does the athletic training outreach program generate resources for the sports medicine clinic? Direct income (eg, contracts, specific services)? Indirect income (eg, referrals, physician visits, physical therapy)?**
- Discuss how these essential programs and services could be done more efficiently, or with fewer resources.
    - How could streamlining or technology make them more efficient?
    - Are there best practices to learn from others?
    - What opportunities are there for partnering, restructuring, or consolidation?
- What are ways we might generate additional revenues? Are there ways we might shift funding sources?
    - **What additional revenue can the outreach program generate? Restructuring of contracts? Increase referrals? Offer other services?**
- Identify functions, programs, services, or units that could possibly be reduced, restructured, or eliminated. Consider the following criteria in deciding which to do:
    - Potential savings: time, cost, results. Short term. Long term.
    - Impact on services. On whom?
    - External perceptions. Political implications
    - Quality/effectiveness sustained or improved
    - Complexity—How hard is it to do?
    - Unintended negative effects on climate, costs

Note: These criteria can also be helpful in discussing bullet #3.

THE PURCHASING PROCESS

Purchasing is the process of acquiring goods and services on behalf of an organization for the purpose of fulfilling specific goals and objectives. While purchasing items can be fairly straightforward, it gets a bit more complicated due to the necessary guidelines put in place by institutions and organizations. While many an athletic trainer laments the steps he or she may need to take to get something purchased, those same steps are designed to insure judicious and cost effective spending habits. Purchasing is an exercise in trust. You are being entrusted to carefully spend other people's money in the interest of the needs of your larger program.

To understand purchasing, it is best to start with some terms[7]:

- Bid—A document provided by a vendor for goods or services you may wish to purchase.
- Competitive bids—A group of bids (usually a minimum of 3) that are collected from vendors to determine best price and value for items you wish to purchase.
- Lot—A group of items that vendors bid on in a group. For instance, you may wish to purchase your pre-wrap from the same vendor who delivers your tape, therefore the tape and pre-wrap can be grouped as a lot.
- Requisition—A written document requesting to purchase specific items from a vendor.
- Internal requisition—A written document requesting goods or services from a group or department within your own organization (eg, printing services, professional services).
- Purchase order—A formal agreement to purchase items that have been requisitioned. Usually issued by a purchasing department at an institution or large organization.
- Invitation for bids (IFBs) and request for proposals (RFPs)—A formal invitation by an organization to a variety of vendors to supply bids for specific purchases or services. Usually used for long-term contracts and capital outlays. Many large institutions maintain Web sites with open IFBs and RFPs. In an athletic training setting, construction projects, large purchases, and long-term contracts for expensive items (like tape) may require an IFB.
- Blanket order or open account—An open purchase order that can be used over a period of time for purchases as needed. Most purchase orders are for specific items purchased on a specific date. Open accounts are often written for the length of the fiscal year for items that may need to be purchased quickly and whose use cannot be easily predicted.
- Shipping—Determines how the items will be transported to your location from the vendor.
- Freight on board (FOB), free on board (FOB), and FOB origin—FOB is used not only to signify who pays for shipping a product, but also when title to the goods transfers. Thus, FOB origin states that the buyer is responsible for shipping charges and that title to the goods (and risk of loss) passes at the moment the seller delivers the goods to the appropriate carrier for shipping.[7]
- Receiving—The act of taking possession of purchased items. Receiving should involve

comparing the invoiced items against the items requested.

- Invoice—A request for payment from the vendor to the purchasing organization.
- Terms—The purchasing terms outline how many days the organization has before they must pay the vendor. This can be problematic; many large institutions have terms of 60 to 90 days while companies (particularly smaller ones) wish to be paid in 30 days.
- Purchasing delegate—A purchasing delegate is an individual authorized by the organization to issue purchase orders on behalf of that department. Many athletic trainers will work with a purchasing delegate.
- Specifications or "specs"—A generic description of the items being bid on in a bid process. Many institutions require blind bid processes with no brand names to insure the most fair and accurate bid process. Vendors can be very creative in writing specifications to insure that only their product can fulfill the order.
- Substitutions—The unfortunate act of having one product substituted for the one you requested. Thorough understanding of organization purchasing rules combined with obtaining clear specifications will help you avoid this problem.

While the specifics of the purchasing process will vary among organizations, many concepts are central to the process. Table 3-2 maps 2 common purchasing scenarios for the athletic trainer using many of the terms outlined above.

Working With Vendors

A positive professional working relationship with vendors can greatly aid the athletic training health care manager as he or she navigates the purchasing process. Vendors are very willing to come to your location and show you new products and explain the services they can provide. They can also provide specifications for items you wish to purchase. It is essential that this relationship be completely above board. Never accept gifts from vendors in exchange for purchasing opportunities—this is illegal in most states. Avoid sending vendors bids unless you intend to give them the full opportunity to submit a competitive bid. Make sure competitive bids are truly competitive. The availability of information on the World Wide Web has made working with vendors easier as athletic trainers determine products they wish to review for purchase. Trade shows, like the exhibits at the National Athletic Trainers' Association annual meeting, are a good location to see various products.

General Purchasing Guidelines

- Base purchasing on program needs after conducting an inventory.
- Understand organizational rules. A large state institution may require the following:
  - Items under $2500 require judicious selection of vendor.
  - Items between $5000 and $25,000 require 3 competitive bids.
  - Items over $25,000 require posting of RFP/IFB.
- Use competitive bidding to get the most for the available funds.
- When purchasing, make product safety an overriding consideration.
- When purchasing agents are not available, delegate purchasing responsibilities to competent and interested staff members.
- When purchasing equipment and supplies, consider service and replacement of items purchased.
- Purchase items in advance of need.
- Insure that product specifications are written with care.
- Purchase products at the lowest cost available without sacrificing either safety or quality.
- Do not accept gifts and favors from vendors.
- Purchase from local vendors when possible.

Note: Individual institutions and organizations will have specific purchasing processes that must be followed.

Adapted from Langley TD, Hawkins JD. *Administration for Exercise-Related Professions*. 2nd ed. Belmont, CA: Thomson-Wadsworth; 2004.

INVENTORY

Managing inventory in your athletic training facility begins with a well-conceived purchasing plan. Storage availability often dictates what must be purchased and when. Purchasing multiple cases of supplies and having no place to put them is not efficient. A clear understanding of patterns of use will influence purchase planning. Once items are received, they need to be properly stored and then accounted for as they are used. Inventory tracking will allow you to avoid running out of essential items when you need them most. Developing a system that is simple and easy for all staff to follow is best. The system

Table 3-2

Sample Purchasing Sequence

Simple Purchase

Step	Action
1	Athletic trainer determines need for purchase.
2	Review of items available from vendors.
3	Desired items for purchase are identified and best price obtained.
4	Requisition is requested from departmental purchasing delegate.
5	Purchasing delegate completes requisition based on bid and contacts vendor.
6	A formal purchase order is written and sent to vendor.
7	Vendor agrees to terms and ships item.
8	Item is received and invoice is compared to packaged items.
9	Invoice is presented to purchasing delegate and payment is made.

Purchase of Items Requiring Bids

Step	Action
1	Athletic trainer receives permission to purchase capital item.
2	Athletic trainer contacts vendors to obtain specifications.
3	Specifications are provided to purchasing delegate.
4	Purchasing delegate includes specifications in an invitation for bids (IFB).
5	IFB is posted for potential vendors to respond.
6	Vendors submit bids based on specifications.
7	Purchasing delegate reviews bid results with athletic trainer.
8	Athletic trainer confirms no substitutions have been included.
9	Purchasing delegate completes requisition based on bid and contacts vendor.
10	A formal purchase order is written and sent to vendor.
11	Vendor agrees to terms and ships item.
12	Item is received and invoice is compared to packaged items.
13	Invoice is presented to purchasing delegate and payment is made.

Adapted from University of Wisconsin-Madison. Purchasing policy and procedure. Available at http://www.bussvc.wisc.edu/purch/policyindex.html. Accessed January 27, 2009.

should also be easily viewed for patterns to emerge. Commercial software programs are available but many inventory programs use simple spreadsheets to track supplies. It should not be left to chance; it does no good to spend considerable time with planning and purchasing only to see items wasted and lost due to poor inventory.

Secure storage with limited access is an essential element to avoiding waste and controlling costs. Allowing access to inventory to anyone other than designated staff can lead to problems; supply areas should not be open to general access. In addition, inventory should be monitored to insure that any items that can expire are used in a timely fashion. Programs that consistently have an abundance of expired or unused items should evaluate purchasing processes and adjust accordingly.

SUMMARY

- Describe the 7 steps to the budgeting process.

  The 7 steps in the budgeting process are planning, gathering data, analyzing feedback, presenting a final budget plan, getting approval, implementing the budget, and evaluating the budget plan. This process forms a feedback loop that allows for continuous monitoring and improvement.

- Define the components of a common athletic training budget.

  Two types of budgets are common in the athletic training setting; short-term and long-term budgets. A short-term budget usually lasts for a period of 1 year and covers the day-to-day costs of operating a program. There are 2 types of short-term budgets: operational and equipment/supply. The operational budget includes items like salaries, administrative costs, and office operations and the equipment/supply budget will include the expendable and nonexpendable supplies, equipment, and services. A long-term budget involves budget items that exceed the annual budget. These items may be related to long-term projects (building) or equipment. Such purchases are called capital expenses or capital outlays.

- Differentiate the various budget systems.

  A variety of budget systems and classifications are presented in the chapter, and they are part accounting procedure, part program philosophy, and part organizational tool. Incremental, zero-based, line item, program planning, fixed, variable, limited, and rollover budgets are described in detail and are all used in various forms in both the public and private sector. Budget systems largely vary by organizational type. At the program level the budget type may be dictated by the larger organization.

- Identify common challenges associated with budget administration.

  Understanding the budgeting process, how budgets are organized, and the nuances of purchasing are essential skills in the cost-efficient provision of care. The successful athletic trainer must be aware of the relationship between budgeting and the implementation of program goals and objectives. Athletic trainers have historically identified organization and administration in general, and financial resources specifically, as key continuing education needs. These needs will only increase as athletic trainers branch out and utilize their unique skills in a range of health care settings.

- Describe the purchasing process.

  Purchasing is the process of acquiring goods and services on behalf of an organization for the purpose of fulfilling specific goals and objectives. Organizations put purchasing procedures in place to insure judicious and cost-effective spending habits. Athletic trainers with purchasing responsibilities must recognize that purchasing is an exercise in trust as you make spending decisions on behalf of others.

- Understand the specifics of the competitive bid process.

  Competitive bids are very specific listings of products and services that a program wishes to purchase. Vendors compete to provide the best available pricing. Multiple bids are collected in order to determine both best price and value. Public organizations such as schools, colleges, and universities often have very strict procedures for the competitive bid process. Athletic trainers who fully understand the process will be better able to maximize their budgets.

- Explain the role of inventory control in cost containment.

  The development of a simple inventory control system is an essential element in an overall budget and spending plan. Insuring that supplies are accounted for, not misused, and do not expire will eliminate waste and have a positive budget impact.

ACTIVITIES

The following activities are designed to reinforce material presented in the chapter and to allow for discussion among students and instructors.

THE BUDGET GAME

Congratulations. You have been hired as the head athletic trainer at a small Division III college. Anytown Tech is starting a sports medicine program for the very first time. You have one assistant to assist with managing the sports medicine program. Due to the generosity of many thoughtful alumni, you have a nice new 1500 square foot athletic training facility fully stocked with tables, office equipment, therapeutic modalities, and an ice machine. You will not need to budget for salary of personnel. However, you need to develop a short-term budget for your supplies and services and expendable items. Please develop a line item budget using the zero-based budget technique. Consider the following facts about your program as you develop your budget:

- Anytown offers 12 sports (men's and women's soccer, softball, baseball, men's and women's indoor track and field, men's and women's outdoor track and field, volleyball, wrestling, and men's and women's basketball).
- A total of 250 athletes participate in the sports program.
- You are limited to only $4000.00 for supplies and services.
- Think about everything you will need (tape, bandages, service contracts).

Questions to consider:

- How will you determine amounts for your various purchases?
- How will you determine pricing for each item?
- What office items will you need?
- How will your budget reflect your athletic training program goals?
- What if you had to trim your budget by 10%?

Securing Bids: A Purchasing Activity

Your athletic training staff has recently been the recipient of a generous donation to aid in the purchase of some new therapeutic modalities. The head athletic trainer has asked you to secure 3 competitive bids for a new combination electrotherapy and ultrasound machine. Outline the steps you would take to complete this process.

Items to consider:

- What steps will you take to develop the bid for the modality you want?
- If you are not allowed to identify the exact brand you want to purchase, how can you write specifications to help secure your desired modality?
- How can vendors be of assistance in this process?

REFERENCES

1. Langley TD, Hawkins JD. *Administration for Exercise-Related Professions*. 2nd ed. Belmont, CA: Thomson-Wadsworth; 2004.
2. McGuine TA. Assessing the continuing education needs of Wisconsin athletic trainers: a comparison of three needs assessment methods. The University of Wisconsin-Madison. Available at http://proquest.umi.com. Accessed January 9, 2008.
3. Weidner TG, Vincent WJ. Evaluation of professional preparation in athletic training by employed entry-level athletic trainers. *Journal of Athletic Training*. 1992;27:304-310.
4. Board of Certification. *Role Delineation Study*. 5th ed. Omaha, NE: Board of Certification; 2005.
5. Birnbaum R. *Management Fads in Higher Education: Where They Come From, What They Do, Why They Fail*. San Francisco, CA: Jossey-Bass; 2000.
6. University of Wisconsin Madison Office of Quality Improvement. Discussing budget priorities and reduction. Available at http://www.mbo.wisc.edu/biennial/bienn0305/M07.B.0305.pdf. Accessed December 16, 2007.
7. University of Wisconsin Madison. Purchasing policy and procedure. Available at http://www.bussvc.wisc.edu/purch/policyindex.html. Accessed January 27, 2009.

Chapter 4

HUMAN RESOURCES

Gina M. Delmont, MPA, ATC

OBJECTIVES

At the end of this chapter, the reader will be able to:

- Apply the intent of key employment laws
- Define sexual harassment and explain the 2 most prevalent types of sexual harassment
- Write a job description
- Recognize the different types of employment categories
- Recall legal and illegal questions that may be asked as part of a job interview
- Describe a performance appraisal/evaluation process and its purpose
- Explain the components of a compensation and benefit package

More times than not, certified athletic trainers (ATC) are asked to wear many hats in the job setting. Of these particular hats, the human resources (HR) function shows up in a variety of duties, dictated largely by nature and type of organization. When examined on the basis of organizational culture, organizational behavior, and organizational structure, it becomes apparent that smaller, less structured/formal organizations tend to divide the HR tasks amongst their managers. Dependent upon the organizational structure, an athletic trainer may be asked to participate in particular HR functions from recruiting, interviewing, and hiring personnel to performance evaluation/appraisal and compensation/benefit packages. Large organizations will have an HR department with established policies and procedures that address many of the topics in this chapter. As organizations try to meet the employment laws, they will address employment issues a little differently, thus you must become familiar with your institution's/organization's HR policies and procedures.

The first part of this chapter examines the federal laws that directly impact HR management. The remainder of the chapter addresses 3 primary functions relative to HR management, including recruiting, hiring, and performance evaluations (Figure 4-1). Box 4-1 also lists Web sites that can be useful in negotiating the HR landscape.

EMPLOYMENT LAWS

Most of the employment laws deal with protecting people from discrimination during the application and hiring process and then once they are on the job. It is illegal to discriminate on the basis of a number of factors, including but not limited to race, religion, sex, age, disability, veteran status, pregnancy, and marital status.[1] The Civil Rights Legislation over the years has led to the identification of a number of "protected classes or characteristics." These are traits that the law prohibits employers from considering when making an employment decision as well as state and local laws may also protect additional characteristics (Box 4-2), thus the need to be familiar with state/local law.[2]

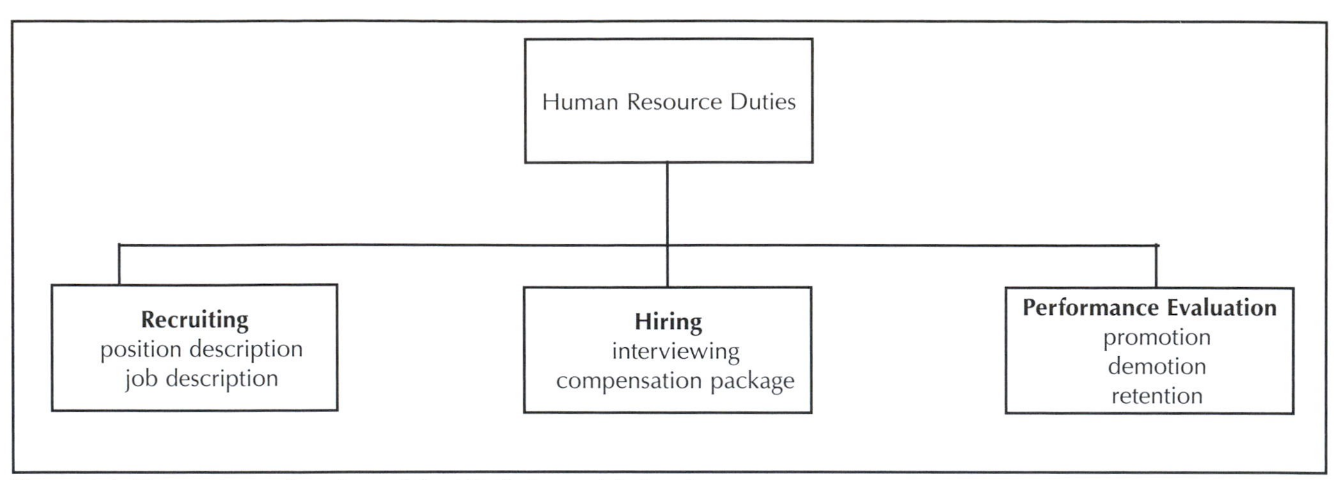

Figure 4-1. Three primary functions of the HR duties and their subcomponents.

Box 4-1

Human Resources-Related Web Sites

Equal Employment Opportunity Commission (EEOC)	www.eeoc.gov
Occupational Safety and Health Administration (OSHA)	www.osha.gov
ELAWS (Employment Laws Assistance for Workers and Small Businesses) Advisor	www.dol.gov/elaws
Americans with Disabilities Act (ADA) Document Center	www.usdoj.gov/crt/ada
Bureau of Labor Statistics (BLS)	www.bls.gov
State Department of Travel	www.travel.state.gov
Society for Human Resource Management (SHRM)	www.shrm.org
WorldatWork	www.worldatwork.org
Workforce Online	www.workforceonline.com

Adapted from Messmer M. *Human Resources Kit for Dummies.* Hoboken, NJ: Wiley Publishing, Inc; 2007.

Box 4-2

Protected Classes/Characteristics

Federal law recognizes these traits as protected classes:

- Sex
- Race
- Color
- National origin
- Religion
- Age
- Disability
- Military status

Additionally, federal or state law may also recognize these as protected characteristics:

- Sexual orientation
- Gender identity
- Marital status
- Creed
- Pregnancy

What Is a Protected Class?

Protected class is a group of people distinguished by the special characteristic(s) that has inhibited its progress: race, color, ethnic identification, national origin, religion, sex, age, disability, and veteran status.

What Is BFOQ?

Bona fide occupational qualification (BFOQ) is a trait that is integral or essential to the job in question.

Adapted from Messmer M. *Human Resources Kit for Dummies.* Hoboken, NJ: Wiley Publishing, Inc; 2007.

The first step in planning for a potential new hire is to determine the vacant position's necessary qualifications.[3] The important consideration in this necessary step is to familiarize yourself with the laws that govern any portion of the employment process.

The Equal Employment Opportunity Commission (EEOC) (www.eeoc.gov) is the federal agency responsible for enforcing federal antidiscrimination laws in employment. It is the EEOC's Uniform Guidelines on Employee Selection Procedures (1979)[4] that should be referred to when beginning to understand what these practices entail. These guidelines present content specific to job postings, questions asked within interviews, employee testing procedures, and other pertinent areas.[4]

It is possible to require specific qualifications that, in effect, disqualify large quantities of individuals. For example, if the position involves working with a team made up of players that speak a foreign language and requires international travel for a majority of the season, it is legal to list the qualification of bilingual within all of the hiring procedures.[5] This legal qualification that does exclude anyone who does not speak the foreign language, for example, is called a bona fide occupational qualification (BFOQ).

There are 6 federal labor laws that directly affect ATCs who are responsible for recruiting, hiring, and performing evaluations/appraisals: Age Discrimination in Employment Act—1967 (ADEA),[4] Americans with Disabilities Act—1990 (ADA),[6] Equal Pay Act (1963),[4] Family and Medical Leave Act—1993,[7] Title VII of the Civil Rights Act (1964),[4] and the Fair Labor Standards Act—1938.[4] Each of these laws is summarized in Table 4-1. Although each is a separate legislative act, these laws all have the common effect of creating "protected classes" (see Box 4-2). Within the legal context, a protected class is a group of people legislators have identified as having suffered from economic discrimination in the past.

Sexual Harassment

Sexual harassment by definition is any form of harassment that has sexual overtones and includes unwelcome sexual advances, requests for sexual favors, and other verbal or physical conduct of a sexual nature.[1] It can involve either situations between males and females or same-sex interactions or advances.[8] There are 2 types of sexual harassment: quid pro quo and hostile work environment.[8]

Quid pro quo is a Latin term meaning "this for that." It involves instances when a manager or supervisor makes it clear to an employee that his or her job and or job benefits are dependent upon an exchange of sexual favors and follows through with the threat in a way that tangibly affects the recipient's employment (ie, loss of job, denied pay increase).[8] Examples of this type of sexual harassment include the following situations[7]:

- A manager promises an employee a promotion if the employee agrees to date him or her, the employee refuses to date, and promotion is subsequently denied.
- A manager threatens to terminate (fire) an employee who refuses his or her sexual advance, and the employee is subsequently terminated.

A sexually hostile work environment is one in which an employee is regularly exposed to offensive sexual comments, jokes, cartoons/pictures, and/or any sexual conduct that makes it difficult for an employee to perform his or her job.[8] A work environment may be considered hostile not only based on sex, but also on other factors, including race, religion, age, disability, and national origin. The inappropriate comments or behaviors that constitute a hostile work environment can be transmitted by words, e-mails, faxes, Internet material, posters, calendars, etc.[8] Generally, conduct that creates a hostile work environment must be[7]:

Table 4-1

Six Important Human Resources–Related Laws

Act	*Purpose*	*Whom the Act Protects*
American Discrimination in Employment Act of 1967 (ADEA)	To promote employment of older persons, to prohibit age discrimination unemployment, and to help employees and workers find ways of meeting problems arising from the impact of age on employment	All persons age 40 or older
Americans with Disabilities Act of 1990 (ADA)	To provide a clear and comprehensive plan for eliminating discrimination against individuals with disabilities and to provide clear, strong, consistent, and enforceable standards addressing discrimination against individuals with disabilities, including the power to enforce the 14th amendment and to regulate commerce with regard to discrimination faced daily by people with disabilities	Must read the act in its entirety
Equal Pay Act of 1963 (EPA)	To prohibit unequal payments to men and women doing the same job, assuming that the jobs require equal skill, effort, and responsibility and that employees perform the jobs under similar conditions	Women
Family and Medical Leave Act of 1993 (FMLA)	To establish minimum standards for employment—namely to: • Balance workplace demands with the needs of families • Promote the stability and security of families • Promote the national interest in preserving family integrity Note: The act is to accomplish those goals by entitling employees to take reasonable unpaid leave of up to 12 weeks in a 12-month period for medical reasons, for the birth or adoption or care of a son or daughter, and for the care of a son or daughter, spouse, or parent who has a serious health condition	Both men and women
Title VII, Civil Rights Act of 1964	To protect constitutional rights, to extend the Commission on Civil Rights, to establish a Commission on Equal Employment Opportunity (EEOC), and for other purposes	People of race or color other than white (now defined by the Supreme Court in terms of the Civil Rights Act of 1866: all ethnic minorities) People of any bona fide religious persuasion Members of either sex People whose national origin is other than the United States
Fair Labor Standards Act (FLSA) of 1938	Establishes the minimum wage, requires overtime for certain employees, provides restrictions on the employment of children and requires certain forms for record-keeping	Most companies

Adapted from Messmer M. *Human Resources Kit for Dummies.* Hoboken, NJ: Wiley Publishing, Inc; 2007.

- Repeated sexual (racial, religious, etc) behavior that pervades the workplace (however, some conduct can be so severe that one occurrence may be sufficient)
- Offensive to a reasonable person
- Offensive to the recipient

The difficulty with sexual harassment legal cases is that the law is open to interpretation (ie, what is offensive to a reasonable person) and if the case goes to trial, it would ultimately be decided by a jury who would also grapple with this interpretation dilemma. As a manager and/or a person in a supervisory position within an organization, it is your responsibility and duty to report allegations of sexual harassment to the HR department (or through the organization's reporting structure for this type of complaint) for investigation. Given the proliferation of sexual harassment court cases in the workplace, most organizations will have a policy on sexual harassment and a mechanism for reporting these complaints. The complaint of an employee who tells you he or she does not want to get anyone in trouble or cause a big mess over this type of complaint must be investigated, otherwise, why would he or she tell you, his or her supervisor, about it if he or she did not want something done? If this same person walked in and told you that someone had a gun in the workplace but did not want to make a big deal out of it, would you still do nothing? Probably not. The same logic and rationale applies to sexual harassment complaints.

Athletics is not immune to this federal law and with male and female student and certified athletic trainers, coaches, and athletes in close proximity to each other complaints of sexual harassment can occur. The athletic arena is no different from any other workplace.

RECRUITING

Recruiting an employee is a planned process and certain steps must be followed to insure labor law compliance.[3] A position/job description is one of those steps and should be written before actually advertising a position vacancy. A well thought-out and developed job description will result in the following benefits[1]:

- Ensures that everyone who has a say in the hiring decision is on the same page with respect to what the job entails.
- Serves as the basis for key hiring criteria.
- Ensures that candidates have a clear idea of what to expect if, indeed, you hire them.
- Serves as a reference tool during the evaluation process.
- Serves as a benchmark for performance after you hire the candidate.

The job description should communicate as specifically but concisely as possible what responsibilities and tasks the job entails and indicate the key qualifications of the job and if possible the attributes that underlie superior performance.[1] Tasks in a job description describe what the person actually does, while qualifications are the skills, attributes, or credentials a person needs to perform each task.[1] At a minimum, the job description should include position title, department (if applicable), who the position directly reports to, responsibilities, necessary skills, and experience required. An example of a job description appears in Box 4-3.

What Is a Job Description?

Job descriptions are action-oriented documents that clearly and concisely state the primary duties performed, responsibilities carried out, and requirements in a particular job or position. They are not meant to be an encyclopedia of every task performed. Job/position descriptions are the foundation of a sound compensation system and should be used for hiring, evaluation and classification, market pricing, performance appraisal, career pathing, and third-party defensibility.

Adapted from The Human Resources Office at Massachusetts Institute of Technology. Available at http://web.mit.edu/hr/compensation/descriptions.html

The job description will actually help the athletic trainer in exercising due diligence in screening applicants based on job requirements rather than personal characteristics. Beyond being "legal," this will also lead to higher employee retention as it heightens the chances that the best individual has been hired for a given position.[9] The process of hiring an employee is expensive for any organization.

The job setting that often aligns with the organizational culture, behavior, and structure either necessitates or negates these formal job descriptions. However, even though a small clinic setting may not require the formal written descriptions, the same laws must be followed when hiring an employee.[10] Therefore, in a court of law it is a better defense if these written and followed job descriptions can be produced as evidence. Traditionally, processes of hiring within school districts (middle school and high school), college/university, academic program

Box 4-3

Sample Job Description

Job Title: Head Athletic Trainer

Reports To: Athletic Director
Assistant Athletic Director

Supervises: Associate Athletic Trainers
Assistant Athletic Trainers
Graduate Assistant Athletic Trainers
Athletic Training Students

Occupational Summary

Develop, coordinate, and administer a comprehensive sports medical program for University intercollegiate sports. The head athletic trainer will also perform professional and administrative services essential for the successful implementation and development of the program.

Primary Responsibilities

- Develop overall sports medicine program for the University, including injury prevention programs, injury evaluations, injury management, injury treatment and rehabilitation, educational programs, and counseling for student-athletes
- Provide athletic training services for the University's athletic department, including attendance at scheduled team practices and home and away competitions as necessary
- Coordinate and schedule physical examinations and medical referrals for student-athletes to determine their ability to practice and compete
- Responsible for the formation of the University's athletic training staff, including hiring, training, and supervision of assistant/associate athletic trainers, graduate assistant athletic trainers
- Supervision of students majoring in athletic training
- Work in conjunction with the strength and conditioning staff to ensure safety in the design and implementation of fitness, nutrition, and conditioning programs customized to meet individual student-athlete needs
- Schedule and coordinate athletic training staff and students for coverage of all team practices and athletic competitions
- Assist Athletic Director and Business Manager in the development of the sports medical program budget
- Evaluate and recommend new techniques and equipment that would enhance the benefit of the sports medical program
- Recordkeeping and documentation

Required Qualifications

- Bachelor's degree in appropriate area of specialization and 4 to 5 years professional experience. Master's degree preferred, 2 to 3 years professional experience
- Certified by the National Athletic Trainers' Association Board of Certification (NATABOC)
- State athletic training licensure
- Familiarity with NCAA, NAIA, or NJCAA governing rules

For more examples of job descriptions of Certified Athletic Trainers according to setting, see www.nata.org.employment/jobdescriptions.htm

Table 4-2

Applicable Laws According to Number of Employees

Law	Applicability
ADEA (1967)	Applies to all private sector employers with 20 or more employees who work 20 or more weeks per year
ADA (1990)	Applies to all private employers with 15 or more employees
EPA (1963)	Applies to all private employers who have 2 or more employees
FMLA (1993)	Applies to all private employers with 50 or more employees within a 75-mile radius
Title VII of Civil Rights (1964)	Applies to employers with 15 or more employees, as well as virtually all government institutions, employment agencies, and labor unions

settings, and industrial settings are required to follow strict recruiting, selecting, and hiring policies mandated and directed by their HR department.

Clinical and clinic-outreach positions have tended to remain more informal about the hiring process. The organization's total number of employees plays a key role in determining which laws and regulations must be followed. Laws and regulatory issues (some 35,000 and counting) do not apply uniformly to all businesses. These laws and which ones apply to what type of business can be attributed much of the time to 2 evolving factors: the total number of employees within an organization and the demographics of the workforce. Of the 6 laws that most often apply to ATCs in any kind of HR capacity, each law is applicable based on the total number of employees within the organization (Table 4-2).

Beyond specific laws, other more subtle factors have a great deal of influence on the administrative culture specifically related to hiring and firing. One of the subtle factors is the dynamic nature of workplace demographics. In the past, athletic training positions were fairly easy to "pigeon hole" (classify). Antiquated language referred to the "traditional" setting that meant an athletic training position that was associated with a college or high school. The "non-traditional" setting referred to positions that were tied to clinics or hospitals. The scope of athletic training employment opportunities has evolved tremendously! Individuals engaged in filling a vacant athletic training position must also consider, at least to an extent, the general demographics of the pool of potential employees. All administrators or managers would do well to closely examine the demographics of the workplace and consider how these demographics are changing and also consider how the demographics of the job candidates have changed (Table 4-3).

There are several classifications of employees, including full-time, regular part-time, per diem, temporary, and contract. Each organization will have different types of job classifications. The reason that these classifications are important is that it affects salary, payroll taxes, and benefits administration. Full-time employees work a full week, regardless of what they do for the company, where they work, or who they work for. They are generally eligible for all benefits offered by the organization. The organization is also required by law to withhold applicable state, federal, and local taxes.[1] Regular part-time employees work less than 40 hours a week but have a regular schedule, perform a prescribed set of tasks, and have a fixed place where they do their work.[1] They also enjoy the same benefits as full-time employees, including being eligible for benefits. Per diem employees work when they are needed by the organization. Their hours are not regular and they are not generally eligible for benefits. Finally, temporary and/or contract employees are contracted to the organization, typically from a third party but there are independent contractors. Agencies that offer temporary help for entry-level positions as well as those that provide nurses and physical therapists fit this category.

The contingent employee is the latest trend in employee classification in athletic training. The contingent employee instead of having one full-time job with a single employer, may work part-time or on a contract or project basis for a variety of companies in a given year. As evidenced on the Position Vacancy Notice (PVN) on the National Athletic Trainers' Association (NATA) Web site, a "seasonal" vacancy for summer sports/cheerleading camps, "visiting" professorships, and outreach positions are growing in number. These "seasonal" vacancies fit the profile definition of the contingent employee. Virtual offices have and will only increase in athletic training. The outreach positions whereby a clinic employs the certified athletic trainer (ATC) to provide athletic training services to a school/team and does not require the

Table 4-3

Dynamic Demographics of Workforce

Demographic Trends	*Description*
Generational trends	Silent generation Composed of people born before World War II Baby Boomers Composed of people born between 1946 to 1964 Need flexible benefits to accommodate for simultaneously caring for their children and parents Gen-Xers Composed of people born between 1965 to 1980 Generation Y Composed of people born in the early 1980s "Millennials" "Netsters"
Minority/gender trends	"Women and minorities will make-up 70 percent of all new entrants to the workforce in 2008" (Bureau of Labor Statistics prediction)
Information technology trends	Telecommuter/virtual office These employees, although not physically present at a specific building or piece of real estate owned by the company, still count as FTE, thus must be regulated under the same laws as if they were working physically from the business' operational headquarters
Employee classification trends	Temporary employee Contingent employee Contract employee Leased employee

person's physical presence for any number of hours inside the physical plant of the clinic fits the profile of contingent employees.

In 1993, the NATA stepped in to help ATCs by proposing a ratio of full-time equivalents (FTE) to number of athletes. This specifically impacted the intercollegiate athletics setting when the NATA published the *Recommendations and Guidelines for Appropriate Medical Coverage for Intercollegiate Athletics.*[11] This statement aids in proposing more FTE in a sports medicine program based upon the number of athletes along with various other factors.

Full-Time Equivalent

Full-time equivalent (FTE) refers to employee classification. An FTE is a combination of part-time employees whose combined hours are the equivalent of a full-time position, as defined by the employer. This classification system is important to the federal government because it affects salary, payroll taxes, and benefits administration.

In athletic training positions, for example, the FTE might be 50% academic, 50% intercollegiate responsibilities; 50% clinical, 50% outreach services; 50% management, 50% provider; etc.

ADVERTISING

Effectively advertising a position vacancy saves both time and money. Athletic trainers in charge of hiring other athletic trainers are at a natural advantage in this process. Think about where you would look if you were searching for a new job. As a benefit to its members, the NATA hosts a "Career Center" on its Web site at www.nata.org.[12] The career center located on-line also specifies job setting. Job seekers are able to use this site with current membership status at no additional charge. Employers are able to fill out an online form, submit a reasonable advertising fee for a selected amount of time, and reach a targeted population of over 22,000 certified members.

National Athletic Trainers' Association Job Categories

- All other (full time)
- All other (part time)
- Clinic
- Clinic-outreach
- College—academic, educational, and dual appointment
- College—part time
- College—professional staff/athletics/clinic
- Industrial/occupational/corporate
- International
- Professional sports
- Secondary school
- Secondary school (part time)

Reprinted from National Athletic Trainers' Association. Available at http://www.nata.org/members1/careercenter/index.cfm. Accessed January 27, 2009.

Other potentially effective ad placement sites tend to be more setting-sensitive (Box 4-4). For example, if you are advertising for a college/university position working with intercollegiate and/or intramural athletics, the National Collegiate Athletic Association (NCAA) would be an appropriate organization to advertise with. In fact, the NCAA publishes and distributes a biweekly newspaper, *NCAA News*, as well as an online classifieds section devoted to position openings (including athletic trainers) at the college/university intercollegiate/intramural athletic level. The nominal fee involved with placing the ad makes it an effective tool for reaching the target population.

Other venues of advertising specifically for ATC are NATA district and state Web sites, the American College of Sports Medicine (ACSM), and the many listservs that exist. Independent schools (Pre K through 12) often advertise position vacancies in their professional association's newspapers and Web sites.

Box 4-4

Strategic Advertising Places for Recruiting Certified Athletic Trainers

Organization	Web Site
National Athletic Trainers' Association (NATA)	www.nata.org
National Collegiate Athletic Association (NCAA)	www.ncaa.org
District/State Athletic Training Associations	www.nata.org/districts/index.htm
National Association of Independent Schools (NAIS)	www.nais.org
American College of Sports Medicine (ACSM)	www.acsm.org

INTERVIEWING

Interviewing candidates is an expensive and time-consuming task. However, taking the interview for granted can cost the company much more money in the long run at the expense of poor employee retention.[3] Therefore, invest the time, effort, and attention to detail that the interview process requires.

High Cost of Turnover

The Employment Policy Foundation (EPF), a government agency, cited in 2004 an average cost of turnover of 25% of an employee's salary. The exact percentage was different for particular industries.

Adapted from Employment Policy Foundation. Employee turnover is expensive. Available at www.super-solutions.com/pdfs/EmployeeTurnoverExpense2004.pdf. Accessed August 17, 2008.

Messmer[1] lists 4 tasks that the interview process enables you to perform in relation to the candidate.

1. Obtain first-hand information about the candidate's background, work experiences, and skill level and confirm that information with the candidate's resume and/or previous interviews.
2. Get a general sense of the candidate's overall intelligence, aptitude, enthusiasm, and attitudes and how these qualities match up in relationship to the job requirements.
3. Obtain a better sense of the candidate's basic personality traits and motivation for the job.
4. Estimate the candidate's ability to assimilate (fit into) the organization's work culture/environment.

Interviewing is considered any verbal exchange that takes place between a candidate and an employer. However, the interview process begins with the written application if applicable.[5] An application, like an interview, should ask only for information that will help you when considering several candidates for the same position and help you to make the best choice in the hiring decision. To be safe, all questions on a job application or in any interview should only ask for job-related information. Again, do not ask in any form about any protected characteristics unless the characteristics to perform the job are BFOQ (see Box 4-2).

The US Department of Labor—Bureau of Labor Statistics (DOL-BLS)[7] contains a section on employment as an athletic trainer. It is a great resource for not only writing job descriptions but also guiding interview questions. The specifications of certain job settings in athletic training may require certain personal characteristics that would imply a BFOQ and can be asked in the interview process.

Telephone Interview

When narrowing down the "pool" of candidates, the last stage before inviting a candidate for a face-to-face interview should be a telephone interview. Before calling a candidate, it is important to review the resume or curriculum vitae (CV) and cover letter carefully, noting areas of relevance to the position opening that you may want to investigate. Estimate how long you will need to effectively conduct a telephone interview (keeping in mind, the telephone interview is a much shorter conversation). Typically, these can last anywhere between 15 to 30 minutes in length. It is important to communicate the length of the telephone interview beforehand when it is initially scheduled as well as when it begins to stay on-task. Remember, a good rule of thumb is to ask the same questions of each candidate in each telephone interview. Having a list of questions you want to ask both in the phone and face-to-face interview will not only keep the questions consistent from candidate to candidate but also help keep the interview itself more time-efficient (Box 4-5 and Appendix A).

Box 4-5

Questions Suggested in the Telephone Interview

"Tell me a little about yourself and your work history."

"What interests you about this particular job?"

"What unique skills can you bring to this job?"

"What sort of work environment brings out your best performance?"

Face-to-Face Interviews

After the telephone interviewing process, the candidate pool should be reduced to between 3 and 5 candidates invited for a face-to-face interview. There are many ways to structure the face-to-face interview, and depending on the job setting and parameters in place by the hiring organization, the interview may be carried out by the athletic trainer manager or may be completed by a committee in the case of a college/university setting. Whatever the structure and whoever conducts the interview, the questions asked and the activities planned must remain consistent from candidate to candidate.

Questioning

There are several types of interviewing questions that will be addressed below, but amongst these question types there are questions that are not permissible to ask. Again, questions pertaining to protected classes/characteristics (see Box 4-2) are unacceptable and perhaps illegal if not considered a BFOQ. This same warning applies to both interview questions and application questions.[13] Box 4-6 provides some examples of legal and illegal questions.

Generally, interviewing questions can be divided into 4 categories of questions: closed-ended, open-ended, theoretical, and leading.[1] Table 4-4 defines each type of question, when to use it, and examples of each. These questions can be further subcategorized around questions addressing technical and performance skills. Technical skills are those skills that require specific technical knowledge or experience, such as using specific kinds of machines or equipment, using specific kinds of computer hardware or software, and manipulating tools in prescribed and

Box 4-6

Examples of Legal and Illegal Interview Questions

Age Discrimination	
Legal Questions	**Illegal Questions**
Are you over the age of 18? Can you, after employment, provide proof of age?	How old are you? When is your birthday? In what year were you born? In what year did you graduate from college/high school?
Marital/Family Status	
Legal Questions	**Illegal Questions**
Would you be willing to relocate if necessary? Travel is an important part of the job. Do you have any restrictions on your ability to travel? Do you have responsibilities or commitments that will prevent you from meeting specified work schedules? Do you anticipate any absences from work on a regular basis? If so, please explain the circumstances.	Are you married or do you have a permanent partner? With whom do you live? How many children do you have? Are you pregnant? Do you expect to become pregnant and have a family? When? How many children will you have? What are your child care arrangements?
Personal	
Legal Questions	**Illegal Questions**
Are you able lift a 50-pound weight and carry it 100 yards, as that is part of your job?	How tall are you? How much do you weigh? (Questions about height and weight are always illegal unless it can be proven that there are minimum requirements to do the job.)
Disabilities	
Legal Questions	**Illegal Questions**
Are you able to perform the essential functions of this job with or without reasonable accommodations? (Legal if the interviewer thoroughly described the job.) Will you be able to carry out in a safe manner all job assignments necessary for this position? Are you able to lift a 50-pound weight and carry it 100 yards, as that is part of the job?	Do you have any disabilities? Have you had any recent illness or operations? Please complete this medical questionnaire. What was the date of your last physical exam? How is your families' health? When did you lose your eyesight/leg/hearing/etc?

(continued)

Box 4-6 (continued)

Examples of Legal and Illegal Interview Questions

National Origin/Citizenship	
Legal Questions	**Illegal Questions**
Do you have any language abilities that would be helpful in doing this job? (Legal if language ability is directly relevant to job performance.) Are you authorized to work in the United States?	Where were you/your parents born? What is your native language? What is your country or citizenship? Are you a US citizen?
Social Affiliations	
Legal Questions	**Illegal Questions**
List any professional or trade groups or other organizations that you belong to that you consider relevant to your ability to perform this job.	What clubs or social organizations do you belong to? Do you go to church?
Race/Color/Religion	
Legal Questions	**Illegal Questions**
Are you available for work on Saturday and Sunday?	All questions are illegal.

precise ways.[1] Performance skills are the tasks and responsibilities assigned to the position that may relate to managing other employees, making and being responsible for decisions, following established guidelines, following policies and procedures, dealing with other departments, dealing with the public, and receiving an assignment and reporting its results when completed.[1]

If you do not get the answer you were looking for from your question, either rephrase the question or ask a probing question to the candidate, such as "Can you say more about that?" "How did you respond to that?" or "What was the final outcome?" (see Chapter 10 under listening regarding probing questions). Finally, allow for silence particularly with open-ended and behavioral (see below) types of questions. Sometimes a candidate will simply have trouble thinking of a specific instance of the kind of behavior you are interested in and will sit for a moment or two in silence. Do not hesitate to let the person know that silence is okay and that you do not mind waiting while he or she tries to formulate the best example.

Behavioral Interviewing

Behavioral interviewing is a structured interviewing strategy built on the premise that past behaviors and performance are the best predictors of future behavior and performance. Because of this, you want to get the candidate talking about how he or she handled situations similar to those that will be experienced on the new job instead of asking hypothetical questions about how the candidate might handle some future task. Typically, these are open-ended type questions that could take a candidate 30 to 60 seconds to formulate an answer, so allow for silence. Box 4-7 contains some examples of behavioral interviewing questions, as does Appendix A.

Box 4-7

Examples of Behavioral Interviewing Questions

- Tell me about a time when your work or an idea of yours was criticized.
- Describe a difficult problem at work that you have had to deal with and how you resolved it.
- Describe a situation in which you were required to work under pressure and how you reacted.
- Describe a time that you showed initiative.
- Tell me about a time when you put your foot in your mouth at work.
- Describe a situation when you found yourself challenged. How did it work out?

Table 4-4

Types of Questions

Question Type	*Definition*	*When to Use*	*Examples*
Theoretical	Questions that place you in a hypothetical situation.	Useful when framed in the context of actual job situations. More likely to test the candidate's skill at answering questions rather than in doing a good job.	"How would you organize your team to begin work?" "What kind of change would you implement in this department?"
Leading	Questions that hint at the answer the interviewer is seeking by the way they are phrased.	Rarely, if ever.	"Working on your own does not bother you, does it?" "This is a stressful position with constant deadlines. How are you with deadlines?"
Closed-ended	Require a "yes" or "no" answer.	Used mostly to verify or confirm information.	"You have an master's degree, is that correct?" "Do you like working with people?" "Did you like your last job?"
Open-ended	These require more than a "yes" or "no" response. They get the candidate to talk about how he or she solved a problem, handled a specific responsibility, or carried out a task. They often begin with, "Tell me...", "Describe...", "When...". These questions should be prepared around the technical and performance skills needed to be successful in the job.	Most of the time.	"When is it okay to break the rules?" "Describe a time you had to be flexible in planning a workload." "What does it take to challenge you?" "What kind of people annoy you?" "If I call your references, what will they say about you?"

Peer Interviewing

Peer interviewing involves the candidate's potential future coworkers interviewing the candidate for the job. Peer interviewing can be done either one-on-one or with several employees and the candidate at one time with people taking turns asking questions. It is generally a good idea with a group interview of this type to discuss beforehand what questions will be asked by whom. It is also not a bad idea for the manager to review the questions with the group to be sure all of the questions are legal. This type of process allows for the employees' input into the candidate selection process and allows the candidate to meet the employees as well. This type of interview is typically done without management present.

COMPENSATION AND BENEFITS

The organization's overall compensation package plays a major role in your ability to recruit and retain employees.[14] Unless the athletic trainer either owns or manages the business, he or she may not have any control over the structure of the compensation package he or she can offer a candidate. The compensation package refers to all the rewards that an employee receives in exchange for his or her work, including base salary or hourly pay, raises, bonuses/incentives, and benefits. Within the compensation package, it is beneficial to align base salary to a national average or in the case of athletic training, setting appropriate. Raises are justified increases in pay that should be documented through a performance appraisal/evaluation. Bonuses/incentives are inherent to the nature of the organization—it may be natural to be on a bonus/incentive plan if the athletic trainer worked as a sales representative for an orthotic company, but not be offered that same type of plan when working in the high school setting. Benefits such as holiday/vacation time or accrual, health insurance, tuition/continuing education unit (CEU) reimbursement, and paid membership dues/licensure fees change frequently. Box 4-8 summarizes some of the items to look for in a benefit package.

Box 4-8

What to Look for in a Benefit Package

- Health insurance and the type (indemnity plan, HMO, PPO, etc)
- Dental insurance
- Vision insurance
- Long-term disability
- Short-term disability
- Retirement/pension plan
- 401k (or 401b) plan
- Tax shelter annuity match with 401k plan
- Incentives/bonuses
- Long-term care insurance
- Day care for children
- Medical spending accounts/reimbursement accounts
- Time off, leaves of absence, sick days—how is this all accrued
- Employee assistance program
- Payment of membership/licensure dues
- Continuing education reimbursement

Note: Depending on the organization, some of these benefits could be employee pay all, organization pay all, or employee and organization split some of the cost.

It is the benefits portion of the compensation package that is important for the employer to "sell" the organization to the candidate.[8] Some intangible benefits athletic trainers are often able to offer and are often eager to receive include close contact with physicians of the sports medicine team, surgical observations, and professional development.

What Is COBRA?

The Consolidated Omnibus Budget Reconciliation Act (COBRA) gives workers and their families who lose their health benefits the right to choose to continue group health benefits provided by their group health plan for limited periods of time under certain circumstances such as voluntary or involuntary job loss, reduction in the hours worked, transition between jobs, death, divorce, and other life events. Qualified individuals may be required to pay the entire premium for coverage up to 102% of the cost to the plan.

COBRA generally requires that group health plans sponsored by employers with 20 or more employees in the prior year offer employees and their families the opportunity for a temporary extension of health coverage (called continuation coverage) in certain instances where coverage under the plan would otherwise end.

COBRA outlines how employees and family members may elect continuation coverage. It also requires employers and plans to provide notice.

Reprinted from U.S. Department of Labor. Health plans & benefits: continuation of health coverage—COBRA. Available at http://www.dol.gov/dol/topic/health-plans/cobra.htm. Accessed December 22, 2008.

What Is FMLA?

Family Medical Leave Act (FMLA) requires covered employers to grant an eligible employee a total of 12 workweeks of unpaid leave during any 12-month period for one or more of the following reasons:

- For the birth and care of the newborn child of the employee
- For placement with the employee of a son or daughter for adoption or foster care
- To care for an immediate family member (spouse, child, or parent) with a serious health condition
- To take medical leave when the employee is unable to work because of a serious health condition.

The employee's job and benefits are protected during this period. See Table 4-1 for additional information.

Adapted from U.S. Department of Labor: Employment Standards Administration. Family and Medical Leave Act. Available at http://www.dol.gov/esa/whd/fmla. Accessed December 22, 2008.

Base Salary

Salary laws are governed under the Federal Labor Standards Act (FLSA). An athletic trainer's base salary is the salary before deductions and other incentives that employee receives in return for the work he or she performs. Although the more awareness that exists with regard to pay scales within athletic training job settings, the more consistent the compensation packages become between jobs.[14] To be competitive in the marketplace as an employer, you should educate the organization as to relative salaries for the different job settings in athletic training. The 2005 NATA Salary Survey is available to members at www.nata.org.[8] The US Department of Labor—Bureau of Labor Statistics[15] also cites a salary range for athletic trainers, but it is not specific to the job setting. The Equal Pay Act of 1963 prohibits pay differences between men and women performing the same work. Managers must examine their organization's compensation system to ensure compliance with the laws (Box 4-9).

Box 4-9

Self-Assessment Questions on Equal Pay Act (1963)

- How does pay compare for positions with similar grades/titles/responsibilities within your company?
- On average, are women and minorities paid similarly to men and nonminorities within the same jobs?
- How long do men, women, and minorities stay within one job classification before promotion occurs? Do all workers have equal opportunity for advancement?

Exempt and Nonexempt Status

Jobs are either classified as exempt or nonexempt positions. Exempt positions define employees who perform certain types of duties and receive salaries and are thus ineligible for overtime pay. Exempt positions are excluded from minimum wage, overtime regulations, and other rights and protections afforded to nonexempt workers.[16] Typically, only executive, supervisory, professional, or outside sales positions are exempt positions, but there are can be exceptions.[16] Nonexempt workers are paid an hourly wage that must be at least the federal minimum wage, entitled to overtime pay of not less than one-and-a-half times their hourly rate for any hours worked beyond 40 each week, and are covered by the provisions of the Fair Labor Standards Act (FLSA) and comparable state laws.[1,16-18] The criteria for determining if a position is exempt or nonexempt is complex but includes taking into account the salary amount, how the worker is paid, and what kind of work he or she performs. To be exempt an employee must be paid at least $23,600 per year, be paid on a salary basis, and perform exempt job duties.[17] Most employees must meet all 3 of these "tests" to be exempt. Typically, the "tests" for exemption get a little murky when considering "performing exempt job duties" and may require help from an experienced HR person or a wage and hour/labor attorney. Generally, exempt employees are paid more than nonexempt employees because they are expected to complete tasks regardless of the hours required to do them.[1,16]

HIRING/MAKING THE OFFER

Extending an offer to a candidate may be the easiest part of the hiring process. In some instances the candidate will counteroffer, usually wanting more money, since in most instances benefits are set by the organization as a whole and not negotiable. Generally, in large organizations an offer is made on a pay grade/range that is commensurate with experience and degree. However, if you have a master's degree and the position only calls for a bachelor's degree, it does not guarantee you will get credit for a master's degree on the pay grade scale since the job does not call for master's degree to do the job. In essence, you may be overqualified for the job. When a candidate asks for more money than the original offer, the organization must consider if the pay would be significantly out of line with existing pay levels for comparable positions in the organization. The larger the organization, the more this can become a central issue. The lack of a reasonable degree of internal equity in compensation levels can impact employee morale and ultimately retention.[1] Some organizations attempt to offset this request for more money by offering a signing bonus, which is an up-front lump-sum payment to the candidate. These can come with some stipulations based on job performance and length of tenure. For instance, if you voluntarily leave (or are terminated from) the organization within 1 year, you would be required to pay back all or part of the signing bonus.

Whatever has been agreed to in the hiring process should be placed in an "official" job offer letter to the candidate. This will result in reduced confusion and protects both the candidate and the organization if a dispute arises. Finally, most job offers are contingent on the passing of a drug test and physical. While reference checks are still done, background checks take the process further. Background checks are used to increase the probability that the candidate being hired is holding him- or herself out to be the person he or she says he or she is. Typically, background checks include criminal background check, education records/academic degree verification, and certifications and licenses. Other checks may be performed depending on the organization. Typically, the reference and background checks are done before the offer is made; however, if not completed, the job offer would be pending successful clearance in these areas.

PERFORMANCE APPRAISAL/ EVALUATION

An important human resource function completed by athletic trainers in charge of other athletic trainers is the performance appraisal/evaluation. This is a key factor in employee retention.[19,20] Performance appraisals/evaluations are also a critical component of reinforcing appropriate behaviors and of helping employees understand how to avoid inappropriate behaviors within the organization.[20] Athletic trainers' behaviors are traditionally aligned with the NATA Code of Ethics; however, beyond that an organization may have more in-depth rules/policies inherent to its culture. Please refer to www.nata.org/codeofethics/code_of_ethics.pdf for a complete review of the NATA Code of Ethics (also see Chapter 5).

Employers are natural targets for lawsuits in this litigious society. Federal and state laws prohibiting employment discrimination are the main sources of legal concern for performance appraisals.[3] However, properly administered and well-documented performance appraisals/evaluations can serve as a paper trail and aid in developing a good legal defense in the event of a discrimination lawsuit. These lawsuits are filed by an individual and followed up by a branch of the federal government such as the EEOC. Wrongful discharge is the most common claim for litigation and the performance appraisal plays a key role in these cases. Therefore, it is as important to be very detail oriented with performing and documenting the performance appraisal as it is when conducting the interview.

The performance appraisal is usually an annual event whereby the employee expects a raise to be given.[21] If for some reason the employee is terminated or does not receive a raise, the performance appraisal must support the decision in a legally defensible way.

Many of the laws protecting classes of people from discrimination also have an impact on how you should complete the performance appraisals and give pay grade raises. Title VII of the Civil Rights Act of 1964, the EPA (1963), FMLA (1993), ADA (1960), and the ADEA (1967) are all legislative acts that can impact promotion, demotion, and retention of employees (Box 4-10). Furthermore, the Equal Pay Act of 1963 prohibits pay differences between men and women performing the same work. Athletic trainers must make sure there is a consistent method of evaluating performance for all ATCs on staff, regardless of their gender. Although there are several different types and methods of completing performance appraisals, managers should keep in mind several tips to reduce legal exposure (Box 4-11).

Box 4-10

How to Avoid Legal Pitfalls of Performance Appraisals

- Do not use subjective criteria to produce a disparate impact on minorities and other protected classes.
- Do not use a promotion-from-within policy to discriminate against minorities and other protected classes.
- Do not misuse objective records to discriminate.
- Do not "build a file" (ie, writing up your documentation after the fact)
- Do not use a performance appraisal to retaliate for some perceived harm, such as filing an EEOC complaint or worker's compensation claim.

SUMMARY

- Apply the intent of key employment laws.

  Most of the employment laws deal with protecting people from discrimination during the application and hiring process and then once they are on the job. It is illegal to discriminate on the basis of a number of factors, including but not limited to race, religion, sex, age, disability, veteran status, pregnancy, and martial status.[1] The Civil Rights Legislation over the years has led to the identification of a number of "protected classes or characteristics." These are traits the law prohibits employers from considering when making an employment decision.

Box 4-11

Performance Appraisal Tips for Managers

- To minimize exposure to employee litigation, employers should develop a checklist of items that are necessary for the enforcement of fair, consistent, and legally sound performance appraisal systems.
- Apprise employees of performance standards in advance. When a new employee is hired or when new standards are adopted, supervisors should amend job descriptions and performance evaluation forms and copies should be given to all affected employees.
- Document all performance problems regularly on appropriate appraisal or progressive discipline forms. Provide the employee with a copy immediately. A precise format for conducting an evaluation leads to more thorough, accurate recording of information. Informality, on the other hand, may lead to claims of discrimination.
- Provide employees with relevant feedback. Vague, generalized, or subjective evaluations may lead to litigation.
- Promptly evaluate nonproductive employees. When managers tolerate an employee with a performance problem for months and then suddenly give him or her a negative evaluation and terminate him or her, the employee may claim that the action was arbitrary or discriminatory and may be able to show that no opportunity for improvement was given.
- Give the employee an opportunity to comment on or dispute the performance appraisal. This will support the fact that you provided the employee with notice.
- Train supervisors in how to evaluate employee performance and how to administer the company's appraisal system.
- Establish a review audit system to prevent manager bias or personal feelings from impacting on the appraisal.
- Develop written policy statements approving only a specified procedure for conducting appraisals.
- Document through performance files as well as job-related testing, rating systems, appraisal forms, and signed memoranda.

- Define sexual harassment and explain the 2 most common types of sexual harassment.

  By definition, sexual harassment is any form of harassment that has sexual overtones and includes unwelcome sexual advances, requests for sexual favors, and other verbal or physical conduct of a sexual nature.[1] It can involve situations between males and females or same-sex interactions or advances.[8] There are 2 types of sexual harassment: quid pro quo and hostile work environment.[7] Quid pro quo involves instances when a manager or supervisor makes it clear to an employee that his or her job and/or job benefits are dependent upon an exchange of sexual favors and follows through with the threat in a way that tangibly affects the recipient's employment (ie, loss of job, denied pay increase).[8] A sexually hostile work environment is one in which an employee is regularly exposed to offensive sexual comments, jokes, cartoon/pictures, and/or any sexual conduct that make it difficult for an employee to perform his or her job.[8] A work environment may be considered hostile not only based on sex, but also on other factors, including race, religion, age, disability, color, and national origin.

- Write a job description.

  The job description should communicate as specifically but concisely as possible what responsibilities and tasks the job entails and indicate the key qualifications of the job and if possible the attributes that underlie superior performance.[1] Tasks in a job description describe what the person actually does, while qualifications are the skills, attributes, or credentials a person needs to perform each task.[1] The job description should include at a minimum position title, department (if applicable), who the position directly reports to, responsibilities, necessary skills, and experience required.

- Recognize the different types of employment categories.

  There are several different types of employment categories used to classify employees. They can be considered full-time, regular part-time, per diem, or temporary/contract. A full-time employee works 40 hours a week while a regular part-time employee works less than 40 hours per week and both are eligible for benefits. A per-diem employee works when needed, and a temporary or contract employee is not on the organization's payroll and could be paid through a third party.

Jobs are also either classified as exempt or nonexempt positions. Exempt positions define employees who perform certain types of duties and receive salaries and are thus ineligible for overtime pay. Exempt positions are excluded from minimum wage, overtime regulations, and other rights and protections afforded to nonexempt workers.[16] Typically, only executive, supervisory, professional, or outside sales positions are exempt positions, but there are can be exceptions.[16] Nonexempt workers are paid an hourly wage that must be at least the federal minimum wage, entitled to overtime pay of not less then 1.5 times their hourly rate for any hours worked beyond 40 each week, and are covered by the provisions of the Fair Labor Standards Act (FLSA) and comparable state laws.[1,16-18]

- Recall legal and illegal questions that can be asked as part of a job interview.

  There are certain types of questions that cannot be asked in an interview or on an application. Typically, these question types center around protected classes, which include sex, race, color, national origin, religion, age, disability, and military status.

- Describe a performance appraisal/evaluation process and its purpose.

  The performance appraisal is usually an annual event and is generally attached to a pay raise. The purpose of a performance evaluation is to assess the employee's performance against a standard and set goals that not only help the organization achieve its vision and mission but also further develop the employee's skills.

- Explain the components of a compensation and benefits package.

  The organization's overall compensation package plays a major role in its ability to recruit and retain employees.[14] The compensation package refers to all the rewards that an employee receives in exchange for his or her work, including base salary or hourly pay, raises, bonuses/incentives, and benefits. Benefits include holiday/vacation time or accrual, health insurance, tuition/continuing education unit (CEU) reimbursement, and paid membership dues/licensure fees.

ACTIVITIES

The following case studies are designed to reinforce material presented in the chapter and to allow for discussion among students and instructors; case scenarios are based on actual events.

Inappropriate Comments During a Job Interview

Bill was pleased that his new position at Anytown University was going so well. He was starting his second year on the job as an assistant athletic trainer and had adjusted well to his new surroundings and coworkers. He enjoyed the vibrant atmosphere offered by the large urban campus and the surrounding city. It was mid-summer and the only pressing issue was to hire a new staff member at Anytown. The entire staff was excited about the new position and the potential it had to help improve services to their student-athletes. Bill was happy to volunteer to escort a visiting job candidate to a local eatery while the search committee shared notes from the morning's interviews. The head athletic trainer had indicated in private that this candidate had been very strong during the interview so Bill should not be afraid to talk about how much he enjoyed living in the city and working at Anytown U. She seemed to have the leg up.

Somewhere between the salad and the sandwich, Bill was making small talk and asked why she had decided to pursue the job at Anytown. She nonchalantly admitted that there were just getting too be too many people in her current town that did not look like her. Bill nearly choked on his food and asked, "What do you mean?" What followed was a blatantly racist remark. Bill sheepishly said, "Well, this is a very diverse community. I don't know how you will feel about living here." Bill kept replaying the conversation in his mind. Did her really hear her correctly?

Questions to consider: Should Bill have reacted more strongly to the initial comment? What should he say to the head athletic trainer who was so high on this candidate? Would you follow up with the people who wrote recommendations for this candidate? What would you say if you heard someone in your organization was considering hiring this person?

Position Vacancy Exercise

- Visit the NATA Career Center at www.nata.org and review samples of job postings.
- Write a position vacancy listing for a hypothetical athletic training position offered in the following employment settings:
  - High school
  - College or university
  - Corporate industrial workplace
  - Performing arts

  How would these position listings differ? What commonalities would they contain?

Appropriate Interview Questions

- Write a list of 10 interview questions for a hypothetical job interview. Make sure that at least half of them are behavioral-style interview questions.
- Write a list of 10 questions you are NOT allowed to ask in the interview process. Explain why these questions are illegal.

REFERENCES

1. Messmer M. *Human Resources Kit for Dummies*. Hoboken, NJ: Wiley Publishing, Inc.; 2007.
2. The University of Chicago Human Resources. Key concept learning: protected classes. Available at www.hr.uchicago.edu/train/EEO-AATUTORIAL/pdfs/EEO-AA%20Tutorial.pdf. Accessed August 17, 2008.
3. Mueller LM, Dunleavy EM, Buonasera AK. Analyzing personnel selection decisions in employment discrimination settings. *New Directions for Institutional Research*. 2008;138(17):67.
4. United States Equal Employment Opportunity Commission. Available at http://www.eeoc.gov/. Accessed July 31, 2008.
5. Choon-Hwa L, Winter R, Chan C. Cross cultural interviewing in the hiring process: challenges and strategies. *Career Development Quarterly*. 2006;54(3):4.
6. Dutton G. The ADA at 10. *Workforce*. 2000;79(12):5.
7. U.S. Department of Labor Employment Standards Administration. Available at http://www.dol.gov/esa/whd/fmla/. Accessed July 31, 2008.
8. Employment Learning Innovations. *Civil Treatment for Managers: Fair Employment Rights and Responsibilities*. Atlanta, GA: Employment Learning Innovations, Inc; 1998.
9. Oss M. Eight strategies for human resources development. *Behavioral Health Management*. 2004;24(2):4.
10. Hartley D. Job analysis of reality. *Training and Development*. 2004;58(9):3.
11. National Athletic Trainer's Association. Recommendations and guidelines for appropriate medical coverage for intercollegiate athletics. June 2007. Available at http://www.nata.org/statements/support/AMCIARecsandGuides.pdf. Accessed August 7, 2008.
12. National Athletic Trainer's Association. National Athletic Trainer's Association Career Center Web site. Available at http://www.nata.org/careercenter/welcome.htm. Accessed August 7, 2008.
13. Conklin J. Turning the table: six questions to ask your interviewer. *Quality Progress*. 2007;40(11):1.
14. Hansen F. Currents in compensation and benefits. *Compensation and Benefits Review*. 2007;39(5):6.
15. U.S. Bureau of Labor Statistics. Occupational outlook handbook, 2008-2009 edition. Available at www.bls.gov/olo/ocos294.htm. Accessed August 17, 2007.
16. Barada PW. What's the difference between exempt and nonexempt workers? Available at www.career-advice.monstor.com/salary-trends/Whats-the-Difference-Between-Exempt/home.aspx. Accessed August 17, 2008.
17. Chamberlin J, Kaufman AS, Jones, RA. Coverage under the FLSA. Available at www.flsa.com/coverage.html. Accessed August 17, 2008.
18. U.S. Department of Labor: Wage and Hour Division. Fact sheets. Available at www.dol.gov/esa/whd/fact-sheets-index.htm. Accessed August 17, 2008.
19. Den-Hertog D, Belschak F. Personal initiative, commitment and affect at work. *Journal of Occupation and Organizational Psychology*. 2007;80(4):22.
20. Mollerman E, Vander der VG. The performance evaluation for novices: the importance of competence in specific work activity clusters. *Journal of Occupational and Organizational Psychology*. 2007;80(3):20.
21. Roch S, McNall L. An investigation of factors influencing accountability and performance ratings. *J Psychol*. 2007;141(5):25.

Chapter 5

ETHICAL PRACTICE IN ATHLETIC TRAINING

OBJECTIVES

At the end of this chapter, the reader will be able to:

- Recall the 3 categories of ethics
- Compare and contrast the 3 areas of ethics
- Summarize the ethical issues commonly seen in health care
- Explain the key points related to the National Athletic Trainers' Association (NATA) Code of Ethics

What does it mean to be ethical? Taken a step further, what is meant by ethics? Most would point to the behavior or decision-making process of an individual that demonstrates high moral and professional standards. A common misconception is that ethics is synonymous with good or proper behavior. Ethics has almost become a "trash can" term in which multiple "things" such as morals, professional behavior, a system of beliefs, and proper actions are placed. A prime example of this is the frequent reference to an individual with a strong "work ethic" when what is actually meant is that the individual values work and works diligently as a result. In truth, ethics is a branch of philosophy that is sometimes referred to as moral philosophy. It is more than a belief system; it is the study of that belief system and how the belief system came into being. This chapter presents an introduction to the foundations of the study of ethics and examines current standards of practice and professional behavior in athletic training from that foundation.

ETHICS: DEFINED

The field of ethics is generally divided into 3 separate, but on occasion overlapping, areas of study: metaethics, normative ethics, and applied ethics.

METAETHICS

Metaethics is a global study of ethical thought, or more specifically, the origin of ethical thought. One concern of metaethics is determining whether or not moral values exist outside of the human realm. Some would argue that moral values do indeed exist outside of human thought. Plato is a prime example of this. He likened moral thought to mathematical relationships. Consider a number such as 2. Man did not create the number 2 nor does man have anything to do with the fact that 2, when doubled, becomes 4. A number, according to Plato and those that espouse a supernatural perspective of moral values, is an abstract entity beyond the reach of human influence. The logical progression for this train of thought is toward an eternal law that exists, like numbers, beyond human influence. Carrying the progression a step further, William of Ockham, medieval philosopher, believed moral principles or values came from God and were revealed to man through moral conscience and scripture.[1]

Other philosophers such as Sextus Empiricus argued that moral values are inventions of the human mind.[2] This school of thought was the spawning ground for the thoughts of Friedrich Nietzsche concerning moral relativism. Individual relativism supports the concept that individuals create their own moral standards. In other words, what a given individual perceives as moral is strictly relative to him or her as an individual. Cultural relativism is an interesting companion theory to individual relativism. Cultural relativism is also based on a denial of the absolute nature of moral values. While individual relativism is based on the moral values of the individual, cultural relativism is based on the moral values of an entire society or culture.

Case Study 5-1

Cultural Relativism

Case. According to the theory of cultural relativism, moral values are based on cultural norms. The values of a particular society dictate what is and is not morally acceptable. Most readers would agree it is morally wrong to steal. Consider a culture of remote village people that have been largely isolated from the outside world. Any interaction between the members of this village and the outside world are few and far between. A unique aspect of this culture is that they have no concept of ownership. Within this village, it is impossible to own livestock, possessions, or land. It is impossible to own a home because everyone in the village lives in the same large communal dwelling.

Debriefing Questions

- Is it possible to steal within this culture?

Let us take the scenario a step further and imagine that a member of the village had to travel into the closest town on a legitimate errand for members of the village. While in town, the villager became hungry and ate some fruit from a merchant's cart. Of course, he could not pay as he does not understand the concept of money and he is promptly arrested.

- Is it morally right to charge this person of the crime of theft when he has no understanding of property ownership?

Why should you obey the speed limit? Several responses come immediately to mind. Perhaps the most immediate is to avoid getting a costly speeding ticket. You may also have a sincere wish to drive safely and avoid causing an accident. The issue of what motivates people to follow laws or rules or act in a moral fashion is, not surprisingly, of concern in metaethics. Several different theories exist to explain why people make decisions and choices that follow moral values. One theory is based on the ego of the individual making the decision. If someone gives to a charity, according to the theory of psychological egoism, he or she is doing so because it makes him or her feel good to give. The person is making the contribution to gain a sense of self-worth or self-importance, not to help the charity. The rather cynical psychological egoism theory is countered by psychological altruism. Psychological altruism contends there is an inherent desire to be benevolent and the contributor is simply satisfying this desire. Another important ingredient in decision making is the presence or absence of emotion. The presence of emotion becomes much more important when you consider that most philosophers contend that reason and emotion do not both exist within a given decision. Emotion is removed from the equation to facilitate the dominance of reason or vice versa.

Normative Ethics

A second area of study in ethics is normative ethics, which focuses on the principles or moral criteria upon which individuals make decisions. Normative ethics function as the standards for determining what is right or wrong and what is appropriate or correct action or behavior in light of that fact. An excellent example of a principle that fits into this category is the Golden Rule, "Do unto others as you would have them do unto you." If the Golden Rule is the basis for decision making, then making a contribution to help a local charity feed homeless people would be an appropriate decision because you would want someone to help care for your needs if you found yourself missing not only a home but meals as well. There are several theoretical sets of normative principles and a complete discussion of those is beyond the scope of this text. However, 3 of the most common systems or sets of theories will be discussed in order to help develop a basic understanding of the foundations of ethical decision making. These include virtue theories, duty theories, and consequentialist theories.

Virtue Theories

Virtue theories are among the oldest theory sets within the study of ethics. Plato originally identified 4 virtues or characteristics: wisdom, courage, temperance, and justice. The basic premise in virtue theory ethics is that the decision maker chooses action based upon his or her own character or virtue. While good decisions are based on virtues, bad decisions are the result of vices. Simply put, vices are bad characteristics such as cowardice, insensibility, injustice, and vanity. Interestingly enough, Aristotle theorized that all characteristics exist on a continuum and the identification of each as a virtue or a vice is determined by where each falls on that continuum. As an example, courage would be considered by most to be a virtue. However, if courage is carried to an extreme, it becomes rashness, which may not be a virtue at all and would be considered by many to be a vice. Likewise, the opposite end of the courage continuum could be considered cowardice, which is certainly not a virtue.

Consider the following scenario within the context of an athletic training setting. During the championship game, a player injures her knee severely enough to make you question whether or not she should return to play. The chances of her return to play resulting in further injury are substantial. Unfortunately, it is unlikely that the team will win the game if this player is sitting on the bench. The coach is adamant that the player be returned to play and becomes very angry and confrontational during the exchange. You stand your ground and the player is held from competition. Analyzed within the context of virtue theory, you made your decision and stood by it because of some virtue you possess. You defended your decision under duress because you possess courage.

Duty Theories

Duty theories are based on a fundamental and unarguable obligation. Duty theories are sometimes referred to as nonconsequentialist theories because the duty or obligation exists without regard for the consequences. Although, once again, a complete discussion of the topic is beyond the scope of this text, there are several duty theories that merit discussion here. Three general areas of duty were identified early in the development of duty theories, those being duty to God, a duty to one's self, and a duty to others. Specific duties exist within these areas, some of which are relative and some are absolute. One example of an absolute duty would be treating people as equals.

The rights of an individual act as the source of another theory of duty ethics. It is quite logical to relate rights to duties because a given right of one person is typically manifested as the duty of a second person. For example, if you enter the hospital, you have the right to expect that your medical records will not be broadcast on the 6:00 news. This right translates to a duty to maintain the confidentiality of patient records on the part of hospital personnel. In his Second Treatise of Government, British-born philosopher and physician John Locke identified the duty to refrain from taking away the life, liberty, or property of a fellow man.[3,4] Thomas Jefferson built upon these thoughts when he wrote the Declaration of Independence, which recognizes the foundational rights of life, liberty, and the pursuit of happiness. In effect, the framework of the United States of America can be traced back to duty theory ethics.

Consider the previously mentioned scenario in which the injured player is held from competition. Within a duty-based theory, the decision to do so is quite understandable. You as a certified athletic trainer have a duty to provide the highest level of athletic health care possible. Your duty in this particular case is to prevent the player from further injury regardless of the consequences. As such, the probable loss to the team is irrelevant as you make your decision.

Consequentialist Theories

Consequentialist or teleological theories are based on the concept of letting the consequences of a decision determine the appropriateness of that decision. In essence, the action is ethically "right" if the consequences of the decision are more positive than negative. There are 3 basic subdivisions of consequentialist theories, each differing according to whose perspective is taken when determining whether an outcome is good or bad (Table 5-1). Ethical egoism is one of the subdivisions and is typified by examination of whether the outcome is good or bad for only the individual making the decision. In contrast, ethical altruism contends that any given decision is good or bad depending on how the outcome affects everyone except the person making the decision. Somewhere in the middle lies the third subdivision, utilitarianism, which requires that the action or decision produce positive results for everyone in order to be considered a correct or ethical decision. The problem with consequentialist theories is readily apparent in that it all depends upon the question of which party is benefiting from the action or outcome. Whose perspective is considered when making the decision?

Once again consider the scenario where you are faced with making the decision to hold an injured athlete from participation or allowing her to continue to play. Recall the probable outcome of not allowing the athlete to continue to play will be losing a championship game. Instead of going home with a big win and a championship trophy, the team will return home with only a big loss. It is difficult to see a "big loss" being considered a positive outcome for anyone involved in this scenario. Within the context of ethical egoism, the outcome is considered in terms of how beneficial or, conversely, harmful, the outcome is to the certified athletic trainer making the decision not to allow the athlete to continue the play. Ethical altruism, on the other hand, considers the same outcome relative to how it benefits everyone except the certified athletic trainer. If the certified athletic trainer followed a utilitarian model, he or she would have had to consider all options and selected a plan of action that resulted in a positive outcome for everyone. Unfortunately, it is seldom possible to reach a decision that is ultimately positive for all stakeholders in a situation.

Table 5-1
Summary Table of Consequentialist Theories

Theory	Perspective	Example
Ethical egoism	The individual making the decision	Making decisions strictly on the basis of what benefits YOU as the decision maker
Ethical altruism	Everyone EXCEPT the individual making the decision	Making decisions with complete disregard for how the outcome will affect YOU as the decision maker
Utilitarianism	Everyone	Making decisions on the basis of how the outcome affects the most individuals in a positive way

Applied Ethics

Applied ethics is the branch of ethics that deals with specific issues. These issues are current and almost always controversial. A few examples of current issues in general health care include euthanasia, stem cell research, and abortion. Most of these issues carry an associated level of emotional involvement, which can serve to complicate the process of reaching a resolution. Fortunately, stem cell research and euthanasia fall outside the scope of everyday practice for athletic trainers.

According to Wadsworth, an issue must meet 2 requirements to be considered an applied ethical issue. In order for an issue to fall into the applied ethical realm, it must first be controversial. The issue of anabolic steroids is quite controversial, but that in and of itself is not sufficient to merit labeling it as an applied ethical issue. The second element that must be present is a moral element. The issue must be a moral issue. If examined within the context of morality, anabolic steroids, as an applied ethical issue, fails to meet the mark. Using anabolic steroids is a practice few, if any, could condone as being morally right thus there is no real moral issue. Using steroids is wrong on many different levels, one of which happens to be the moral level.

COMMON ETHICAL ISSUES IN HEALTH CARE

Up to this point, the ethics discussion has been very academic and maybe somewhat difficult to apply directly to athletic training. A look at general health care ethics can prove useful here. There are certain issues that are identified by Edge and Groves[5] as basic tenets of health care ethics. These include, but are not limited to, confidentiality, veracity, beneficence, benevolence, and role fidelity (Table 5-2). These basic tenets can provide insight into ethical behavior within athletic training and as such merit further discussion.

Confidentiality

Confidentiality is paramount in health care regardless of the area or branch of health care being considered. It is not only unethical but also illegal to breach confidentiality. The opportunities for such a breach are often present in an athletic training room or clinic. Consider the athletic trainer working with a NCAA Division I basketball team playing in the final four of the NCAA tournament. The starting center, and leading scorer, sprained his knee during the last game. At this point, virtually the whole world wants to know the status of the injured player. Is this not a situation that begs for the breach of confidential information? You do not have to be in a high visibility position to encounter the issue of confidentiality. Athletes in a high school deserve the same level of consideration that high profile collegiate or professional athletes deserve. The content of a medical file, specific information relative to the diagnosis and prognosis of a patient/client/athlete, as well as personal information (eg, social security number) is confidential and must be treated as such.

While no one will argue the need to maintain confidentiality, it must be stated here that confidentiality is not absolute. There are several specific situations in which it is in fact illegal to maintain confidentiality. Like other health care providers, certified athletic trainers are in a position of trust relative to the individual under their care. As such, it is not uncommon for an athlete to divulge information of a very sensitive nature nor is it uncommon that this information is such that it must be brought to the attention of proper authorities. Generally speaking, the following situations listed in Box 5-1 mandate breaking confidentiality.[6]

Table 5-2

Basic Tenets of Health Care Ethics

Confidentiality	Maintaining the privacy status of medical records and personal information of the patient/client/athlete
Role fidelity	Refraining from engaging in activities that are outside of your legal scope of practice; respecting the role of other members of the health care team
Veracity	Being truthful in all communications with the patient/client/athlete
Beneficence/nonmaleficence	Performing only those actions that promote the well being of the patient/client/athlete; refraining from those actions that do not promote the well being of the patient/client/athlete
Autonomy	Recognition of the patient/client/athlete as an individual with a will to make decisions relative to his or her own health and well being; respect for the patient/client/athlete as a human being with inherent value

Adapted from Edge RS, Groves JR. *Ethics of Health Care: A Guide for Clinical Practice.* 3rd ed. Florence: Thomson Delmar Learning; 2005.

Box 5-1

Situations Where Confidentiality Cannot Be Maintained

- Child abuse
- Drug abuse
- Communicable disease
- Injuries with guns or knives
- Blood transfusion reactions
- Poison and industrial accidents
- Misadministration of radioactive materials

While it is highly unlikely that a certified athletic trainer will encounter the misadministration of radioactive material (see Box 5-1), it is not that unlikely that he or she might encounter drug use or even child abuse depending on the patient population he or she is working with. The underlying principle within each of the above exceptions is the harm principle. If maintaining confidentiality will result in harm to the patient or someone else, a breach of confidentiality is indicated. The harm principle is clearly depicted in a case involving a patient under psychological treatment in California. The patient shared with his psychologist that he intended to kill a woman who had rejected him as a suitor. The psychologist recommended that his patient be detained for observation, but the patient managed to convince authorities he would stay away from the woman. Tragically, the patient made good on his threat to kill the woman and the victim's family subsequently held the same authorities responsible. The Supreme Court of California agreed and held the authorities liable for the death of the young woman.[7]

Case Study 5-2

Confidentiality

Case. You are employed as an athletic trainer by a hospital that provides athletic training services to local high schools. During a treatment session with a high school athlete, you become concerned because this particular athlete, usually bright and cheerful, seems despondent. You ask the athlete some general questions about how he is feeling and the athlete asks if he can share something with you in confidence. After you agree, the athlete tells you he has experienced several emotionally traumatic events in the past year and he simply does not think he wants to be alive anymore. He has considered taking his own life.

Debriefing Questions

- Is it right to breach confidentiality in this situation?
- What principle comes into play here?

Role Fidelity

Role fidelity is a term that implies an individual will remain consistent with the expectations of the professional role he or she plays. In the case of athletic training, this means the individual will perform the duties of an athletic trainer and nothing else. More specifically, the term implies that the individual will not venture beyond the scope of athletic training practice. Role fidelity issues may arise as a certified athletic trainer is working as part of a team that delivers health care to the patient/client/athlete. It may be easy for the lines of distinction between professional to become blurred. If such a situation arises, the athletic trainer must remember his or her role as outlined by the NATA[8]:

> *Certified athletic trainers are health care professionals who specialize in preventing, recognizing, managing and rehabilitating injuries that result from physical activity. As part of a complete health care team, the certified athletic trainer works under the direction of a licensed physician and in cooperation with other health care professionals, athletics administrators, coaches and parents.*

While it is difficult to imagine an athletic trainer simply deciding he or she is qualified to practice pharmacy and subsequently begin dispensing prescription medications from the athletic training room, there are other, much more subtle situations in which role fidelity issues are encountered. Role fidelity implies more than restricting your practice to that which a certified athletic trainer can legally do in the particular state where you reside. Role fidelity also means respecting the role of other professionals on the health care team. It means acting in a professional manner when relating to other members of the team and interacting with patients/clients/athletes.

Veracity

Veracity is more than truthfulness. Veracity is behaving in a manner that is truthful at all times. The importance of veracity in the relationship between the certified athletic trainer and the patient/client/athlete is readily apparent. It must also be mentioned here that veracity is very much a two-way issue. It is as important for the person receiving treatment to be completely honest with the athletic trainer as it is for the athletic trainer to be completely honest with the individual being treated.

Taken a step further, a certified athletic trainer can actually improve the treatment outcome if efforts are taken to make the individual being treated aware of what is happening in his or her treatment plan and why specific measures are being taken. A very significant factor in compliance with a rehabilitation program, according to Duda,[9] is how the athlete perceives the rehabilitation program. Athletes that perceive the program as highly valuable displayed more compliant behavior. How an athlete perceives a rehabilitation program or treatment plan is greatly influenced by what he or she knows, or does not know, about that program. An ethical certified athletic trainer recognizes this and in doing so is acknowledging the value of being completely truthful with the athlete and explaining all aspects of the rehabilitation or treatment plan to him or her.

Case Study 5-3

Role Fidelity

Case. While you are working with a knee rehabilitation patient in the outpatient clinic, you struggle to regain full extension of the involved knee. You have suspected for several weeks that the result of the surgery was not quite as good as the patient believes. In fact, you suspect the surgery resulted in less than optimal graft placement and the patient will most likely never fully recover her range of motion without additional surgery. The patient shares with you that a friend of hers had the same surgery done and that this individual had much better results. The patient begins to ask questions about recovering full range of motion and eventually asks you, "Did the physician mess up my knee?"

Debriefing Questions

- What do you tell this patient?
- Beyond dealing with the patient's immediate question, what other steps or actions can you take that would be appropriate?

Beneficence/Nonmaleficence

Beneficence alludes to doing what is beneficial for others. The concept of nonmaleficence is almost a negative restatement of beneficence because the term means "to refrain from harming another."[5] Both are vital to the ethical practice of any health care profession. The scenario that appeared earlier in the chapter in which the star athlete was held from participation lends itself very well to exemplification of beneficence and nonmaleficence. Adhering to the concept of beneficence, the athlete is not allowed to participate and is protected from further aggravation of the injury or additional harm. Likewise, a decision to allow the athlete to continue is placing him or her at risk and is in direct conflict with the concept of nonmaleficence.

AUTONOMY

Regardless of which branch or health care field is under discussion, the autonomy of the individual being treated must be respected. Respect for patient autonomy implies that the patient will be treated as an individual with a mind and a will and an inherent right to exercise that will. The patient is not merely a case or number or "an ACL patient." The patient should be part of the decision-making process relative to the selection of treatment options. Few, if any, practitioners would deny the importance of patient autonomy.

Like role fidelity, the problems that rise relative to patient autonomy are quite likely to be more subtle than frank and obvious. Case Study 5-4 illustrates this subtly. In this case, simply forbidding the athlete from returning home to have the surgery performed is behavior that ignores the autonomy of the athlete. Such actions would certainly be avoided by ethical practitioners! A much better strategy would be to discuss the situation with the athlete and tell her exactly why you want her to have the surgery and rehabilitation done by the team physician group. By doing this, you are treating the athlete as an individual with the will and intellect to make a decision. In explaining your position, you enable the athlete to make an informed decision. In a very real sense, you are respecting the autonomy of the athlete (see Table 5-2).

PRACTICE SPECIFIC ETHICS

Most health care professions have adopted their own separate code of ethics. While the particular professions adopting the individual code vary tremendously, there are elements that are common to all. The source of some of this commonality can be traced back to the Hippocratic Oath. Although many aspects of the original Hippocratic Oath are no longer congruent with either modern society or modern medicine, there are still parts of that original document that remain valid. As an example, the oath specifically mentions confidentiality in the following verbiage[10]:

> *All that may come to my knowledge in the exercise of my profession or in daily commerce with men, which ought not to be spread abroad, I will keep secret and will never reveal."*

For modern readers one of the most potentially confusing sections of the oath mentions "cut for stone." This odd wording refers to kidney stones, which were a frequently seen malady in the days of Hippocrates due primarily to diet and living conditions.[10] Fortunately, the treatment of kidney stones has progressed along with the rest of medicine! However, the underlying principle behind the statement is still very applicable. In swearing not to "cut for stone," Hippocrates was demonstrating role fidelity. The difference between a physician and a surgeon was substantial in the days of Hippocrates. Specific mention of refraining from the practice of surgery is direct acknowledgement of that fact and further acknowledges intent to remain true to the role and practice of a physician and avoid venturing into another's area of practice.

Case Study 5-4

Autonomy

Case. An athlete under your care at a small university needs to have shoulder surgery. This athlete is going home for the summer and wants to have the surgery performed at home by a physician who is a long-time friend of the family. Your concern is that the recovery may not progress as you would like if the rehabilitation is done while the athlete is off campus. Respect for the autonomy of the athlete demands that she be allowed to do as she feels is in her best interest. However, you have a legitimate stake in the outcome as you will be responsible for helping this athlete continue the rehabilitation program and eventually return to play.

Debriefing Questions

- Is it ethical for you to forbid this athlete to have the surgery done at home and insist that she remain in town over the summer and have the procedure performed by the team physician group?
- How could you resolve this situation while maintaining respect for the athlete's autonomy AND ensuring the very best possible outcome from rehabilitation?

Hippocratic Oath

I swear by Æsculapius, Hygeia, and Panacea, and I take to witness all the gods, all the goddesses, to keep according to my ability and my judgement, the following Oath.

To consider dear to me as my parents him who taught me this art; to live in common with him and if necessary to share my goods with him; To look upon his children as my own brothers, to teach them this art if they so desire without fee or written promise; to impart to my sons and the sons of the master who taught me and the disciples who have enrolled themselves and have agreed to the rules of the profession, but to these alone the precepts and the instruction.

I will prescribe regimens for the good of my patients according to my ability and my judgment and never do harm to anyone.

To please no one will I prescribe a deadly drug nor give advice which may cause his death.

Nor will I give a woman a pessary to procure abortion.

But I will preserve the purity of my life and my arts.

I will not cut for stone, even for patients in whom the disease is manifest; I will leave this operation to be performed by practitioners, specialists in this art.

In every house where I come I will enter only for the good of my patients, keeping myself far from all intentional ill-doing and all seduction and especially from the pleasures of love with women or with men, be they free or slaves.

All that may come to my knowledge in the exercise of my profession or in daily commerce with men, which ought not to be spread abroad, I will keep secret and will never reveal.

If I keep this oath faithfully, may I enjoy my life and practice my art, respected by all men and in all times; but if I swerve from it or violate it, may the reverse be my lot.

Reprinted from Carrick P. *Medical Ethics in the Ancient World.* Georgetown: Georgetown University Press; 2001.

National Athletic Trainers' Association Code of Ethics

Athletic training has a code of ethics designed to guide practitioners in the decision-making process. The NATA has published a Code of Ethics[11] that is designed to guide and direct athletic trainers as practitioners and health care administrators. The NATA Code of Ethics is a well-designed document that, when examined in close detail, is quite compatible with those common tenets of health care ethics previously cited by Edge and Groves.

The preamble to the NATA Code of Ethics sets the stage for the document (Box 5-2). The preamble establishes the scope of the document and clearly indicates that the document cannot be construed as addressing each and every situation that a certified athletic trainer will encounter in the course of his or her career. Even with those limitations, the document is remarkably applicable to any practice setting.

Principle 1

The first principle articulated in the NATA Code of Ethics involves a directive to respect the patient or client without discrimination (see Box 5-2) The issue of confidentiality is specifically addressed in Principle 1. Subpoint 1.3 admonishes practitioners to respect the confidentiality. As previously mentioned, confidentiality is a basic component of ethical practice in all health care professions. The sentence mentions a situation many athletic trainers have found themselves facing relative to releasing medical records without a release. A detailed discussion of HIPAA is beyond the scope of this chapter, but the compatibility of Principle 1, subpoint 1.3 with the spirit of HIPAA is immediately apparent. The latter part of the last sentence also fits well with case law relative to breaching confidentiality.[7]

Principle 2

The second principle that appears in the NATA Code of Ethics addresses the practice of athletic training relative to laws and regulatory statutes (see Box 5-2). Although licensure laws or practice acts as we understand them did not exist in the time of Hippocrates, the Hippocratic Oath does indeed mention "rules of the profession." Reference to regulatory agencies and laws is directly related to role fidelity, one of the previously mentioned tenets of health care ethics. In this manner, the implementation and refinement of individual state laws governing the practice of athletic training, or any other health care profession, are essential to ethical practice.

Box 5-2

National Athletic Trainers' Association Code of Ethics

PREAMBLE

The National Athletic Trainers' Association Code of Ethics states the principles of ethical behavior that should be followed in the practice of athletic training. It is intended to establish and maintain high standards and professionalism for the athletic training profession.

The principles do not cover every situation encountered by the practicing athletic trainer, but are representative of the spirit with which athletic trainers should make decisions. The principles are written generally; the circumstances of a situation will determine the interpretation and application of a given principle and of the Code as a whole. When a conflict exists between the Code and the law, the law prevails.

PRINCIPLE 1:

Members shall respect the rights, welfare and dignity of all.

1.1 Members shall not discriminate against any legally protected class.

1.2 Members shall be committed to providing competent care.

1.3 Members shall preserve the confidentiality of privileged information and shall not release such information to a third party not involved in the patient's care without a release unless required by law.

PRINCIPLE 2:

Members shall comply with the laws and regulations governing the practice of athletic training.

2.1 Members shall comply with applicable local, state, and federal laws and institutional guide lines.

2.2 Members shall be familiar with and abide by all National Athletic Trainers' Association standards, rules and regulations.

2.3 Members shall report illegal or unethical practices related to athletic training to the appropriate person or authority.

2.4 Members shall avoid substance abuse and, when necessary, seek rehabilitation for chemical dependency.

PRINCIPLE 3:

Members shall maintain and promote high standards in their provision of services.

3.1 Members shall not misrepresent, either directly or indirectly, their skills, training, professional credentials, identity or services.

3.2 Members shall provide only those services for which they are qualified through education or experience and which are allowed by their practice acts and other pertinent regulation.

3.3 Members shall provide services, make referrals, and seek compensation only for those services that are necessary.

3.4 Members shall recognize the need for continuing education and participate in educational activities that enhance their skills and knowledge.

3.5 Members shall educate those whom they supervise in the practice of athletic training about the Code of Ethics and stress the importance of adherence.

3.6 Members who are researchers or educators should maintain and promote ethical conduct in research and educational activities.

(continued)

Box 5-2 (continued)

National Athletic Trainers' Association Code of Ethics

PRINCIPLE 4:

Members shall not engage in conduct that could be construed as a conflict of interest or that reflects negatively on the profession.

4.1 Members should conduct themselves personally and professionally in a manner that does not compromise their professional responsibilities or the practice of athletic training.

4.2 National Athletic Trainers' Association current or past volunteer leaders shall not use the NATA logo in the endorsement of products or services or exploit their affiliation with the NATA in a manner that reflects badly upon the profession.

4.3 Members shall not place financial gain above the patient's welfare and shall not participate in any arrangement that exploits the patient.

4.4 Members shall not, through direct or indirect means, use information obtained in the course of the practice of athletic training to try to influence the score or outcome of an athletic event, or attempt to induce financial gain through gambling.

If a certified athletic trainer is practicing while struggling with a chemical dependency, he or she is practicing with little regard for the well being or safety of the athlete. The basic tenet of nonmaleficence is in jeopardy of being compromised. As previously mentioned, many of the real life problems faced by athletic trainers are much more subtle.

Principle 3

The third principle contained in the NATA Code of Ethics focuses on promoting and maintaining appropriate levels or standards of care (see Box 5-2). The first 3 subpoints share the commonality or underlying thread of role fidelity. These sub-points direct the clinician to refrain from misrepresentation of his or her credentials and training, provide athletic training services within professionally and legally appropriate parameters, and to refer a patient/client/athlete to another practitioner when proper management of the case falls beyond the scope of athletic training.

The spirit of these sub-points in Principle 3 is supported by both the Hippocratic Oath and well-established ethical tenets such as role fidelity and veracity. The relationship between role fidelity and the avoidance of claiming your credentials qualify you to deliver a service you are not qualified to deliver is readily apparent. In admonishing practitioners to avoid seeking compensation or making referrals for services that are not indicated, the document gets right to the heart of ethical practice. If an athletic trainer is administering treatment or directing a rehabilitation program that is unnecessary, the veracity of the client/clinician relationship has obviously been compromised.

Case Study 5-5

Nonmaleficence

Case. As the assistant athletic trainer at a major university, you are constantly under a great deal of pressure. The hours are long and the stress level is incredibly high. You feel the pressure and stress as an assistant, but you can only imagine how much more pressure and stress is felt by the head athletic trainer. As the year progresses, you begin to suspect the head athletic trainer has some issues with alcohol use. You begin to notice that this individual has been drinking a little more as time goes by. On a few occasions, you are almost sure you can smell alcohol on his breath when he comes back from a lunch break. You choose not to say anything, believing it is not your business. You are several steps down the ladder of authority and do not feel right speaking up.

Debriefing Questions

- Which health care tenets are being violated by the head athletic trainer?
- By remaining silent, are YOU displaying ethical behavior?
- What possible actions should you take in this situation?

Principle 4

The fourth principle of the NATA Code of Ethics is slightly broader than the previous 3 (see Box 5-2). Avoiding conflict of interest is specifically mentioned in the principle as is the more general and broad caution to avoid actions that reflect negatively on the profession. The potential for conflict of interest is inherent in a situation in which the success of your employer (winning a game or championship) conflicts, at least in theory, with making the well being of the athlete the top priority. It is hoped that an educational institution would always place the well being of student athletes ahead of winning or losing and that must almost certainly be the case in all but a very few situations. However, to deny that potential exists is to deny the current mentality of society, sports fans, athletic boosters, and the university itself. It must be noted here that the risk of conflict of interest is certainly not restricted to athletic trainers employed in the intercollegiate athletic setting. Consider the athletic trainer that is providing outreach services of a local hospital. The reality is that the hospital depends upon the athletic trainer to generate revenue. That very fact creates a temptation to increase the number of referrals. A certified athletic trainer working in an industrial setting may be pressured to return an employee to his or her workstation earlier than is ideal to protect production numbers.

The final sentence in Principle 4 addresses the issue of gambling. The awareness of this issue was elevated by a story involving a major college coach that had been involved in something as seemingly harmless as an NCAA basketball championship pool. Granted, there were several factors that contributed to the escalation of this particular situation,[12] but the fact remains that governing agencies in the athletic world are dead serious about gambling. Involvement in gambling, if discovered, can be career suicide.

SUMMARY

- Recall the 3 categories of ethics.

  Ethics is the formal study of the thought process and logic underlying decision making. The study of ethics is typically broken down into 3 areas that include metaethics, normative ethics, and applied ethics. Applied ethics are often of the most interest to health care providers.

- Compare and contrast the 3 areas of ethics.

  Metaethics is the study of the origin of ethical thought. Normative ethics function as the standards for determining what is right or wrong and what is the appropriate or correct action or behavior in light of that fact. Applied ethics is the branch of ethics that deals with specific issues that are current and almost always controversial. Examples of current issues in health care include euthanasia, stem cell research, and abortion.

- Summarize the ethical issues commonly seen in health care.

  Ethical issues commonly encountered in health care include respect for the autonomy and privacy of the patient. Other issues related specifically to the patient/practitioner relationship include veracity, or maintaining truthfulness with the patient, and beneficence, or doing no harm to the patient. Other issues involve the interpractitioner relationship such as role fidelity, or staying within your scope of practice and respecting the scope of practice of other clinicians.

- Explain the key points related to the NATA Code of Ethics.

  The first principle articulated in the NATA Code of Ethics involves a directive to respect the patient or client without discrimination. The second principle that appears in the NATA Code of Ethics addresses the practice of athletic training relative to laws and regulatory statutes. Promotion and maintenance of appropriate levels or standards of care are addressed as the third principle. The fourth principle is broader and speaks to avoiding conflicts of interest and other actions that are a negative reflection on the profession.

REFERENCES

1. Ockham WO. *Philosophical Writings.* Indianapolis, IN: Hackett Publishing Company, Inc; 1990.
2. Empiricus S. *Outlines of Pyrrhonism.* Amherst, MA: Prometheus Books; 1994.
3. Locke J. *Second Treatise of Government.* Indianapolis, IN: Hackett Publishing Company; 1980.
4. Short BW. The healing philosopher: John Locke's medical ethics. *Issues Law Med.* 2004;20(2):103-154.
5. Edge RS, Groves JR. *Ethics of Health Care: A Guide for Clinical Practice.* 3rd ed. Florence, KY: Thomson Delmar Learning; 2005.
6. Pozgar G. *Legal and Ethical Issues for Health Professionals.* Boston, MA: Jones and Bartlett; 2005.
7. *Tarasoff v. Regents of the University of California,* 17 California 3rd 425 (1976).
8. National Athletic Trainers' Association. Website of the National Athletic Trainers' Association. Available at http://www.nata.org/about_AT/whatisat.htm. Accessed February 22, 2007.
9. Duda J, Tappe M. Predictors of adherence in the rehabilitation of athletic injuries: an application of personal investment theory. *Journal of Sport and Exercise Psychology.* 1989;11:367-381.

10. Carrick P. *Medical Ethics in the Ancient World.* Georgetown: Georgetown University Press; 2001.
11. National Athletic Trainers' Association. *Code of ethics*. Available at http://www.nata.org/codeofethics/code_of_ethics.pdf. Accessed August 5, 2008.
12. Neuheisel trying to keep his job. *New York Times.* June 15, 2003:8, 11.

Chapter

ATHLETIC TRAINING ADMINISTRATION
ISSUES IN EDUCATIONAL SETTINGS

OBJECTIVES

At the end of this chapter, the reader will be able to:

- Discuss the use of policies and procedures to guide operational programming
- Explain how the Health Insurance Privacy and Accountability Act (HIPAA) has impacted athletic training health care organizations in educational settings
- Describe the Family Education Rights and Privacy Act of 1974 (FERPA) and explain how it impacts the athletic training organization
- Identify the range of program functions common to athletic training programs in the educational setting
- Describe the considerations for appropriate medical coverage in the intercollegiate and interscholastic athletic settings
- Explain the organization and administration issues facing athletic training educators
- Describe the organization and proper use of medical records
- Identify the various authorizations and consent documentation required to treat patients in an educational venue
- Discuss the organizational and administrative issues inherent to planning and carrying out preparticipation examinations (PPE)
- Define the components of a drug-testing plan
- Explain the key elements of designing an athletic training health care facility

Various chapters in this text address issues that are of importance to athletic training health care organizations serving populations in a variety of employment settings. The organization and administration foundations, applications, and tools found in this text can aid any practicing athletic trainer in these settings. This chapter focuses on the educational environment. The profession of athletic training has deep roots in the educational setting; namely the university system. Some historians believe that the first individuals who held the role of athletic trainer were employed at Ivy League universities (there is some dispute about who was first). Despite this uncertain beginning, the profession has had much of its evolution focused on educational environs. The first collegial meetings and attempts to form a national organization before World War II were aligned with the Penn and Drake relays—collegiate events. The evolution of the various districts still used by the National Athletic Trainers Association evolved around natural athletic conference and regional alignments. Much has transpired since those early days. It is hard to say if the pioneers in this setting could have imagined the need to dedicate entire textbooks and courses to the organization and administration of such programs. While the profession has expanded to a range of work environments (clinics and hospitals, corporate industrial, military, etc), 36.3% are employed in educational settings (college/university and secondary schools) and this setting is the primary clinical educational environment for athletic training students.[1] Given the number of athletic trainers working in this setting, the rich history, and its impact on professional practice and education, exploring organizational and administrative issues facing practitioners in educational environments is a worthy pursuit. This chapter will address the operational nature of managing an athletic training program in the interscholastic and intercollegiate setting.

OPERATIONAL PRACTICES

The tasks, policies, procedures, practices, and standards that require daily consideration when administering an athletic training service program in a high school, college, or university can be thought of as operational practices. Guiding these day-to-day operations are operational plans. Unlike the strategic planning tools found in Chapter 11, operational plans do not look ahead for long-term planning—they are tools that have grown from long-term plans. Operational plans are rarely more than 2 years long. The operational plan is the result of the hard work of strategic planning. It is a chance to build practices that are rooted in your program vision and mission. The most common form of operational plan is policy and procedures.

Policy and Procedures

A review of the Board of Certification Role Delineation Study[2] domain for organization and administration reveals 2 specific areas that focus on policy and procedure:

1. Establish policies and procedures for the delivery of health care services following accepted guidelines to promote safe participation, timely care, and legal compliance.
2. Establish policies and procedures for the management of health care facilities and activity areas by referring to accepted guidelines, standards, and regulations to promote safe and legal compliance.

Clearly, the need to understand and be able to develop policy and procedure manuals is required for all athletic training professionals. A policy is a clear and accurate written statement that identifies the basic rules and principles used to control and expedite decision-making.[3] Procedures describe the steps that should be followed—the processes—of how something should be done. Table 6-1 outlines some common policies found in an intercollegiate sports medicine environment. Policy and procedure guides are useful tools that provide athletic training staff, physicians, administrators, and coaches a clear

Organization and Administration Considerations for Athletic Training Educators

The athletic training educator must possess specific organizational and administrative skills to shape and manage the athletic training education program. Many similarities exist between the educational program and the provision of clinical services. The most striking similarity is the need for operational procedures. Educational programs must have a mechanism to explain how the program is structured and how the program operates. Admission policies, technical standards, program progress, clinical requirements, costs, and academic guidelines are just a sample of items that must be explained to prospective and current students.

The ATEP program director must be an excellent communicator in order to work closely with students, clinical instructors, and other faculty that make up the courses in the program. The ATEP program director must keep abreast of the Commission on Accreditation of Athletic Training Education (CAATE) Standards and Guidelines for Athletic Training Education and insure that the program is in compliance. In addition, he or she must know the NATA Educational Competencies for Athletic Training Education inside and out in order to insure he or she is instructed in the curriculum. Program directors must maintain program documents to be used in annual reports, program self-studies, and site visits. Much like their clinical counterparts, program coordinators must keep specific program and clinical files and insure that they are kept and protected to comply with FERPA laws.

Above all, the ATEP program director must represent the educational program to his or her home department and the campus community. Strong communication skills, a desire to promote learning among students, and genuine enthusiasm will go a long way to program success.

Table 6-1

Examples of Policy and Procedure Topics: Intercollegiate Athletics

- Athletic-related dental care and mouth guards
- Athletic training coverage by sport
- Blood-borne pathogens
- Catastrophic injury insurance
- Chiropractic services
- Coordination of event medical coverage for spirit squad
- Dietary supplement policy
- Distribution of medications
- Emergency department use/urgent care clinic use
- Event coverage
- Illnesses
- Influence vaccine
- Insurance coverage, medical bills, and payment of bills
- Medical record archiving
- Orthopedic appliances, orthotics, and braces
- Outside services/second opinions
- Payment of outside rehabilitation services
- Performance-related blood evaluations
- Physician clinics at the sports medicine center
- Pre-participation physical exams (PPEs)
- Psychiatric and psychological services and resources
    - Emergency and nonemergency guidelines
- Referral to specialty clinics
- Reporting injuries and illnesses
- Restorative sport massage therapy
- Short-term tryouts
- Sports medicine center operations
- Sports nutrition/dietician referral
- staff PT/ATC services
- Summer camp coverage
- Therapeutic sport massage therapy
- Vision correction lens policy
- Visiting teams
- Weight control policy

Adapted from Sports Medicine Policies and Procedures Guide 2006-2007. University of Wisconsin-Madison. Copyright 2006, University of Wisconsin Board of Regents. Used with permission.

understanding of specific program functions. They also provide a foundation for continuity of care and a uniform guide for daily operations. An athletic training staff with diverse backgrounds and approaches can create a dynamic and positive work environment. However, having written policies and procedures provides uniformity to the program, establishes fair and equitable practices, and allows for greater shared vision in the application of the program's vision. When assembling a policy and procedure manual, each topic can be broken down into 4 key areas (Box 6-1):

1. Policy—Basic rules and principles
2. Purpose—Explain the need for the policy
3. Procedures—Steps to follow the policy
4. Documentation—How we document and provide evidence that the policy and procedures have been followed

Samples of areas addressed in the policy and procedures manual include:

- Delivery of health care services. How are the athletes served by your program provided care? What responsibilities do they have to the process? How are injuries and illnesses reported? Who had the final decision on playability? How can an athlete obtain a second opinion? What is the policy on distributing over-the-counter medications?
- Management of health care facilities. What level of staffing will each team require? What are the hours of operation for our facilities?

ATHLETIC TRAINING PROGRAM FUNCTIONS

A variety of program functions require attention that extends beyond the policy and procedures manual. They may require additional planning, specific documentation, and greater attention to implementation. Several of these organizational and administrative program functions carried out in the athletic training setting are done to comply with governing regulations and in the interest of medical-legal responsibilities. A review of recent legislation from the National Collegiate Athletic Association (NCAA) involving health and safety issues reveals many items related to these important program functions (Table 6-2). These areas include emergency planning, PPE, drug testing, information management, management of physicians' clinics, and handling of medications.

Keep in mind that this is not a complete list of administrative program functions. Other chapters address key concepts for the athletic training health

Box 6-1

Sample Policy and Procedures

Policy for Influenza Vaccine

Policy

Influenza vaccinations are provided for student-athletes, coaches, and athletic trainers who have competitions and training through the winter influenza season. Student-athletes with chronic illnesses (ie, asthma, diabetes, heart conditions) should receive the vaccination. Coaches and student-athletes should discuss influenza vaccinations with their staff athletic trainer or Division-designated team physician.

Purpose

To provide influenza vaccinations for student-athletes, coaches, and support staff, when appropriate, during the peak winter influenza season.

Procedures

- Vaccinations are set up on a team basis. Group vaccination times are coordinated through the staff athletic trainer responsible for the sport.
- The medical staff will make the vaccine available during the fall based upon annual recommendations of the Centers for Disease Control and Prevention (CDC).
- At the time of the inoculation, the student-athlete will fill out a vaccine screening form.

Documentation

The vaccine screening form will be put into the student-athlete's file.

Sports Medicine Center Hours of Operation

Policy

The Sports Medicine Center is the central location for the athletic training staff and for all clinical visits for all intercollegiate sports teams. The Sports Medicine Center business hours of operation are 9 a.m. to 5 p.m. August 15th to May 31st, Monday through Friday. Hours from June 1st to August 14th are 10 a.m. to 12 p.m. and 1 p.m. to 5:30 p.m., Monday through Friday. Exceptions to posted hours will be available for scheduled practices and competitions. Satellite rooms will be open for pre-practice and post-practice care only.

Purpose

To provide a central area to assure access to all student-athletes for medical services.

Procedures

- Student-athletes with illnesses should contact their staff athletic trainer so that an evaluation can be performed and a referral to a physician be made if necessary.
- Satellite sports medicine facilities are used for pre-practice preparation and post-practice care only.
- Rehabilitation in the afternoon is reserved for special appointments set up by the staff athletic trainer in charge of the sport.
- Staff athletic trainers can be reached in the McClain Sports Medicine Center during the morning hours. If the staff athletic trainer is not present, a message can be left or another staff athletic trainer will be available to assist student-athletes or coaches.
- Staff athletic trainers should coordinate lunch times and adjust them throughout the year as the season dictates. This allows the rest of the staff to regularly plan daily activities and appointments to assure coverage of the room.

(continued)

Box 6-1 (continued)

Sample Policy and Procedures

Documentation

Messages will be placed in the staff athletic trainer's mailbox. The message should include the name of the caller, the date and time of the call, the message, and the name of the person taking the message, or the caller can be referred to the staff athletic trainer's voice mail.

Treatments and rehabilitation procedures will be logged into the Sports Medicine Database in each Sports Medicine Facility by the athletic trainer providing the service.

Adapted from Sports Medicine Policies and Procedures Guide 2006-2007. University of Wisconsin-Madison.

Table 6-2

NCAA Legislation Involving Health and Safety

Topic	*Issue*
Banned drugs	List of banned substances Drugs and procedures subject to restriction Effect on eligibility Effect on championship eligibility Transfer while ineligible due to positive drug test Knowledge of use of banned drugs
Drug testing	Banned drugs and drug testing methods Consent forms: prior to practice/administration/nonrecruited student-athlete/failure to properly administer Effect of non-NCAA positive drug tests
Drug rehabilitation	Drug rehabilitation program expenses Travel to and from drug rehabilitation program
Nutritional supplements	Permissible supplements Impermissible supplements
Tobacco use	Restricted advertising and sponsorship Tobacco use at member institution Tobacco ban summer baseball
Medical expenses	Permissible medical expenses Eating disorders Transportation for medical treatment Summer conditioning—football
Medical waivers	Hardship waiver Five-year rule waiver
Medical records and consent forms	HIPAA/Buckley amendment consent forms

Adapted from The National Collegiate Athletic Association. *NCAA Sports Medicine Handbook* 18th ed. Indianapolis, IN: Author; 2006. Available at http://www.ncaa.org. Accessed February 24, 2007.

care administrator: budget (Chapter 3), insurance and reimbursement (Chapter 9), human resources (Chapter 4), and risk management (Chapter 2) are all key program functions that extend into all athletic training environments.

Emergency Planning

The Board of Certification Role Delineation Study[2] states that the ability to establish action plans for response to injury or illness using available resources to provide the required range of health care services for patients, athletic activities, and events is a component of the organization and administration domain for athletic trainers. All athletic training programs must have emergency action plans. The importance of the emergency action plan is reinforced by the National Athletic Trainers' Association (NATA) position statement specific to emergency planning.[4] A complete listing of NATA statements is provided in Table 6-3. Athletic trainers in educational settings have a heightened responsibility given the broad range of programming and wide variety of facilities that require attention. The NATA position statement on emergency planning in athletics states[4]:

- Institutions that sponsor athletic events must have a written emergency plan. The plan should be comprehensive yet flexible to adapt to many situations.
- The plan must be distributed to key personnel: athletic trainers, team physicians, athletic training students, institutional safety personnel, administrators, and coaches. The plan should be developed in consultation with local emergency medical services (EMS) personnel.
- The plan should identify the personnel responsible for carrying out the plan and the qualifications of those executing the plan. Sports medicine professionals, officials, and coaches should be trained in cardiopulmonary resuscitation, use of an automated external defibrillator, first aid, and prevention of disease transmission.
- The plan should specify the equipment needed to carry out the tasks required in the event of an emergency. The location of the equipment should be identified.
- Establishing a clear mechanism of communication to appropriate emergency care providers and identification of the mode of transportation for the injured participant are critical elements to the plan.
- The emergency plan should be specific to the activity venue.
- Emergency plans should incorporate the emergency care facilities to which injured athletes will be taken. Advance discussion and inclusion of personnel from these facilities in the development of the plan is essential.
- The plan should specify the required documentation supporting the implementation and evaluation of the emergency plan.
- Emergency plans should be reviewed and rehearsed annually (at a minimum).
- All personnel involved with the organization and sponsorship of athletic activities share a professional responsibility to provide for developing and implementing an emergency plan.
- All personnel involved with the organization and sponsorship of athletic activities share a legal duty to develop, implement, and evaluate an emergency plan for all sponsored athletic activities.
- Administrative and legal counsel of the sponsoring organization or institution should review emergency plans.

Multiple organizational and administrative skills are required in the development of an emergency action plan. Implementation of a successful plan requires communication with key players internal and external to the organization, making contacts in the community with EMS personnel and emergency care facilities, documenting key elements of the plan, budgeting and purchasing specific equipment, and systematically reviewing and improving the plan. Chapter 2 addresses the legal responsibility associated with having an emergency action plan. Sample emergency procedures to call 911 are provided in Box 6-2.

Table 6-3

National Athletic Trainers' Association Position Statements

Position Statements

- Emergency planning in athletics
- Exertional heat illnesses
- Fluid replacement for athletes
- Head down contact and spearing in tackle football
- Lightning safety for athletics and recreation
- Management of asthma in athletes
- Management of sport-related concussion

Official Statements

- Automated external defibrillators
- Commotio cordis
- Steroids and performance-enhancing substances
- Full-time, on-site athletic trainer coverage for secondary school athletic programs
- Use of qualified athletic trainers in secondary schools
- Community-acquired MRSA infections
- Youth football and heat-related illness

Consensus Statements

- Appropriate medical care for secondary school-age athletes
- Executive summary: Recommendations on emergency preparedness and management of sudden cardiac arrest in high school and college athletic programs
- Inter-association task force on exertional heat illnesses
- Prehospital care of the spine-injured athlete

Support Statements

- The Coalition to Preserve Patient Access to Physical Medicine and Rehabilitation Services
- American Academy of Family Physicians' support of athletic trainers for high school athletes
- American Medical Association's support of athletic trainers in secondary schools
- Appropriate medical care for secondary school-age athletes
- Endorsement of NATA Lightning Position Statement by the American Academy of Pediatrics
- Recommendations and guidelines for appropriate medical coverage of intercollegiate athletics
    - NCAA support of recommendations and guidelines for appropriate medical coverage of intercollegiate athletics

Adapted from National Athletic Trainers' Association. NATA position statements. Available at http://www.nata.org/statements/index.htm. Accessed February 11, 2007.

Preparing for the Worst: An Administrative Reality

Chapter 11 in this text deals with strategic planning and a form of "outside the box" thinking called scenario planning. Scenario planning deals with a series of "what if?" questions that allow administrators to examine a course of action for a variety of possibilities. One scenario that is often overlooked is the need to have a planned response in the event of a catastrophic incident in the athletic setting. While catastrophes are rare, an event that leads to the disability or death of a student-athlete, coach, or staff member can create uncertainty and confusion for the institution and organization. Guidelines for response to

(continued)

Preparing for the Worst: An Administrative Reality (continued)

a catastrophic event (Catastrophic Incident Guidelines) help provide information and support necessary to family members, teammates, coaches, and staff following a catastrophe. Establishing a plan for this response can help centralize the flow of information and insure that appropriate and accurate details are being properly handled. Athletic training staff will often be called upon to assist with such processes. Components of such a plan should include:

- Define a catastrophic incident—Incident plans are usually written to respond to a catastrophe such as the sudden death of a coach, student-athlete, or staff member from any cause, or a disabling and/or quality of life-altering injury. They may also be expanded to coordinate response to a public safety issue (eg, national emergency, travel and safety issue, natural disaster) or other issues as determined by the individual institution.
- A management team—Identify a select group of administrative personnel to receive all the facts pertaining to the incident. This team works to officially communicate information to the appropriate parties.
- Immediate action plan—At the moment of the catastrophe, a checklist of whom to call and immediate steps to secure facts and offering support are items to include in the action plan. Other essential items should identify who will speak on behalf of the organization to insure uniform communication of the facts. This should identify internal and external audiences.
- Chain of command and role delineation—Specific duties should be outlined for each individual's responsibility during the aftermath of a catastrophe.
- Cooperation with law enforcement—Organizations should outline how they will collaborate with university, local, and state law officials.
- Away contest responsibilities—Planning should include how to respond to an incident that takes place out of town.
- Phone list and flow chart—Phone numbers of all key individuals involved in the management of the catastrophe should be listed and kept current. A flow chart of persons to be contacted in the event of a catastrophe is also useful in coordinating communication.
- Incident record—A written chronology by the management team of the catastrophe is recommended to critique the process and provide a basis for reviewing the efficacy of the procedures.

Adapted from the NCAA Sports Medicine Handbook 18th Ed. The National Collegiate Athletic Association. 2005-06. Indianapolis. Available at www.ncaa.org. Accessed February 24, 2007.

Box 6-2

Sample Telephone Instructions For Emergency Plan Activation

- Be sure you are aware of 911 access issues. Some schools and universities still require special dialing (eg, outside line 9-911).
- Provide the dispatcher with the following information:
  - Your name and position (eg, Joe Smith, Athletic Training Student at State U).
  - The name and exact location of the emergency (I am at the Student Center Arena on the main floor).
  - A brief description of the emergency (Our coach has lost consciousness and is having trouble breathing).
  - Current care being rendered and by whom (One of our staff athletic trainers is monitoring his vitals and prepared for further rescue action if needed).
  - Location of the injured person (We are located on the main gym floor at the Student Center Arena).
  - Directions for easy medical personnel access (You can enter the arena through the loading ramp on the east side of the building off of Main St.).

(continued)

Box 6-2 (continued)

Sample Telephone Instructions For Emergency Plan Activation

- Telephone number from which you are calling (555-1212).
- Tell them someone will meet them at the entrance if there is someone available to do so (I will meet you at the doors after we hang up from this call).
- Be ready to review all the information you have provided.
- Only hang up when the dispatcher indicates that you should.

Preparticipation Physical Examinations

Governing bodies in both the secondary school (National Federation of State High School Associations [NFHS]) and collegiate settings (National College Athletic Association [NCAA] and National Association of Intercollegiate Athletics [NAIA]) have recommendations and guidelines for preparticipation medical examinations. In the secondary school setting, the NFHS Sports Medicine Advisory Committee states that preparticipation physical evaluations for high school student-athletes are a necessary and desirable precondition to interscholastic athletic practice and competition. The NFHS can only make recommendations since state organizations govern the high school participation. The Wisconsin Interscholastic Athletic Association[5] rules for PPE in the high school setting state:

> *Article VII—Health and Behavior. Section I Physical Examination.*
>
> *A. A student may not practice for or participate in interscholastic athletics until the school has written evidence on file in its office attesting to (a) parental permission each school year and (b) current physical fitness to participate in sports as determined by a licensed physician or Advanced Practice Nurse Prescriber (APNP) no less than every other school year with April 1 the earliest date of examination.*

The NCAA guideline for medical evaluations states:

> *NCAA Guideline 1b. Medical Evaluations*
>
> *A preparticipation medical evaluation should be required upon a student-athlete's entrance into the institution's intercollegiate athletics program. This initial evaluation should include a comprehensive health history, immunization history and defined by current Centers of Disease Control and Prevention guidelines and a relevant physical exam with strong emphasis on the cardiovascular, neurologic and musculoskeletal evaluation. Subsequent to the initial medical evaluation, an updated history should be performed annually.*

These rules may address the requirements for the PPE but they do not address reasons for conducting the PPE. In addition to the legal requirements for the exam, Lombardo and Badolato[6] state that the primary goal of the PPE is to detect any conditions that may limit an athlete's participation and predispose the athlete or others to injuries or illness during competition. Secondary goals are to determine the general health of the individual, assess fitness level, and counsel the athlete on health-related issues. The PPE is often the only involvement many student-athletes have with the health care system; it is important that examiners make this encounter as comprehensive as possible. An important function of the exam is to identify athletes who are not only at risk for general medicine and orthopedic conditions but also for psychosocial problems involving sexuality, substance abuse, violence, or any other emotional or psychological factors.

Student-athletes may be concerned about disqualification from competition because of the PPE. However, actual disqualification numbers are less than 2% and those requiring follow-up evaluations range from 3.2% to 13.5%. Most PPEs are performed by physicians (MDs and DOs); however, some high school associations allow for other care providers (eg, nurse practitioner) to sign off on the PPE form.

Exam Timing and Type

Ideally, the PPE should be held 6 weeks prior to the start of the athletic season. This allows for additional diagnostic tests, consultation, and any needed rehabilitation prior to the start of the practice season. There are 2 primary styles of PPE that can be arranged: the office-based examination and the station-based examination. In the high school setting, many athletes will see their personal physician for their PPE. However, given the range of insurance coverage and economic needs of many students, it is equally common for local high schools or sports medicine clinics to sponsor station-based exams as a community service. The station-based exam is common in the intercollegiate setting given the number of athletes reviewed annually. In organizing the PPE, the intercollegiate athletic trainer must work closely with the general medicine

Table 6-4

Station-Based and Office-Based Preparticipation Exams: Advantages and Disadvantages

Exam Type	Advantages	Disadvantages
Station-based	Cost-effective Efficient Able to utilize skills and expertise of various personnel Better communication between coaches, athletes, and medical team	Can be noisy and confusing if not well organized May compromise continuity of care Lack of time and privacy
Office-based	Better continuity of care Improves physician-patient relationship Greater opportunity to discuss sensitive issues	Athlete may lack primary care physician Increased cost Lack of communication between coaches, athletes, and medical team Physician may be uncomfortable in determining clearance to participate

team physician since the team physician will have final say over potential disqualification from participation. Many decisions must be made (eg, how to collect the medical history, what forms should be used, what style of examination will be conducted, and how many allied health and medical staff will be needed).

The station-based examination is used to examine a large number of people in a fairly short period of time. In station-based exams, athletes move from station to station (in separate rooms for the sake of privacy) to complete the exam. The station exam is cost-effective and efficient and allows for more access, improved communication, and the use of specialized physicians. The station-based exam usually concludes with a team physician reviewing all medical history and examination form with the athlete in a "check out" arrangement. In the intercollegiate setting, this is helpful and allows for good communication between the athletic trainer and the physician regarding the athletes in their care. The disadvantages of the station-based exam include possible noise and confusion, possible compromised care, and lack of privacy. Good organization and using a location that promotes privacy can help address many of the disadvantages.

The office-based examination allows the athlete to see his or her personal physician in the privacy of the physician's office. This is advantageous since the physician is familiar with the patient and has more time to address sensitive issues. Identifying adolescent stressors surrounding peer relationships, drugs and alcohol, sex, safety, and family can more easily be done in the office-based PPE. In addition, Landry and Bernhardt[7] suggest the private setting will allow for greater attention to anticipatory guidance such as identifying overbearing parents, providing fitness and nutritional counseling, and spending time discussing injury prevention. Table 6-4 summarizes the advantages and disadvantages of the office-based and station-based examinations. Table 6-5 details the various stations and the specialized personnel required for the station-based examination.

Medical History and Exam Content

Collecting a complete medical history in advance of the PPE is one of the most important organizational tasks in the athletic health care setting. A complete and accurate medical history is the cornerstone of the PPE. The history should give special focus to cardiovascular and musculoskeletal anomalies since these 2 areas are most likely to result in disqualification or require patient follow-up prior to clearance to participate. In a Mayo Clinic study of athletes not cleared for participation from a station-based exam, 18.9% had cardiac issues and 43.4% had musculoskeletal issues.[8] Symptoms of chest discomfort, palpitations, syncope, or near syncope with exercise should be noted. A history of hypertension or cardiac murmur must also be elicited.[6] The medical history form should elicit information on family history of premature death (sudden or otherwise) or significant disability from cardiovascular disease in close relatives younger than 50. Knowledge of hypertrophic cardiomyopathy, Marfan syndrome, or other related conditions must be asked on the medical history form. Nontraumatic sudden cardiac death in young adults usually results from unknown cardiac disease. Unfortunately, the first

Table 6-5

Stations and Personnel for Preparticipation Examination

Stations	*Personnel / Specialist*
Vital signs	Nurse, medical assistant, athletic trainers, or students in any of these areas
Vision	Same as above + ophthalmologist if available
History	Nurse to review forms, including immunizations
Medical Head, eyes, ears, nose, and throat (HEENT) Heart/lung Abdomen (includes hernia check for males)	Physician, nurse practitioner, or physician's assistant
Orthopedic	Physician, athletic trainer, or physical therapist
Lab testing (optional)	Phlebotomist
Fitness testing (optional) Endurance testing Strength Body fat Aerobic capacity	Coach, exercise specialist, athletic trainer

Adapted from Landry GL, Bernhardt DT. *Essentials of Primary Care Sports Medicine*. Champaign, IL: Human Kinetics; 2003.

indication of this underlying disease is the catastrophic event of collapse and death. Studies have recently examined the use of echocardiograms (ECHOS) to detect athletes at risk for sudden cardiac death. CITE examined nearly 3000 high school athletes, integrating ECHO into a station-based PPE. The results found a poor correlation between ECHO findings and the history/physical exam. This study found no abnormalities that precluded participation. Widespread use of ECHOS as a PPE screening tool may not be a reasonable choice given the high cost, low prevalence of cardiovascular disease in the athletic population, and low predictive value of the ECHO in predicting cardiovascular disease. Those responsible for organizing PPEs must be familiar with the American Heart Association (AHA) Screening Recommendations for history and physical examination (Table 6-6).[9,10] Any concerns on the medical history or findings on physical examination should then be referred to a cardiovascular specialist for review prior to clearance.

An orthopedic history is of particular importance as well. Gomez et al[11] reported that 92% of all injuries can be detected by history alone. Of particular importance are previous injuries that limit the athlete's ability to participate in sports and any injury associated with chronic discomfort, swelling, weakness, or that causes the athlete to compensate by changing his or her mechanics, position on the field, or duration of intensity of play.

The athletic training health care administrator assisting with the organization of the PPE must have a clear understanding of each of the components of the exam. Referrals for further testing, additional diagnostic evaluations, and documentation of PPE outcomes will often be the responsibility of the athletic trainer. The physical exam should include the following[12]:

- Height, weight, and vital signs
    - A seated blood pressure must be accessed in context of the age, height, and sex of the patient. Proper fit of the blood pressure cuff will avoid inaccurate measurements.
- Eyes, ears, nose, and throat
    - Visual acuity should be assessed as well as a general examination of the ears, nose, throat, and oral cavity. Poor dental health may be an indicator of an eating disorder. A high arched palate may be a sign of Marfan syndrome.
- Heart
    - Refer to the AHA guidelines in Table 6-6.
- Pulmonary auscultation
    - Observe for accessory muscle use, prolonged expiration, and auscultate for wheezing. Signs of exercise-induced distress will not be present at rest.

Table 6-6

Recommendation for Cardiovascular Screening During Preparticipation Examination

A health care worker with requisite training, medical skills, and background to reliably obtain a detailed cardiovascular history, perform a physical examination, and recognize heart disease should perform screening for athletes.

The cardiovascular screening should include a complete medical history and physical examination that includes brachial artery blood pressure measurement.

The cardiovascular history should include questions that determine a history of the following:

- Exertional chest pain or discomfort
- Syncope or near syncope
- Excessive, unexpected, and unexplained shortness of breath with exercise
- The past detection of a heart murmur or elevated blood pressure
- A family history of premature death (sudden or otherwise)
- Significant disability from cardiovascular disease in close relatives younger than 50 years of age
- Specific knowledge of the occurrence of hypertrophic cardiomyopathy, Marfan syndrome, arrhythmias, long QT syndrome, or dilated cardiomyopathy

Parental involvement in completing the history portion should be encouraged.

The cardiovascular examination should emphasize assessment of the following:

- Femoral artery pulses to exclude coarctation of the aorta
- Precordial auscultation in the supine and standing positions to identify heart murmurs consistent with dynamic left ventricle outflow obstruction
- Recognition of the physical stigmata of Marfan syndrome
- Brachial blood pressure measurement in the sitting position

Adapted from Maron BJ, Thomson PD, Puffer JC, et al. Cardiovascular preparticipation screen of competitive athletes: a statement for health professionals from the Sudden Death Committee and Congenital Cardiac Defects Committee, American Heart Association. *Circulation*. 1996;94:850-856 (addendum published in *Circulation*. 1998; 97:2294).

- Abdominal palpation
    - Assess for hepatic or splenic enlargement.
- Genitalia
    - Assess for single testicle, hernia, varicoceles, and undescended testicles.
- Skin
    - Evaluate for rashes, infections, and infestations.
- Musculoskeletal system
    - If the history indicates previous injury, an examination specific to that problem should be performed. If no history of injury is indicated, a general exam (eg, 2-minute orthopedic examination) should be used.
- Neurologic examination
    - A neurologic exam should only be performed if the musculoskeletal examination is abnormal or if the patient has a history of concussion with symptoms.
- Lab testing
    - Lab testing is optional and should only be ordered when history and physical examination warrant further evaluation.

A sample medical history form is provided in Figure 6-1, and a sample PPE examination form can be found in Figure 6-2.

Drug Testing

The beginnings of drug testing in athletics grew out of the 1960s. During that decade, a number of deaths were attributed to amphetamine abuse; this coupled with a greater recognition of anabolic steroid abuse lead the International Olympic Committee (IOC) to commission a drug-testing program. The IOC piloted a testing program at the 1968 Olympics

Name: ______________________ Birth Date: ________________ Exam Date: ____________

Address: __________________________________ City: ________________ Zip: __________

Phone: ____________________ Sport: ______________________________

		Yes	No	Medical History
1	a.	❐	❐	Have you had any illness/injury recently, or do you have an illness/injury now?
	b.	❐	❐	Have you had a medical problem, illness or injury since your last exam?
	c.	❐	❐	Do you have an ongoing medical condition (like diabetes or asthma)?
	d.	❐	❐	Have you ever had any illness lasting more than a week?
	e.	❐	❐	Have you ever been hospitalized overnight?
	f.	❐	❐	Have you had any surgery other than tonsillectomy?
	g.	❐	❐	Have you ever had any injuries requiring treatment by a physician?
	h.	❐	❐	Do you have any organ missing other than tonsils (appendix, eye, kidney, testicle, etc.)?
2.		❐	❐	Are you presently taking ANY medications (including birth control pill, vitamin, aspirin, etc.)?
3.		❐	❐	Do you have ANY allergies (medicines, bees, foods, or other factors)?
4	a.	❐	❐	Have you ever had chest pain, dizziness, fainting, passing out during or after exercise?
	b.	❐	❐	Do you tire more easily or quickly than your friends during exercise?
	c.	❐	❐	Have you ever had any problem with your blood pressure or your heart?
	d.	❐	❐	Have any close relatives had heart problems, heart attack or sudden death before they were age 50?
5.		❐	❐	Do you have any skin problems (acne, itching, rashes, etc.)?
6	a.	❐	❐	Have you ever had fainting, convulsions, seizures or severe dizziness?
	b.	❐	❐	Do you have frequent severe headaches?
	c.	❐	❐	Have you ever had a "stinger" or "burner" or "pinched nerve"?
	d.	❐	❐	Have you ever been "knocked out" or "passed out"?
	e.	❐	❐	Have you ever had a neck or head injury?
7.		❐	❐	Have you ever had heat exhaustion, heat stroke, heat cramps or similar heat-related problems?
8.		❐	❐	Have you had asthma, or trouble breathing, or cough during or after exercise?
9	a.	❐	❐	Do you wear eyeglasses, contact lenses or protective eye wear?
	b.	❐	❐	Have you had any problem with your eyes or vision?
10.		❐	❐	Do you wear any dental appliance such as braces, bridge, plate, retainer?
11	a.	❐	❐	Have you ever had a knee injury?
	b.	❐	❐	Have you ever had an ankle injury?
	c.	❐	❐	Have you ever injured any other joint (shoulder, wrist, fingers, etc.)?
	d.	❐	❐	Have you ever had a broken bone (fracture)?
	e.	❐	❐	Have you ever had a cast, splint, or had to use crutches?
	f.	❐	❐	Must you use special equipment for competition (pads, braces, neck roll, etc.)?
12.		❐	❐	Has it been more than 5 years since your last tetanus booster shot?
13.		❐	❐	Are you worried about your weight?
14.		❐	❐	Females: Have you had any menstrual problems?
15.		❐	❐	Do you have any medical concerns about participating in your sport?

I hereby state that, to the best of my knowledge, I have answered the above questions correctly.

Signature of athlete: ______________________________________

Signature of parent or guardian ______________________________________

Date: ____________________

***** ATHLETE SHOULD NOT WRITE BELOW THIS LINE *****

EXAMINER'S COMMENTS ON ALL "YES" ANSWERS (refer to question number):

____

____

____

____

Figure 6-1. Sample preparticipation history and physical examination form.

Name: ______________________________

Age: __________ Pulse: __________

Height: __________ Blood Pressure: __________

Weight: __________ Visual Acuity: Left 20/__________
Right 20/__________

Optional

Urinalysis:

Body Fat %:

HCT:

Est VO_2 Max:

Audiometry:

Follow up/Sensitive Issues (asked by examiner):

	Yes	No
1. Do you feel stressed out or under a lot of pressure?	❐	❐
2. Do you ever feel so sad or hopeless that you stop doing some of your usual activities for more than a few days?	❐	❐
3. Do you feel safe?	❐	❐
4. Have you ever tried cigarette smoking, even 1 or 2 puffs? Do you currently smoke?	❐	❐
5. During the past 30 days, did you use chewing tobacco, snuff, or dip?	❐	❐
6. During the past 30 days, have you had a least 1 drink of alcohol?	❐	❐
7. Have you ever taken steroid pills or shots without a doctor's prescription?	❐	❐
8. Have you ever taken any supplements to improve your performance?	❐	❐

Normal		Abnormal	Comments/Abnormal Findings	Initials*
❐	1. Head	❐	______	______
❐	2. Eyes (pupils), ENT	❐	______	______
❐	3. Teeth	❐	______	______
❐	4. Lymph Nodes	❐	______	______
❐	5. Lungs	❐	______	______
❐	6. Heart	❐	______	______
❐	7 Murmurs	❐	______	______
❐	8. Pulses	❐	______	______
❐	7. Abdomen	❐	______	______
❐	8. Genitourinary (Males Only+)	❐	______	______
❐	9. Neurologic	❐	______	______
❐	10. Skin	❐	______	______
❐	11. Physical Maturity	❐	______	______
❐	12. Spine, Back	❐	______	______
❐	13. Shoulders, Upper extremities	❐	______	______
❐	14. Lower extremities	❐	______	______

+ Having a third party present is recommended *Initials from examiners if using station-based system

Assessment: ❐ Full participation
❐ Limited participation (describe limitations, restrictions):

____

❐ Participation contraindicated (list reasons):

____

DATE: __________ EXAMINER'S SIGNATURE: ______________________________

EXAMINER'S PHONE: __________ PRINT EXAMINER'S NAME: ______________________________

Figure 6-2. Sample physical examination form.

in Mexico City and began a comprehensive program of testing during the 1972 games in Munich.[7] Drug testing has become commonplace in collegiate athletics. The NCAA conducts drug testing at sponsored championships, football bowl games, and random on-site school testing for football and track and field. Individual colleges and universities (and some high schools) have adopted testing programs of their own. The development of an institutional drug-testing program will require input from administration, coaches, legal counsel, and health care providers to determine the scope and nature of the program. Most drug-screening programs are designed to detect illicit drug use, enforce a banned substance list, and punish offenders of the ban.[7]

Drug-testing programs are screening tools that allow practitioners to identify evidence of drug use. Like most screening tools, further evaluation and follow-up with the patient are needed to determine the nature of an underlying problem. While a drug test may indicate a person has used a particular substance, it provides no diagnosis of an underlying disease. Drug testing may be a useful identifier of those with a drug dependency, but assumptions about drug dependence cannot be ascertained from one positive drug test. While drug-testing programs may have consequences for those who test positive, a program solely based on punitive measures without addressing the problem from a medical treatment point of view could place health care providers in a challenging situation when dealing with their patients on this issue. A drug-testing program should not be constructed in such a way as to cast the athletic trainer or team physician in the role of "police officer." Athletic training health care administrators can fulfill a needed role by using the drug testing process as an educational tool for the student-athlete. The program can educate them on what to expect at the NCAA championship level. The program can educate them about substances that can cause false-positives (eg, teas, over-the-counter medicines). A drug-screening program can also serve as an opportunity to provide factual information about the risks associated with illicit drug use. Programs with strong educational goals that are grounded in the medical model can serve their stated goals without placing the patient-care provider relationship at risk.

Developing a Drug-Screening Program

This section deals with the organization and administrative aspects of planning a drug-testing program. A discussion of the biochemistry behind the specific testing techniques and the associated issues of determining positive results and avoiding false positives are beyond the administrative scope of this discussion and better reserved for pharmacology and general medicine courses. The NCAA has developed guidelines for consideration by individual institutions wishing to develop a drug-testing program.[13] These guidelines state the following:

- Institutions considering drug testing for student-athletes should consult with institutional legal counsel early in the development process. This is of particular importance in protecting right-to-privacy statutes, which may differ from one state and locale to another. Drug testing is considered legally acceptable when proper safeguards are followed; however, legal aspects must be evaluated at each individual institution.
- Prior to initiating a drug-testing activity, a specific written policy on drug testing should be developed, distributed, and publicized. The policy should include such information as (a) a clear explanation of the purposes of the drug-testing program; (b) who will be tested and by what methods; (c) the drugs to be tested for, how often, and under what conditions (ie, announced, unannounced, or both), and (d) the actions, if any, to be taken against those who test positive. It is advised that a copy of the drug-testing program be given to all student-athletes entering the institution's intercollegiate athletics program and that they confirm in writing that they have received and read the policy. This written confirmation should be kept on file by the athletics department.
- At many institutions, student-athletes sign waiver forms regarding access to academic and medical records (see p. 108). It is recommended that specific language be added to such waiver forms wherein the student-athlete agrees to submit to drug testing at the request of the institution in accordance to published guidelines. The written confirmation form discussed in guideline number 2 can also serve as an agreement to submit to testing under the publicized program guidelines. NCAA drug-testing consent forms cover NCAA-sponsored testing only.
- Institutions considering a drug-testing program must develop a list of banned substances. The NCAA list of banned substances could be used as a guide.
- Institutions considering a drug-testing program will need to address several logistical, technical, and economic issues, including:
    - When and how samples will be collected, secured, and transported
    - Laboratory(ies) to be used
    - How samples will be stored and for how long before analysis

  - Analytical procedures to be used in the laboratory
  - Cost
  - Accuracy of tests and the false-positive (the test is ruled positive when the athlete is actually clean) and false-negative (the test yields a negative result even though the athlete has used drugs) rates. These rates will vary from lab to lab and from one type of test to another
  - How false positives will be identified and handled
  - Who will get the results and how the results will be used
- The NCAA recommends that each institution considering drug testing of student-athletes appoint a committee of representatives from various relevant academic departments and disciplines (eg, pharmacology, pharmacy, chemistry, medicine) to address various issues in the program.
- The question of where the samples will be analyzed is critical. No matter where the analysis is done, data on false-positive and false-negative rates for specific tests should be provided. If the laboratory cannot provide such information, another laboratory should be considered. Institutions should use labs that are certified and/or accredited. Listings of laboratories are available from the National Center for Drug Free Sport (www.drugfreesport.com).
- Institutions should establish a policy for confirming positive results. No matter what initial screen method is used, including thin-layer chromatography and radioimmunoassay, there is a finite probability of a false-positive test. Institutions are urged to confirm test results with gas chromatography/mass spectrometry, with the latter test providing the definitive result. This is crucial based on the possible disciplinary actions that may be imposed on the student-athlete.
- The NCAA continues to monitor guidelines and protocol in an effort to share new developments regarding drug testing with its member institutions.

The National Federation of State High School Associations (NFHS), National Interscholastic Athletic Administrators Association (NIAAA), and the National Center for Drug Free Sport, Inc conducted an online survey of high school athletic directors in 2003. The results showed that 13% of the nation's high schools have a drug-testing policy in place to test illegal and prohibited substances. Sixty-three percent of those programs with a drug-testing policy test student-athletes, while 20% test all students. In addition to the 13% currently testing, 17% of schools indicated they were interested in pursuing a program. The most common reasons given for not pursuing a program were budget constraints, lack of school board support, and legal considerations.

Beyond these factors, many interscholastic programs indicated that they believe monies were better spent on education and prevention programs.[14] While testing at the secondary school level has shown a decrease in drug use using a past 30 days index; Goldberg et al[15] cautioned that some drug-use risk factors (eg, norms of use, belief in lower risk of drugs, and poorer attitudes about school) actually increased among those athletes being tested. Some states are testing such a small number of athletes that many are uncertain of the actual efficacy of these programs. The American Academy of Pediatrics has said that testing programs at the high school level are impractical because the high cost of testing limits the number of students that can be tested.

The role of the athletic trainer in the drug-testing program must be very carefully considered. Nine percent of the high school programs performing drug testing had the athletic trainer responsible for the testing.[14] If the athletic trainer is viewed as the "cop" trying to find wrong doing, it can compromise his or her role as a health care provider. Efforts should be taken to create a program that is grounded in prevention and education and an avenue for proper care should an athlete have a substance abuse issue. If the program is primarily punitive and the athletic trainer's role is not clearly defined, it may create an atmosphere of distrust and may compromise good care.

Managing Physician Clinics

Athletic training health care administrators will often arrange for team physicians to hold clinics in their athletic training facility rather than transporting athletes to an off-campus destination. The purpose of this clinic arrangement is to provide convenient access to the medical staff for the student-athlete. These patient encounters should be organized and the results of those appointments properly documented and placed in the patients' medical record. Organizing when to hold these appointments, how to schedule athletes to attend, how to document the results, and how to staff these physician clinics are key organization and administration considerations.

Programs are encouraged to develop specific policies and procedures surrounding physician clinics that address the following:

- When physician clinics will be held

- How all student-athletes can be provided access to the physician and notified of appointments
- How athletic training staff will assist during the physician clinic
- How any specific referrals or ordered diagnostic tests will be handled following the clinic
- What information from the clinic visit can be appropriately shared with other athletic training staff for the purpose of coordinating further care
- How notes and referrals will be documented and appropriately filed in the medical record
- How the organization will address missed appointments

Establishing access to team physician clinics will vary widely by institution. Some campus models place the athletic training staff in close proximity to campus health service programs; others are fully separate and independent organizations. Access to quality sports medicine care should be afforded to all student-athletes at the institution, not just those in the most visible sports.

Athletic training health care administrators and institutional administrators must carefully negotiate with team physicians their expectations as they develop position descriptions for the team physician. Establishing how athletes will be seen, where and how often clinics will be held, and any fiscal ramifications for the physician time must be addressed and clearly understood by all parties. This will prevent misunderstandings and foster a positive working relationship among the sports medicine team. Team physicians provide supervision and guidance for athletic trainers as they practice athletic training. A positive cooperative relationship with open communication can only enhance the care provided to your patients in the educational setting.

Medications

Research investigating the dispensing and administering of medication in athletic training environments has shown varying levels of adherence to state and federal laws. Kahanov et al[16] found that individuals other than those legally authorized to dispense medications have provided prescription medications to student-athletes. In addition, state and federal regulations regarding packaging, labeling, record keeping, and storage were not universally adhered to in the intercollegiate athletic training settings. Improper adherence to such guidelines may put patients at risk and expose organizations to undue legal consequences.

The *NCAA Sports Medicine Handbook*[13] provides guidelines for the prescription medications in the athletic training setting. When considering guidelines for medications in the athletic training setting, it is important to distinguish between dispensing a medication and the administering of a medication. Administration generally refers to the direct application of a single dose of a drug. Dispensing is defined as preparing, packaging, and labeling a prescription drug or device for subsequent use by a patient. Distribution deals with how medications are provided to the patient. Physicians cannot delegate to athletic trainers the authority for dispensing prescription medications. Athletic trainers are not authorized under any circumstance to dispense medications. If athletic training health care organizations choose to keep medications (prescription and over the counter [OTC]) on site in their facility they must be able to comply with applicable state and federal laws. It is recommended that these institutions consult with legal counsel in order to insure full compliance in this setting.

The following guidelines constitute a minimal framework for an appropriate drug distribution program in an intercollegiate setting[13]:

- Drug-dispensing practices are subject to and should be in compliance with all state, federal, and Drug Enforcement Agency (DEA) regulations. Relevant areas identified in these laws include packaging, labeling, counseling and education, record keeping, and accountability for all medications.
- Certified athletic trainers should NOT be assigned duties that may only be performed by physicians and pharmacists. These duties cannot be delegated to unqualified personnel.
- Drug-distribution records should be created and maintained where distribution occurs in accordance to appropriate legal guidelines. These records should be up-to-date and easily accessible.
- All prescription and OTC medications should be stored in designated areas at proper temperatures under lock and key.
- All drug stocks should be examined at regular intervals for removal of any outdated, deteriorating, or recalled medications.
- All emergency and travel kits containing prescription and OTC medications should be inspected routinely.
- Individuals receiving medication should be properly informed about what they are taking and how they should take it. Drug allergies, chronic medical conditions, and concurrent medication use should be documented in the student-athlete's medical record and readily retrievable if needed.

- Follow-up should be performed to be sure student-athletes are complying with the drug regimen and to ensure that drug therapy is effective.

Mangus and Miller[17] recommend specific guidelines to avoid legal liability when dealing with medications in the athletic training setting. Documentation of all medications (prescription and OTC) should be logged with the following information:

- Name of the athlete/patient
- Sport
- Age of the athlete/patient
- Name of the drug
- Dose given
- Quantity prescribed
- Indication (ie, why the drug was prescribed)
- Manufacturer
- Lot number
- Drug expiration date
- How the drug was dispensed
- Date that the drug was given

In addition to the above list, the name of the prescribing physician should be included with all non-OTC medications. A sample policy and procedure for handling medications in an intercollegiate athletic training facility is provided in Box 6-3.

INFORMATION MANAGEMENT

Information management takes on many shapes in the athletic training health care organization. Proper information management will require a thorough knowledge of the standards and practices for athletic training care; knowledge of applicable federal and state laws; and an understanding of the necessary medical records, medical documentation (see Chapter 8), and consent and authorization needs for specific educational settings.

MEDICAL RECORDS

Keeping records for patients is a significant responsibility for any athletic training health care organization. Athletic training health care administrators in any setting must adhere to stringent guidelines for the maintaining of proper records. Records maintained in an athletic training facility are medical records and therefore subject to state and federal laws with regard to confidentiality and content (see HIPAA on p. 111). In the intercollegiate setting, the NCAA guidelines[13] recommend that medical records be maintained during the student-athlete's collegiate career. These records should include several items. A record of injuries, illnesses, new medications or allergies, pregnancies, and operations, whether sustained during the competitive season or off-season. The medical record should contain referral for and feedback from consultation, treatment, or rehabilitation. Subsequent care and clearances for participation should also be documented. The record must contain a comprehensive entry-year health status questionnaire and an updated health status questionnaire each year thereafter. Components of the questionnaire should consider recommendations from the American Heart Association (see Table 6-6). Immunization records should be kept in the medical chart; these will often be collected with the medical history. It is recommended that college-age athletes be immunized for measles, mumps, and rubella (MMR); hepatitis B; diphtheria; tetanus (and boosters when appropriate); and meningitis. Medical records must also contain specific permission and consent forms. Consent to treat and authorization for the release of information are most common (see Authorizations and Consent Forms below).

Many factors must be considered when considering items to included in the medical record, or how to document in the athletic training setting. While the NCAA guidelines provide sound advice for the athletic training administrator, practicing athletic trainers must abide by the laws that govern athletic training practice in their state and the Standards and Practices put forth by the Board of Certification (BOC) when it comes to medical records and documentation practices.

> *Standard 7: Organization and Administration states: All services are documented in writing by the athletic trainer and are part of the patient's permanent record. The athletic trainer accepts responsibility for recording details of the patient's health status.*

A complete copy of the BOC Standards of Practice is provided in Appendix K.

AUTHORIZATIONS AND CONSENT FORMS

The annual ritual of obtaining written authorizations and consent forms from student-athletes at the start of a new academic year may seem like a mere formality. However, the process of gathering permissions, statements of understanding, and consent can set the boundaries for proper care, acknowledges the athlete's role in sport safety, establishes the policy for drug testing, and clarifies how specific information can be used. These documents are essential for compliance with state and federal regulation and

Box 6-3

A Sample Policy for Distribution of Medications in an Intercollegiate Setting

Policy

All prescription medications stocked at the State U Sports Medicine Center are pre-dispensed and labeled. Medications will ONLY be distributed by team physicians or dentists with a written prescription. Medications unavailable in the State U Sports Medicine Center will be referred by written prescription to the University Outpatient Pharmacy or to a designated pharmacy in the community. Nonprescription medications will be distributed by the staff athletic trainer following the standard protocol of the team physician and under the guidelines of the state license. State U will only assume financial responsibility for medications prescribed by designated team physicians and dentists for sport/competition-related illness or injury (as governed by NCAA rules).

Purpose

To have commonly prescribed medications available for immediate distribution to the student-athlete upon prescription from the physician or dentist.

Procedures

- Athletic training students must receive permission from the staff athletic trainer to distribute over-the-counter medication to a student-athlete.
- Prior to distributing medication, the team physicians or dentists will inform the student-athlete of concerns while taking the medication, including NCAA rules regarding the use of the medication.
- Medications that are related to athletic participation are the financial responsibility of the State U and purchased at a pharmacy other than University Pharmacy will require a pre-pay. In order to be reimbursed for this payment, an itemized receipt must be presented to the staff athletic trainer of the sport for proper reporting procedure.
- The team physician will determine the need for iontophoresis treatments for a student-athlete's injury and prescribe accordingly. The treatment protocol will be described by the team physician to the student-athlete. This protocol includes application of the treatment by a licensed athletic trainer.

Documentation

- After distribution of the prescription medication to the student-athlete, the licensed athletic trainer will stamp the prescription with a sequential number. That number will be entered into the medication database. The prescription will be filed in sequential order in the physician's office.
- The licensed athletic trainer is responsible for entering all physician-authorized refills into the medication database. This must occur immediately following the distribution of the medication to the student-athlete.
- For iontophoresis treatments, the team physician will write a prescription for the medication needed and will document the treatment (including frequency and duration) in the student-athlete's medical chart.

are the foundation for the care relationship between the sports medicine staff and the student-athlete. Common authorizations and consent forms used in the educational setting include consent to provide medical care, statement of understanding for drug testing, statement of shared responsibility for sport safety, and authorization for the release of information.

Consent to treat is established by a medical consent form that should be on file with the athlete's medical chart of other specific program information. Figure 6-3 provides an example of a medical consent form. These forms allow the athletic trainers under the guidance of their supervising physicians to render preventative, first aid, rehabilitative, or emergency treatment that they deem necessary for the health and well being of the student-athlete. This form can also grant consent to hospitalization and treatment at an appropriate accredited medical facility.

Instructions: If the student-athlete is not a minor, the student-athlete should sign the top half of this form.
If the student-athlete is a minor (ie, under 18 years old), parents or guardian and student-athlete should sign the bottom half of this form.

MEDICAL CONSENT

I hereby grant permission to the State U team physicians and/or their consulting physicians to render any treatment or medical or surgical care that they deem reasonably necessary for my health and well being.

I also hereby authorize the athletic trainers at the State U, who are under the direction and guidance of the State U team physicians, to render any preventive, first aid, rehabilitative or emergency treatment that they deem reasonably necessary for my health and well being. Also, when necessary for executing such care, I grant permission for hospitalization at an accredited hospital.

DATE: ____________________ ATHLETE'S NAME ______________________________
(print)

ATHLETE'S SIGNATURE ______________________________

MEDICAL CONSENT FOR MINOR

I hereby grant permission to the State U team physicians and/or their consulting physicians to render to my son or daughter any treatment or medical or surgical care that they deem reasonably necessary to the health and well being of my child.

I also hereby authorize the athletic trainers at the State U, who are under the direction and guidance of the State U team physicians, to render to my son or daughter any preventive, first aid, rehabilitative or emergency treatment that they deem reasonably necessary to the health and well being of my child. I grant permission for hospitalization at an accredited hospital.

DATE: ____________________ PARENT OR GUARDIAN SIGNATURE ______________________________

DATE OF BIRTH: ___________ ATHLETE'S NAME ______________________________
(print)

ATHLETE'S SIGNATURE ______________________________

NOTE: Signatures on this form are in effect during their status as a student-athlete with the Division of Intercollegiate Athletics. This consent can be withdrawn at any time, by the student-athlete, in writing.

Figure 6-3. Sample medical consent form.

A signed statement of shared responsibility for sport safety is a form of "acceptance of risk" document that all athletes should sign. An example of a shared responsibility form is found in Figure 6-4. Such forms establish that both the institution and the athlete have a responsibility for safety. They also provide that participation in sport requires the acceptance of risk of injury and that the injury may be severe. This form can also establish guidelines for withholding a participant from activity and establish that the institution cannot be held responsible for previous injuries (both detected and undetected) that an individual may have.

As mentioned previously in the chapter, it is recommended that institutions with a drug-testing program have student-athletes sign a consent form that acknowledges their understanding of the guidelines of the testing program and their consent to be tested.

The last authorization that must be obtained is the authorization for the release of information. This authorization is required in order to be in compliance with The Health Insurance Privacy and Accountability

Participation in sport requires an acceptance of risk of injury. Athletes rightfully assume that those who are responsible for the conduct of sport have taken reasonable precaution to minimize such risk and that their peers participating in the sport will not intentionally inflict injury upon them.

Periodic analysis of injury patterns leads to refinements in the rules and other safety decisions. However, to legislate safety via a rulebook and equipment standards, while often necessary, seldom is effective by itself. Also, to rely on officials to enforce compliance with the rulebook is as insufficient as to rely on warning labels to produce compliance with safety guidelines. "Compliance" means respect on everyone's part for the intent and purpose of a rule or guideline.

I have read the above shared responsibility statement. I understand that there are certain inherent risks involved in participating in intercollegiate athletics. I acknowledge the fact that these risks exist, and am willing to assume responsibility for such risks while participating at the State U.

DATE: ____________________ ATHLETE'S NAME ______________________________
(print)

ATHLETE'S SIGNATURE ______________________________

The undersigned, herewith,

A. Understand that I must refrain from practice or play during medical treatment until I am discharged from treatment or given permission by the team physician or licensed athletic trainer to restart participation while continuing treatment.

B. Understand that having passed the physical examination does not necessarily mean that I am physically qualified to engage in athletics at the State U, but only that the evaluator(s) did not find a medical reason to disqualify me at the time of the examination.

C. Fully realize the State U cannot be held responsible for any previous medical condition(s) that I might have.

DATE: ____________________ ATHLETE'S NAME ______________________________
(print)

ATHLETE'S SIGNATURE ______________________________

NOTE: Signatures on this form are in effect during their status as a student/athlete with the Division of Intercollegiate Athletics. This consent can be withdrawn at any time, by the student-athlete, in writing.

Figure 6-4. Sample athlete shared responsibility for sport safety.

Act (HIPAA) and the Family Education Rights and Privacy Act of 1974 (FERPA). Both of these laws and their impact on the athletic training health care organization are discussed.

Health Insurance Privacy and Accountability Act and Family Education Rights and Privacy Act

The element of protection of an individual's right to privacy is at the heart of both the HIPAA and FERPA laws. The HIPAA law focuses, in part, on the protection of medical records and information. The FERPA law surrounds the rights of students in educational settings to review and inspect educational records, to have their educational records amended or corrected, and to control the disclosure of certain portions of their educational records.

HIPAA was passed into law in 1996 and went into full effect in 2003. The HIPAA law regulates how a patient's private health information (PHI) can be shared. HIPAA limits the ways that health plans, pharmacies, hospitals, and other covered entities can use a patient's personal medical information. The provisions of HIPAA protect medical records and other individually identifiable health information, whether it is communicated in writing, electronically, or orally.[18] Key provisions of HIPAA include the following:

- Access to medical records—Patients have the rights to obtain copies of their medical records and request corrections should they find errors. This access should be provided within 30 days.
- Notice of privacy practices—A health care provider must provide notice to patients on how they plan to use personal medical information as well as restrict the use or disclosure of their medical information. In athletic training environments, this disclosure usually takes the form of an authorization (Box 6-4 and Figure 6-5). An authorization can be collected at the start of the year rather than on a per-injury basis. This will provide a framework on how information is disclosed to other care providers for the purposes of assessing the athlete's ability to participate, how information is disclosed to coaches regarding playability status, and how information is released publicly (eg, to the media).

Box 6-4

Guidelines for HIPAA Authorization Form

The HIPAA disclosure authorization should contain the following:

- Description of information to be disclosed
- Identification of the persons or class of persons authorized to make use of the protected information
- Identification of the persons or class of persons to whom the covered entity is authorized to provide or disclose
- A description of each purpose of the use or disclosure
- An expiration date or event
- The individual's signature and date
- If signed by a personal representative, a description of his or her authority to act for the individual

- Limits on the use of medical information—Personal identifiable health information generally may not be used for purposes not related to health care. Health care providers are not allowed to disclose health information to any party without written consent to do so. To promote the best quality of care for patients, the rule does not restrict the ability of doctors and other care providers to share information needed to treat their patients. The athletic trainer can certainly discuss a patient's health information with the team physician responsible for that patient's care. Care providers should not discuss information in any way that would identify the patient. This deidentification allows doctors and other care providers to discuss cases and seek feedback without violating the HIPAA guideline. It also allows for cases to be used in appropriate educational environments, provided the patient cannot be identified.
- Prohibition on marketing—The rule prevents health care providers from using patient information for marketing purposes.
- Confidential communications—Under the privacy rule, patients can request that their doctors, health plans, and other providers take reasonable steps to ensure that their communications with the patient are confidential.

Those groups required to comply with HIPAA regulations are referred to as *covered entities*. A covered entity is defined as one of the following: a health care provider that conducts certain transactions in electronic form, a health care clearinghouse, or a health plan. While many athletic trainers may be working in facilities that are not determined to be covered entities, Konin and Frederick[19] recommend that it is prudent to implement and adhere to the best practices that will protect a patient's/athlete's privacy regarding medical information.

The FERPA law is applied in public educational institutions at all levels (primary, secondary, and postsecondary). It is similar in scope to HIPAA in that it focuses on protecting the student's right to privacy. Educational records under FERPA are determined to be either public or private. When an educational record has been deemed private, it is releasable only to specific parties. Examples of public information could include: your name, major field of study, dates of attendance, and participation in officially recognized activities (eg, a sports team). Examples of private-protected FERPA records would be grades, grade point average, identification number, place of birth, current class schedule, and disciplinary actions. In some instances, it is suggested that medical records be kept as part of the student's educational records. Thus, the student would be protected under FERPA instead of HIPAA.[3] Students, and in some instances their parents (prior to a student turning 18 or attending a postsecondary school), have rights related to reviewing and inspecting educational records, having their educational records amended or corrected, and controlling the disclosure of certain portions of their educational records.

Institutions are encouraged to be compliant with all HIPAA and FERPA guidelines in the interest of protecting the rights and privacy of students. Athletic

I authorize my team doctors and other health care providers (including athletic trainers) who are affiliated with State U and from whom I have received health care treatment to disclose my health information as described below:

I authorize disclosure of the following health information on me for the purpose of enabling them to announce or publicize to the public my medical availability to participate in intercollegiate athletic competition only the following health information:
The fact that I am sick or injured and unable to compete.
If I am injured, the name of the body part injured.
A statement of the time estimated for me to recover and return to athletic competition.

This authorization shall be in force and effect until the termination of my status as a student-athlete at State U.

I am aware that I have the right to revoke this authorization, in writing, at any time by sending my written revocation to the Director of Athletics and to the specific physician(s), team doctor(s) or other health care provider(s) who are affiliated with State U and from whom I have received health care treatment. I am aware that the revocation will not apply to health information that has already been released in response to this authorization and that my revocation of this authorization may, depending on the circumstances of the revocation, prevent me from practicing and competing as a student-athlete.

I am aware that authorizing the disclosure of this health information is voluntary and that my physicians and other health care providers may not refuse to provide me treatment if I do not sign this form. I can refuse to sign this authorization. I am also aware that the disclosure of this health information carries with it the potential for re-disclosure by any recipients who are not subject to health privacy laws and that my health information, once disclosed, may no longer be protected by federal or state law. However, I am also aware that if I refuse to sign this authorization, I will not be permitted to participate in intercollegiate athletics at State U.

I am aware that I may have the right to inspect or copy the information whose disclosure I am authorizing, with certain exceptions provided under state and federal law.

____
Student-Athlete's Printed Name

____ ____________________
Signature of Athlete or Legal Representative Date
(if signed by legal representative, indicate representative's relationship to student-athlete)

Figure 6-5. Sample authorization for publication of health status.

trainers in administrative roles should determine how their specific university, college, or school district interprets the FERPA law and how they educate students about these rights.

A gray area exists in determining what guidelines are applicable to employees contracted to school settings, a common practice of athletic training outreach clinics. It is suggested that these athletic trainers follow the HIPAA guidelines for medical information when seeing patients away from a school setting. When seeing patients in the school environment, the FERPA law would prevail. In any case, it may be necessary to establish contractually how the sharing of information between employees of the clinic and employees of the school will take place.

GUIDELINES FOR MEDICAL COVERAGE OF INTERCOLLEGIATE ATHLETICS

The discussion of appropriate medical coverage for the intercollegiate athlete has received much attention in recent years. The NATA Task Force on Appropriate Medical Coverage for Intercollegiate Athletes (AMCIA) was formed in 1998. This task force came into being to address concerns regarding the increased exposure to injury by student-athletes as a result of expanded traditional sport seasons, nontraditional season practices and competitions, skill instruction sessions, and strength and conditioning that extends year round. Athletic training health care administrators must determine how to assign staff to provide appropriate access to medical care for the student-athlete. The NATA Task Force made its initial recommendations in 2000 and followed up with adjusted data in 2003. The task force has put forth information based on relevant published literature, existing guidelines and position statements, detailed injury studies, a 2-year AMCIA specific injury study, NCAA injury surveillance data, and legal settlements specific to athletic injury.

The task force noted that appropriate coverage involves more than just emergency care. While critical to have an emergency action plan, appropriate medical coverage required daily ongoing interaction with student-athletes (eg, determining readiness to participate, treatment and rehabilitation, risk management and injury prevention, psychosocial intervention and referral, nutritional aspects of illness and injury).

The results are a formula-based approach that attempts to quantify the appropriate coverage needed for any given intercollegiate sport by creating a health care index. This index determines the number of athletic trainers needed to provide appropriate coverage for that sport based upon injury rates and therefore the risk of injury for a given sport, potential for catastrophic injury, and the actual exposures to injury for a given sport (determined by numbers of athletes and numbers of total days for a season). Football, ice hockey, and gymnastics are examples of high-risk sports; tennis, swimming, and softball are examples of low-risk sports. This risk is determined by injury rates and potential for catastrophic injury.[20] While an athletic trainer available for every sport practice and competition may be ideal, it is likely not feasible in most settings. Appropriate coverage for a low-risk sport practice and competition may be the presence of an emergency plan and coaching and personnel trained in CPR; moderate-risk sports may need the ability of an athletic trainer to respond in a short time period (<4 minutes), while high-risk activities need athletic training personnel present at all times. No matter the level of coverage provided at practices and competitions, all student-athletes should have an athletic trainer and team physician designated for ongoing health care needs.

Individual institutions must look at all available data and the NATA Task Force recommendations to determine how these can assist them in their specific setting. All student-athletes are entitled to appropriate medical coverage, and the health and safety of the participants must be paramount in determining staffing needs. Athletic training administrators may have to balance specific administrative expectations for sport coverage with the realities of injury rates and potential risk for catastrophic injury. As the health care expectations in the intercollegiate setting grow with changes in the amount of injury exposures outside the traditional season, colleges and universities may find themselves at a liability risk if they cannot, or will not, provide adequate medical coverage. Athletic trainers in consultation with their medical teams and campus administration must use available injury data and available resources to provide the most logical medical coverage possible in their setting.

RECOMMENDATIONS FOR APPROPRIATE MEDICAL CARE IN THE SECONDARY SCHOOL SETTING

The importance of the athletic trainer to the secondary school setting has been reinforced by many professional organizations. The American Medical Association (AMA)[21] has stated that certified athletic trainers should be used as part of a high school's medical team. The American Academy of Family Physicians[22] agrees and states that, "the AAFP encourages high schools to have, whenever possible, a BOC certified or registered/licensed athletic trainer as an integral part of the high school athletic program." The original AMA statement makes clear that many secondary school settings do not have the resources to hire adequate athletic training staff and must make sure that all coaches and staff who work in the high school athletic setting are properly trained in CPR and first aid. Athletic trainers should work closely with administrative and medical staff to develop care that is based on prevailing sports injury data, risk of participation, local needs, resources, available personnel, and state and local regulations. Many large secondary school athletic programs would be well served by more than one athletic trainer.

The NATA in conjunction with multiple medical and allied health organizations produced the Consensus Statement on Appropriate Medical Care for Secondary School-Age Athletes.[23] It states that the athletic health care team in the secondary school setting should have a designated athletic health care provider who is educated and qualified to do the following:

- Determine the individual's readiness to participate.
- Promote safe and appropriate practice, competition, and treatment facilities.

- Advise on the selection, fit, function, and maintenance of athletic equipment.
- Develop and implement a comprehensive emergency action plan.
- Establish protocols regarding environmental conditions.
- Develop injury and illness prevention strategies.
- Provide for on-site recognition, evaluation, and immediate treatment of injury and illness, with appropriate referrals.
- Facilitate rehabilitation and reconditioning.
- Provide for psychological consultation and referral.
- Provide scientifically sound nutritional counseling and education.
- Participate in the development and implementation of a comprehensive athletic health care administrative system (eg, personal health information, policies and procedures, insurance, referrals).

These recommendations provide a succinct outline of the duties for an athletic trainer who provides care for the secondary school-aged athlete and reinforces the topics outlined in this chapter.

FACILITY DESIGN

The opportunity to contribute to the design of a new athletic training health care facility is an exciting task that not every athletic trainer will get to perform during his or her career. Those fortunate enough may be able to provide input for a start-to-finish project, work with an architect, and see the construction progress to a finished product. A more common scenario is the chance to participate in the remodel of an existing space. Many high schools have remodeled space to accommodate athletic training facilities as programs continue to take root and grow in this setting. No matter if you are helping design a new state-of-the-art facility on a large university campus or designing a remodel to accommodate a growing interscholastic program, athletic training health care facilities must be designed to reflect the multidimensional nature of the care that takes place in these locations.

When participating in the design of a new facility there are many questions to answer:

- Who will use this facility?
- Where will it be located?
- What design elements need to be addressed?
- What specialized service areas should be included?

Understanding how the facility will be used, how many athletes will use it, and any unique needs of those athletes can help answer many questions during the design process. For example, ice hockey teams have special access needs should a player have to come directly from the ice to the athletic training health care facility while still wearing skates. Taping benches and tables can be adjusted in facilities that serve basketball players to account for their size.

The location of the facility should allow for entrance from the outside and not require passage through a locker room facility. If an injured athlete must be brought into or out of the facility, avoiding multiple doorways will allow for easier passage. Doors and hallways should easily accommodate stretchers and wheelchairs. The facility, like all facilities, should be wheelchair accessible and use ramps instead of stairways. Reasonable proximity to locker rooms allows convenient access for athletes coming in before and after practices. Prentice[3] recommends that since athletic training facilities provide emergency treatment, light, heat, and water sources should be independent from the rest of the building.

Design elements that address safety, mechanical considerations, and ergonomics must be addressed. Half walls to allow supervision of hydrotherapy and treatment areas, nonslip flooring, adequate ceiling heights, and proper illumination are all considerations for proper employee and patient safety. Mechanical elements also overlap with safety elements. Electrical outlets must be equipped with ground fault circuit interrupters (GFI). Proper ventilation and air circulation must be considered; the increased humidity and noise generated in the hydrotherapy area requires careful placement in the facility and additional ventilation. Water fill pipes and drains in the hydrotherapy area should be larger to allow for rapid filling and draining of whirlpools.

Greater attention to ergonomics has taken place in recent years. Ergonomics is the study of human work—specifically, issues related to working environments and physical capabilities of workers as they interact with tools, equipment, work methods, tasks, and work environments. The most common application is office ergonomics, examining the office environment. As computers have become ubiquitous machines found everywhere in work settings, attention to computer set up and work environments has grown proportionally. These details must be addressed when designing workstations in the athletic training environment in order to provide safe working environments. Table 6-7 outlines ergonomic elements to consider when setting up an office workspace.

Table 6-7

Ergonomic Considerations for Office Workspaces

Office Component	Ergonomic Consideration
Computer screen position	Screen position so that the operator looks down at an angle of 5 to 20 degrees from the plane of the eyes
Adjustable copy holder	Same distance as screen from the eyes (1 to 2 feet)
Keyboard support surfaces	Independent height adjustable display and keyboard support surfaces allowing clearance of the legs, elbow angle near 90 degrees, straight neutral wrist, and proper viewing angle to the screen
Chair	The chair should include height adjustable backrest with protruding lumbar support, back tilts forward and back, seat angle tilts forward and back, torso to thigh at least 90 degrees, seat height is adjustable from the floor, and feet rest flat on floor or foot rest.
Noise	Noise control in the office area must be considered. Acoustic covers for printers are recommended.

Athletic training facilities must have specialized areas for injury evaluation, treatment and first aid, rehabilitation, program administration, storage, physician examination, taping and bandaging, and storage. Design considerations for these areas include the following:

- General treatment and evaluation area—This area includes treatment tables, modality carts, various modalities, and stools for use by athletic training staff.
- Rehabilitation therapeutic exercise area—An open area for therapeutic exercise should be included with space to use physiotherapy balls, foam rollers, dumb bells, slide boards, or any functional exercise equipment that requires open space.
- Hydrotherapy area—Hydrotherapy areas have additional drainage and flooring needs. A central floor drain, nonslip flooring, and windows to allow for supervision are required for hydrotherapy areas. GFIs, electrical outlets raised up off the floor, and water mixers to allow for preset temperature filling of whirlpools are needed for safety and convenience.
- Taping and bandaging area—A taping and bandaging area separate from the other areas will allow for better traffic flow and eliminate congestion. Taping tables or a built-in taping bench can also double for storage of supplies. Taping tables can also be adjustable in height to accommodate a variety of users.
- Program administration/office area—The size of the athletic training office area will be dependent upon the number of staff. Office windows should allow for supervision of the facility. Offices and program administration areas that contain program and medical files must be kept under lock and key. These locks should be independent of the general facility locks.
- Physician examination room—A private area for physician clinics and consultations is important. An examination table, sink, work area, and storage cabinets are the basic elements of the examination room. When not in use by the physician, it can serve as a more private location for injury evaluation and private conversations among care providers or between patients and athletic trainers.
- Storage room—Adequate storage for supplies and equipment is at a premium in most athletic training facilities. Judicious use of cabinets, storage provided with taping benches and treatment tables, and designated storage areas can help alleviate this common problem.

Figure 6-6 shows photos of various program function areas in an athletic training health care facility.

Physical Resource Management

Athletic training health care administrators in supervisory positions will need established plans for the maintenance of the facilities they supervise. Chapter 3 addresses specific details about budget, purchasing, and inventory. Having a system to account for all consumable and nonconsumable supplies will allow for proper budgeting and a more judicious use of funds. Often overlooked in the detailed budget is

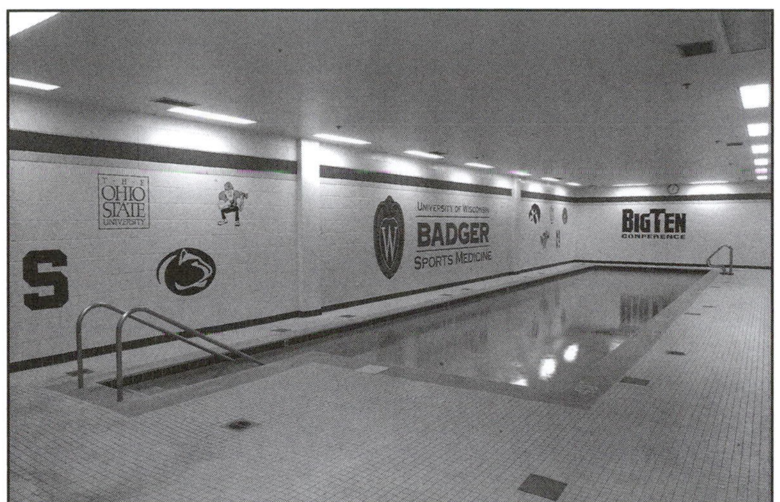

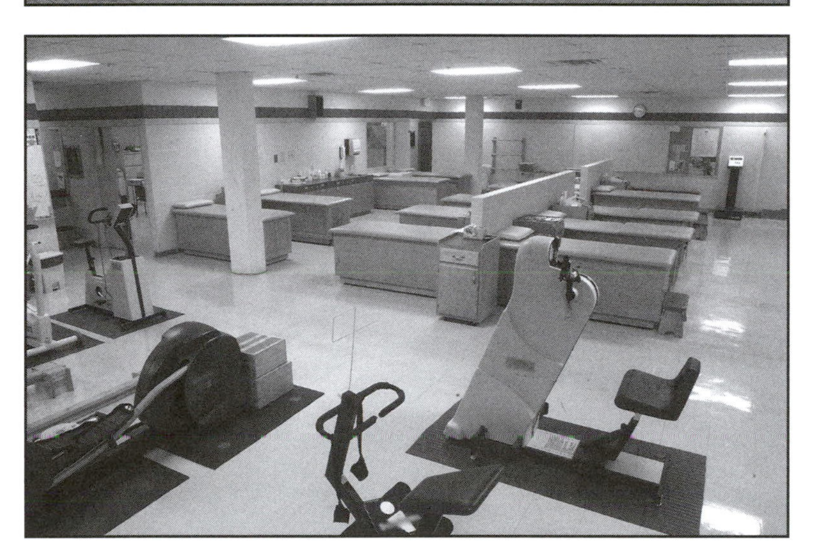

Figure 6-6. A modern athletic training facility includes a variety of program function areas.

funding for repairs and annual upkeep. Modalities, ice machines, and some types of rehabilitation equipment must be calibrated and/or serviced annually. It must also be determined how, how often, and who will clean the athletic training facility on a daily basis. In educational settings, there may be a rotating schedule for cleaning of specific rooms that may not be as frequent as the athletic trainer desires. Athletic trainers may also need specialized disinfectants that are not commonly used by custodial staff. It will also fall to the athletic training administrator to establish proper policies for the discarding of biohazard waste.

SUMMARY

- Discuss the use of policies and procedures to guide operational programming.

  Policy and procedure guides are useful tools to provide athletic training staff, physicians, administrators, and coaches a clear understanding for specific program functions. They also provide a foundation for continuity of care and a uniform guide for daily operations.

- Explain how HIPAA impacts athletic training health care organizations in educational settings.

  HIPAA was passed into law in 1996; however it only went into full effect in 2003. The HIPAA law regulates how a patient's private health information (PHI) can be shared. HIPAA limits the ways that health plans, pharmacies, hospitals, and other covered entities can use a patient's personal medical information. The provisions of HIPAA protect medical records and other individually identifiable health information, whether it is written, electronic, or oral.[18]

- Describe FERPA and explain how it impacts the athletic training organization.

  The FERPA law surrounds the rights of students in educational settings to review and inspect educational records, have their educational records amended or corrected, and control the disclosure of certain portions of their educational records.

- Identify the range of program functions common to athletic training programs in the educational setting.

  A variety of program functions are discussed in the chapter. They generally fall under the categories of delivery of health care services and management of health care facilities. Organizational and administrative considerations for emergency planning, PPE, drug testing, information management, management of physicians' clinics, and handling of medications are discussed in detail.

- Describe the considerations for appropriate medical coverage in the intercollegiate and interscholastic athletic settings.

  Appropriate coverage in all settings involves more than just emergency care. While it is critical to have an emergency action plan, appropriate medical coverage requires daily ongoing interaction with student-athletes (eg, determining readiness to participate, treatment and rehabilitation, risk management and injury prevention, psychosocial intervention and referral, nutritional aspects of illness and injury). The importance of the athletic trainer to the secondary school setting has been reinforced by many professional organizations.

- Explain the organization and administration issues facing athletic training educators.

  The athletic training educator must possess specific organizational and administrative skills to shape and manage the athletic training education program. Educational programs must have a mechanism to explain how the program is structured and how the program operates. Admission policies, technical standards, program progress, clinical requirements, costs, and academic guidelines are just a sample of items that must be explained to prospective and current students.

- Describe the organization and proper use of medical records.

  Keeping records for patients is a significant responsibility for any athletic training health care organization. Athletic training health care administrators must adhere to stringent guidelines for the maintaining of proper records. Records maintained in an athletic training facility are medical records and therefore subject to state and federal laws with regard to confidentiality and content.

- Identify the various authorizations and consent documentation required to treat patients in an educational venue.

  The process of gathering consent and authorization forms helps establish the foundation for the care relationship between the sports medicine staff and the student-athlete. Common authorizations and consent forms used in educational settings include consent to provide medical care, statement of understanding for drug testing, statement of shared responsibility for sport safety, and authorization for the release of information.

- Discuss the organizational and administrative issues inherent to planning and carrying out PPE.

  Governing bodies in both the secondary school and collegiate settings have recommendations and guidelines for preparticipation medical examinations. The primary goal of the PPE is to detect any conditions that may limit an athlete's participation and predispose the athlete or others to injuries or illness during competition. Secondary goals are to determine the general health of the individual, assess fitness level, and counsel the athlete on health-related issues. An overview of station-based and office-based exams is provided.

- Define the components of a drug-testing plan.

  The development of an institutional drug-testing program will require input from administration, coaches, legal counsel, and health care providers to determine the scope and nature of the program. Drug testing programs are screening tools that allow practitioners to identify evidence of drug use. Like most screening tools, further evaluation and follow-up with the patient are needed to determine the nature of an underlying problem. The NCAA has developed guidelines that assist with the appropriate medical legal issues surrounding the implementation of a drug-testing program.

- Explain the key elements of designing an athletic training health care facility.

  Understanding how the facility will be used, how many athletes will use it, and any unique needs of those athletes can help answer many questions during the design process. Athletic training facilities must have specialized areas for injury evaluation, treatment and first aid, rehabilitation, program administration, storage, physician examination, taping and bandaging, and storage.

ACTIVITIES

The following activities are designed to reinforce material presented in the chapter and to allow for discussion among students and instructors.

Policy and Procedure Development

The chapter provides examples of policies and procedures for an intercollegiate athletic training services program. Develop a policy, purpose statement, and procedure for the topics listed below. Remember a policy is a written statement that identifies the basic rules and principles used to control and expedite decision making. Procedures describe the steps that should be followed—the processes—of how something should be done. The purpose statement is a short declarative reason for the policy (see the shaded box examples in the chapter).

Write policies and procedures for the following:

- Blood-borne pathogens (exposures and use of universal precautions)
- Reporting of injuries and illnesses
- Referrals for second opinions
- Coverage of visiting teams

Facility Design

As the head athletic trainer at Everytown High School, you were pleased to hear you can help design the new athletic training facility. Your current athletic training room is obsolete. Thanks to a local fund-raising effort, you will have the chance to remodel to serve the needs of your students. Like most high schools, space is at a premium so you will only have 1000 square feet to work with. Given that your current facility is only 250 square feet (including 50 square feet of storage) you are very excited.

Draw a floor plan schematic for your remodeled facility using the information provided to guide you. The drawing must be to scale (for both the facility and equipment). Include in your finished drawing the location of the required equipment.

- Information on current facility:
    - 250 square feet (that includes a storage room that is about 50 square feet)
    - One 2-person taping bench
    - One whirlpool
    - One small ice machine and one freezer
    - Two treatment tables
    - One stationary bike
    - One stair climbing fitness machine
- Your new space is 1000 square feet (40′ x 25′) and must include the following:
    - Office
    - Storage room
    - Hydro area with whirlpool, ice machine, and freezer
    - Four to 6 treatment tables
    - Three-person taping bench
    - Main and emergency exits
    - One stationary bike
    - One stair climbing fitness machine
    - Other items or program function areas if you feel they can fit

Remember your measurements for equipment must be accurate (do not guess!). It is good to borrow a tape measure and go to your athletic training facility to take some measurements before you begin this assignment. When you are done, share your finished drawings with your classmates and explain your choices for your remodeled facility.

Questions to consider:

- Can I easily move supplies in and out of the facility?
- Where is the storage in relation to the entrance or exit?
- Where is the storage in relation to the wet area?
- Does my space reflect my athletic training philosophy?
- Is there adequate space for rehabilitation activities?
- Is my floor plan open or compartmentalized?

REFERENCES

1. National Athletic Trainers Association. NATA total membership by job setting. Available at http://www.nata.org/membership/MembStats2007_1.htm. Accessed February 11, 2007.
2. Board of Certification. *Role Delineation Study.* 5th ed. Omaha, NE: Board of Certification; 2004.
3. Prentice WE. *Arnheim's Principles of Athletic Training.* 12th ed. New York: McGraw-Hill; 2006.
4. Anderson JC, Courson, RW, Kleiner, DM, McLoda, TA. National Athletic Trainers' Association position statement: emergency planning in athletics. *Journal of Athletic Training.* 2002;37(1):99-104.
5. Wisconsin Interscholastic Athletic Association. Medical policies and procedures. Available at http://www.wiaawi.org/health/medicalprocedures.pdf. Accessed March 1, 2007.
6. Lombardo JA, Badolato SK. The preparticipation physical examination. *Sports Medicine.* 2001;3(1):10-25.
7. Landry GL, Bernhardt DT. *Essentials of Primary Care Sports Medicine.* Champaign, IL: Human Kinetics; 2003.

8. Smith J, Lankowski ER. The preparticipation physical examination: Mayo Clinic experience with 2,729 examinations. *Mayo Clin Proc.* 1998;73:419-429.
9. Maron BJ, Thomason PD, Puffer JC. Cardiovascular preparticipation screen of competitive athletes: a statement for health professionals from the Sudden Death Committee and Congenital Cardiac Defects Committee, American Heart Association. *Circulation.* 1996;94:850-856.
10. Maron BJ, Thomason PD, Puffer JC. Addendum to: Cardiovascular preparticipation screen of competitive athletes: a statement for health professionals from the Sudden Death Committee and Congenital Cardiac Defects Committee, American Heart Association. *Circulation.* 1998;97:2294.
11. Gomez JE, Landry GL, Bernhardt DT. Critical evaluation of the 2-minute orthopedic screening examination. *American Journal of Disabled Children.* 1993;147:1109-1113.
12. Mick TM, Dimeff RJ. What kind of physical examination does a young athlete need before participating in sports? *Cleve Clin J Med.* 2004;71(7):587-597.
13. The National Collegiate Athletic Association. *NCAA Sports Medicine Handbook.* 18th ed. Indianapolis, IN: Author; 2005-06.
14. National Federation of State High School Associations. Sports medicine: high school drug testing programs. Available at http://www.nfhs.org/web/2003/11/sports_mediciine_high_school_drugtesting_programs_august_2003.aspx. Accessed February 27, 2007.
15. Goldberg L, Elliot DL, MacKinnon DP, et al. Drug testing in athletes to prevent substance abuse: background and pilot testing results of the SATURN (student-athlete testing using random notification) study. *J Adolesc Health.* 2003;32:16-25.
16. Kahanov L, Furst D, Johnson S, Roberts J. Adherence to drug-dispensation and drug-administration laws and guidelines in collegiate athletic training rooms. *Journal of Athletic Training.* 2003;38(3):252-258.
17. Mangus BC, Miller MG. *Pharmacology Application in Athletic Training.* Philadelphia, PA: FA Davis; 2005.
18. Department of Health and Human Services. HIPAA fact sheet: Protecting the Privacy of Patient's Health Information. Available at http://www.hhs.gov/news/facts/privacy.html. Accessed March 1, 2007.
19. Konin JG, Frederick MA. *Documentation for Athletic Training.* Thorofare, NJ: SLACK Incorporated; 2005.
20. National Athletic Trainers Association Task Force. Consensus statement on appropriate medical coverage for intercollegiate athletes (AMCIA). Available at http://www.nata.org/statements/support/AMCIARescandGuides.pdf. Accessed March 1, 2007.
21. American Medical Association. Policy H-470.995 Athletic (Sports) Medicine 1998. Available at http://www.ama-assn.org/apps/pf_new/pf_online. Accessed March 8, 2007.
22. American Academy of Family Physicians. Statement on athletic trainers in high schools. Available at http://www.aafp.org/online/en/home/policy/policies/s/sports.html. Accessed March 9, 2007.
23. National Athletic Trainers Association Task Force. Consensus statement on appropriate medical care for secondary school-age athletes. Available at http://www.nata.org/statements/consensus/ConsensusStatement_FinalVersion_Sept02.pdf. Accessed March 2, 2007.

ATHLETIC TRAINING ADMINISTRATION
ISSUES IN CLINICAL SETTINGS

Tim McGuine, PhD, ATC

OBJECTIVES

At the end of this chapter, the reader will be able to:

- Understand the differences between the education and training for employment in the traditional collegiate and clinical settings
- Explain the rationale for employing athletic trainers in the clinical setting
- Describe the various duties of athletic trainers in the clinical setting, including physician extenders, outreach providers, rehabilitation specialists, and supervision performance enhancement programs.
- Understand the importance of marketing and public relations
- Identify programming initiatives
- Describe the advantages and disadvantages of conducting research in the clinical setting
- Summarize contract language necessary to provide athletic training outreach services to schools, institutions, and organizations
- Summarize the position description for a typical clinical/outreach setting

The field of athletic training has grown dramatically since the 1980s. As a result, the employment settings for athletic trainers have shifted dramatically from the collegiate setting to clinic, industrial, and clinic/school-based settings. Athletic trainers in these settings have taken the traditional on-the-field and in-the-stadium approach of sports medicine and extended it to patients who did not traditionally have access to this level of care. The number of athletic trainers in clinical settings has grown substantially. According to the National Athletic Trainers' Association (NATA),[1] approximately 24% of certified athletic trainers employed in the United States work in the clinical setting. This percentage is higher than the percentages of athletic trainers that worked both in the university/collegiate setting (21%) and high school setting (16%) (Figure 7-1).

While some of the administrative and employment skills are the same regardless of employment setting, administrators who work in the clinical setting face challenges that are different from interscholastic and intercollegiate work settings. Administrators employed in these clinics must recognize and deal with these unique challenges to insure their staffs are providing comprehensive health care services to their patients.

THE ATHLETIC TRAINER IN THE CLINICAL SETTING

Athletic trainers often report to a supervisory athletic trainer, athletic director, or academic department

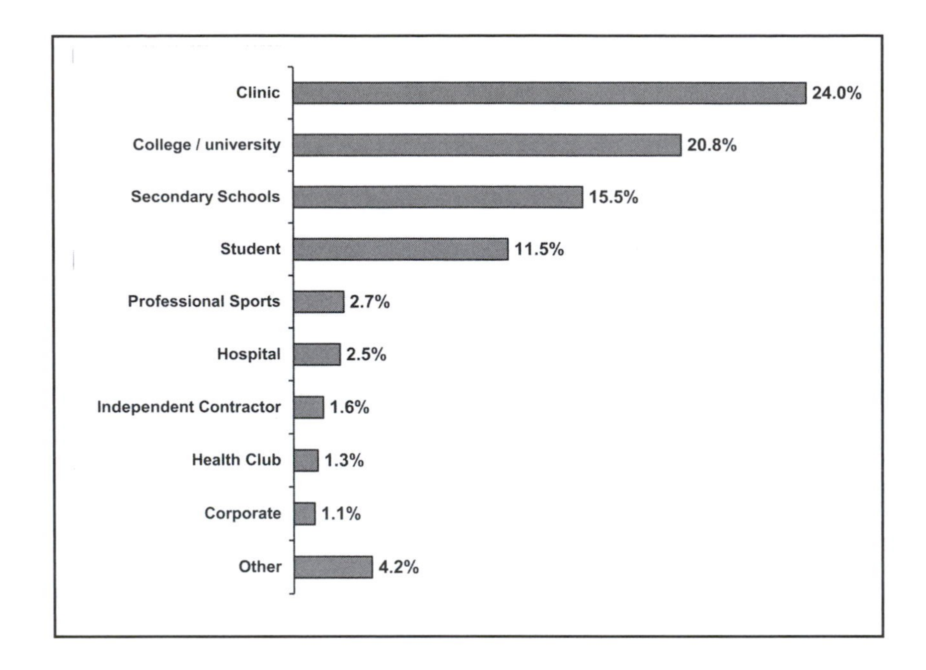

Figure 7-1. Percentage of NATA Certified members in various employment settings. (Source: NATA Site: http://www.nata.org/membership/MembStats/2007_1.htm)

chair in the interscholastic or intercollegiate setting. Their duties can include, providing comprehensive sports medical services to collegiate athletes, instructing athletic training undergraduate and graduate students, developing and maintaining a research program, and taking part in professional or scholarly activities. The educational qualifications for athletic trainers in these roles often include a master's degree and occasionally a doctorate degree in a field related to sports medicine. In addition to NATA-Board of Certification (BOC) certification, a record of prior college level instruction, athletic team care, and supervision of athletic training students is often mandatory. Athletic trainers employed in these setting are expected to work many evening and weekend hours.

In contrast, athletic trainers in the clinical setting often report to a supervisory athletic trainer, clinic manager, or vice president. Their duties often include seeing patients across the age spectrum as a physician extender and in the rehabilitation department alongside physical therapists. In addition, many athletic trainers provide high school and athletic event coverage, as well as design supervision performance enhancement programs for athletes who take part in a variety of athletic activities. Unlike the collegiate settings, clinical positions rarely require a master's or doctorate degree. In addition to NATA-BOC certification, other certifications such as the certified strength and conditioning specialist are desired. Experience working with diverse patient/athlete populations is a plus. Athletic trainers employed in the clinical settings usually have hours similar to other health care providers such as physical therapists, occupational therapists, nurse practitioners, and physician assistants (8:00 am to 5:00 pm Monday through Friday), but they will work evening and weekend hours if they provide outreach services.

ORGANIZATIONAL SKILLS AND ATTRIBUTES

Successful clinic administrators possess organizational skills, attributes, and qualities that help insure the success of their program. A short list of these skills and attributes should include the following:

- Interacting with various medical and administrative personnel (especially those who have little, if any, knowledge of the education, training, and credentials of athletic trainers)
- Negotiating and maintaining contracts
- Dealing with multiple and often competing interests inside and outside the clinic
- Fully understanding the various roles (see below) clinical athletic trainers perform
- Placing personnel with various attributes in the roles that best fit their skill set
- Recognizing and taking advantage of marketing/promotional opportunities

ATHLETIC TRAINING ROLES IN THE CLINICAL SETTING

PHYSICIAN EXTENDERS

One primary role of athletic trainers in the clinical setting is that of physician extender. An athletic trainer in this role utilizes the skills he or she normally uses to work with athletes and applies them to patients seen by physicians in a clinical setting. There are several advantages to employing athletic trainers in this role. First, providing services as a physician extender can provide opportunities for reimbursement. Second, the quality of the medical visit can be enhanced by improving services provided by the physician, including additional knowledge to the physician regarding treatment options and facilitating communication between the patient and physician to insure satisfactory patient outcomes. Finally, the efficiency of the clinic practice can be enhanced.

A recent study[2] reported that athletic trainers employed in an orthopedic sports medicine facility enhanced the overall productivity of the clinic significantly. The athletic trainers spend an average of 25 minutes with each patient performing various physician extender duties. As a result, orthopedists who utilized athletic trainers increased their productivity by 15% to 30%. Primary care physicians who utilized athletic trainers increased their productivity 10% to 20%. The author concluded that the time the athletic trainers spent with the patients enabled the physicians to spend more time with each patient and still see more patients during the normal clinic day. The following are some common tasks an athletic trainer performs in the physician extender role:

- Prior to being examined by the physician:
  - Triage the patient (over the phone) to make sure this is an appropriate referral (a patient who is best served by the medical providers)
  - Room the patient and update medical records for current medication list and drug allergies
  - Obtain a thorough medical history from the patient and perform an initial injury evaluation
  - Screen the patient and order diagnostic tests such as x-rays that will facilitate the initial physician evaluation
- During the physician examination:
  - Document the findings of the physician examination (This documentation will be crucial for dictating the finished provider note for this visit)
  - Assist the physician in the interpretation of diagnostic tests such as x-rays
  - Assist with wound treatment and removal of sutures or wound care following surgery
  - Prepare the patient (clean the area to be injected) for administration of injections
  - Complete paperwork to schedule surgeries or follow-up appointments
  - Provide suggestions for treatment (appropriate rehabilitation, padding or bracing) while the patient is evaluated by the physician
  - Complete workers compensation claims. Give copies of the provider forms to the patient and any case manager present during the exam
- After the physician visit
  - Fit appropriate, noncustom orthotics, braces or casts as ordered by the physician
  - Write referrals for rehabilitative services (this is a good time to explain the benefits of appropriate rehabilitative techniques) and provide the patient with a list of qualified providers in his or her geographic or provider area
  - Answer additional questions from the patient
  - Assist in scheduling follow-up appointments for further physician visits or other diagnostic tests such as magnetic resonance or electromyography
  - Dictate the patient examination note and ask the patient if he or she wants copies sent to his or her primary care provider, the referring physician, or his or her home address
  - Make sure appropriate billing paperwork has been completed and filed (see Chapter 8 for details on appropriate documentation)
  - Be available to answer follow-up questions by the patient after he or she leaves the clinic

An important component in developing an athletic trainers as physician extenders program is to develop a strong working relationship with the physicians in the practice. It is crucial that both parties work together to define the role and the specific duties that the athletic trainer will have in their practice. The duties and responsibilities of the athletic trainer may vary depending on the needs of the MD and experience, qualifications, and certifications of the athletic trainer.

Once these roles and responsibilities have been established, the athletic trainer needs to work with the clinic or hospital billing staff to discuss billing options for these services. Opportunities for reimbursement will be enhanced if the athletic trainer utilizes documentation and reimbursement materials provided by the NATA. In addition, it is wise for the billing department to contact insurance providers and consult other clinics and hospitals that are already successfully billing for these duties (see Chapter 9 for more information on billing and reimbursement).

Case Study 7-1

Facilitating Patient Care

Case. Robin is the athletic training coordinator at Anytown Sports Medicine Clinic. One of his clinic duties is to facilitate care for new patients who seek treatment for their sports injuries. Early one morning, Robin receives a call from a staff athletic trainer notifying him that one of his football players sprained his knee last night and was seen in a local urgent care facility. Today the player's parents called the athletic trainer to see if he could be seen by one of the sports medicine physicians at Anytown Sports Medicine Clinic as soon as possible.

Robin calls and speaks with the player's mother to confirm she wants her son seen at Anytown Sports Medicine Clinic today if possible. During the conversation, he obtains and confirms the player's information (name, birthdate, insurance carrier) from the mother to schedule the appointment. After talking with the mother, Robin looks for openings in the schedules of the physicians seeing patients that day and contacts the clinic schedulers to add the player to be seen that day. Once the appointment is confirmed, Robin calls the mother back to let her know the time the appointment is scheduled. During the call, Robin also reminds the mother to bring along copies of the x-rays taken at the urgent care facility, have information available regarding their insurance carrier, and confirms they know the directions to the clinic.

Once the patient arrives at the clinic, Robin puts the patient in an exam room, obtains the medical history, and examines the x-rays the patient brought. If needed, Robin orders additional x-rays that will assist the clinical decision making of the physician. During the MD examination, the clinical findings indicate a ligament and meniscus tear is suspected. As a result, Robin contacts the radiology department to schedule a magnetic resonance exam later the following day with a follow-up appointment with the physician scheduled after the exam. Before they leave the clinic, Robin instructs the patient on the proper use of crutches and a knee immobilizer. Robin also spends time with the patient and his parents, answering their questions about the tentative diagnosis, treatment options, and long-term prognosis. Robin talks to the patient and his family before they leave the clinic to confirm the follow-up appointments for the magnetic resonance exam and physician visit.

After the patient and family have left the clinic, Robin dictates the clinic provider note detailing the result of the physician examination with a copy sent to the patient's primary care provider. Robin also calls the referring staff athletic trainer to make him aware of the tentative diagnosis and treatment plan.

Outreach Providers

Providing athletic training outreach services is a primary role for many athletic trainers employed in the clinical setting. It is well recognized that certified athletic trainers provide an effective method to help insure the safety of high school athletes. The American Medical Association[3] has stated that certified athletic trainers should be used as part of a high school's medical team. The American Academy of Family Physicians[4] agrees and states on its Web site, "...the AAFP encourages high schools to have, whenever possible, a BOC certified or registered/licensed athletic trainer as an integral part of the high school athletic program."

Most services are provided to high schools and middle schools. Less common are outreach services provided directly to athletic leagues. The benefit to these programs is that they allow athletes from schools and organizations to access excellent sports medicine care without incurring the complete expense of employing an athletic trainer full time.

In many cases, the athletic trainer will travel to an area high school in the afternoon and evening to provide medical coverage for practices and games. During the mornings or off season, these athletic trainers perform other clinical duties such as serving as a physician extender or in a rehabilitation setting within the clinic.

Athletic Training Outreach Program: Sample Mission Statement

The mission of the (ANYTOWN SPORTS MEDICINE CLINIC) Athletic Training Outreach Program is to serve as a sports medicine resource and to provide athletic training services to communities throughout the state. Resource services include education on the prevention, recognition, acute care, and rehabilitation of sports injuries, as well as assistance in obtaining referrals to appropriate specialists. Sports medicine services include providing support activities and athletic training coverage for selected area high schools, colleges, and community sporting events. The primary service areas are youth sports, interscholastic athletics, intercollegiate athletics, recreational athletics, and competitive adult athletics.

Purpose of the Athletic Training Service

- The provision of health care services to area high school, collegiate, and recreational athletes
  - Provide primary evaluation of injuries to athletes.
  - Provide expertise on appropriate treatment and rehabilitation programs.
  - Provide emergency medical coverage of athletic events.
  - Insist on physician intervention when necessary.
- To decrease liability concerns of school administrators and coaches
  - Serve as a consultation service for area high school and collegiate sports coaches on athletic training.
  - Educate coaches, parents, and athletes on methods of injury prevention, injury recognition, and initial care of injuries.
  - Educate and instruct athletes on appropriate methods of enhancing skill performance and decreasing injury susceptibility.
  - Accept responsibility for determining return to play criteria for injured athletes in conjunction with the attending physician.
- Promotion of the presence of the (ANYTOWN SPORTS MEDICINE CLINIC)
  - Publicize the presence of (ANYTOWN SPORTS MEDICINE CLINIC) to (YOUR COMMUNITY) and surrounding counties.
  - Furnish speakers for sports medicine topics as requested by the local sports community.
  - Provide medical coverage for athletic events at the request of local schools, colleges, or organizations.
  - Provide medical services to disadvantaged populations.
- Aggressively promote the expertise of (ANYTOWN SPORTS MEDICINE CLINIC) physician staff for the treatment of sports-related injuries.

It is preferable that there should be an athletic trainer available to student athletes at the school on a daily basis. However, in small schools in rural settings, the school may not be able to afford daily athletic trainer services. In these cases, schools often contract with sports medicine clinics to have athletic trainers visit their school on a 2 to 3 times per week basis, regardless of the services performed.

It is crucial that athletic training outreach services are only provided after a valid contract that describes specific duties and responsibilities for both parties has been signed by the clinic and the school/institution/organization. A set of sample athletic training outreach contracts are provided in Appendix B.

Reimbursement for outreach services is primarily derived from contracts to school/organizations. In some cases, indirect revenues can be calculated based on the referrals to providers who offer treatment and diagnostic and rehabilitative services within the health care system.

Primary duties of outreach athletic trainers include but are not limited to the following:

- Refer injured athletes to other medical providers. When a physician referral is necessary, try to assist in coordinating the initial visit within a reasonable amount of time.
- Facilitate rehabilitation and reconditioning in treatment plans. Often this requires contact with a staff physical therapist to insure the best results.
- Coordinate the care of the medical staff when dealing with injured athletes.
- Determine an athlete's readiness to return to participation. Athletic trainers should include the athlete, parents, and coaches in this decision.

The Danger of Not Having a Signed Contract

In some cases, administrators may be tempted to have their athletic training staff members provide outreach services to individual schools without a valid contract. Administrators may do this in the mistaken belief that providing athletic training services without a valid contract or for "free" will provide them with positive public relations and goodwill in the community and/or schools being served. However, providing athletic training services without a contract is fraught with danger to the clinic as a whole and the athletic trainer as an individual.

Without a valid contract, both the clinic and school may assume the other party is responsible for providing critical emergency equipment such as an electronic defibrillator or less critical equipment such as crutches. A well-written contract should have specific language that outlines the hours of athletic training coverage. This protects the athletic trainer and the clinic if an athletic injury is treated by the school staff before or after the hours the athletic trainer is actually onsite.

- Maintain appropriate medical documents and records and make sure they are completed in an efficient and timely manner.
- Develop working relationships with the local MDs and other medical providers, even those outside your employment environment.
- Develop an action plan to deal with emergencies and respond immediately should an emergency occur.
- Work with the coaches to develop injury and illness prevention strategies.
- Provide appropriate nutritional information and refer athletes to registered dieticians when warranted.
- Promote safe practice and competition facilities. In addition, athletic trainers are encouraged to maintain appropriate equipment.
- Assist in the development of guidelines to deal with inclement weather.
- Assist with pre-season athlete physicals.
- Assist in the development of guidelines to deal with athletes with medical alerts and emergency medications such as bronchial inhalers and Epi-Pens (Dey, LP, Napa, CA).
- Supervise pre-season, in-season, and out-of-season conditioning programs.

Concerns of the Outreach Athletic Trainer

Schools and athletic organizations often find the services of outreach athletic trainers invaluable. As a result, administrators are tempted to contract their outreach athletic trainers to provide services 5 or even 6 days a week throughout the year. This can be especially true in a competitive marketplace (ie, a community or geographic area where multiple clinics and/or hospitals are offering similar athletic training outreach services). An administrator who agrees to provide extensive school or event coverage for little or no cost runs the risk of "burning out" their staff in a short period of time.

Quality administrators make sure that the athletic training staff is provided with the same rights as their other medical staff when performing clinical duties. In addition, they should not be asked to perform extensive "after hours" event coverage duties unless they are compensated over and above their normal salary. Successful sports medicine clinics often require schools/athletic organizations to pay an additional fee ($20 to $30 per hour) for athletic training outreach services provided after 6:00 pm on weekdays or for any coverage on weekends (see sample outreach contracts). These additional fees can be passed on to the outreach staff member providing these services. Outreach athletic trainers enjoy this arrangement because it allows them to be compensated for these "after hours" events and controls the extra amount of work and compensation they accrue.

Some additional rights of the outreach athletic trainers include the following:

- Access to a safe and healthy work environment outside their clinical setting.
- Adequate time to fulfill thorough and accurate patient documentation requirements.
- Prioritizing position description percentage as it relates to employment responsibilities such as clinical duties, athletic training outreach services, public relations events, or game coverage.

Rehabilitation Settings

Sports medicine clinics often utilize a team of physical therapists and athletic trainers to rehabilitate their patients following injury. Rehabilitation of athletic injuries requires the athletic trainers to possess skills that allow them to identify the injuries, control pain, restore range of motion, re-establish muscle strength and endurance, and regain neuromuscular control and proper balance. The same skills athletic trainers

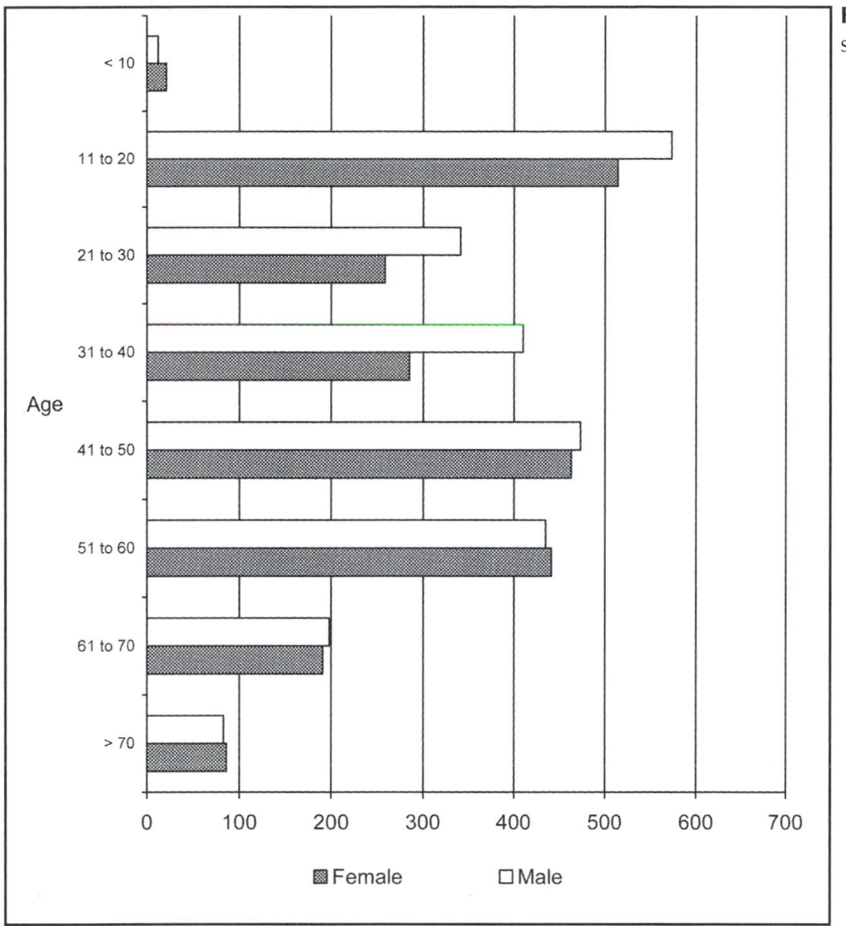

Figure 7-2. Age and sex of patients seen in a sports medicine clinic (1 year).

use to provide care to collegiate athletes provide them with unique perspectives that prove useful to patients during the treatment and rehabilitation process.

However, in the traditional collegiate athletic training setting, the characteristics (age, sport, physical fitness) of the patients are, with few exceptions, quite similar. In contrast, the patients seen by athletic trainers in a clinical setting came from a variety of age groups and often possess varied levels of pre-injury physical fitness. In addition, the athletes being treated may be trying to return to a much wider variety of sports and recreational and fitness activities than collegiate athletes. Figures 7-2 to 7-4 give insight into the wide range of patients, activities, and injuries seen in a hospital-based clinical sports medicine setting.

While both work settings require the athletic trainer to apply rehabilitative skills and use therapeutic modalities in a functional progression, athletic trainers in the clinical settings must be able to integrate practices with the specific age, fitness, and activity demands of a very diverse patient population. Administrators must realize that the majority of athletic trainers currently acquire experience in their undergraduate and graduate settings almost exclusively with collegiate students and athletes. Therefore, the skills necessary to effectively rehabilitate athletes treated in sports medicine clinics are acquired with actual work experience in the clinical setting. Administrators must also realize that reimbursement depends on their state and/or geographic location. Chapters 8 and 9 outline billing and documentation issues in detail.

Performance Enhancement

Many clinical sports medicine settings offer some form of performance enhancement programs for athletes and patients. Due to their extensive education, training, certifications, and licensure requirements, athletic trainers who work in performance enhancement can provide well-rounded programming that provides performance enhancement as one component of a total sports medicine care plan. In addition, many athletic trainers who work in this capacity are certified by the National Strength and Conditioning Association to obtain this certification. Candidates must pass a 4-hour examination to earn the certified strength and conditioning specialist (CSCS) credential. In addition, CSCS credential holders must complete 6 continuing education units within the 3-year reporting period.

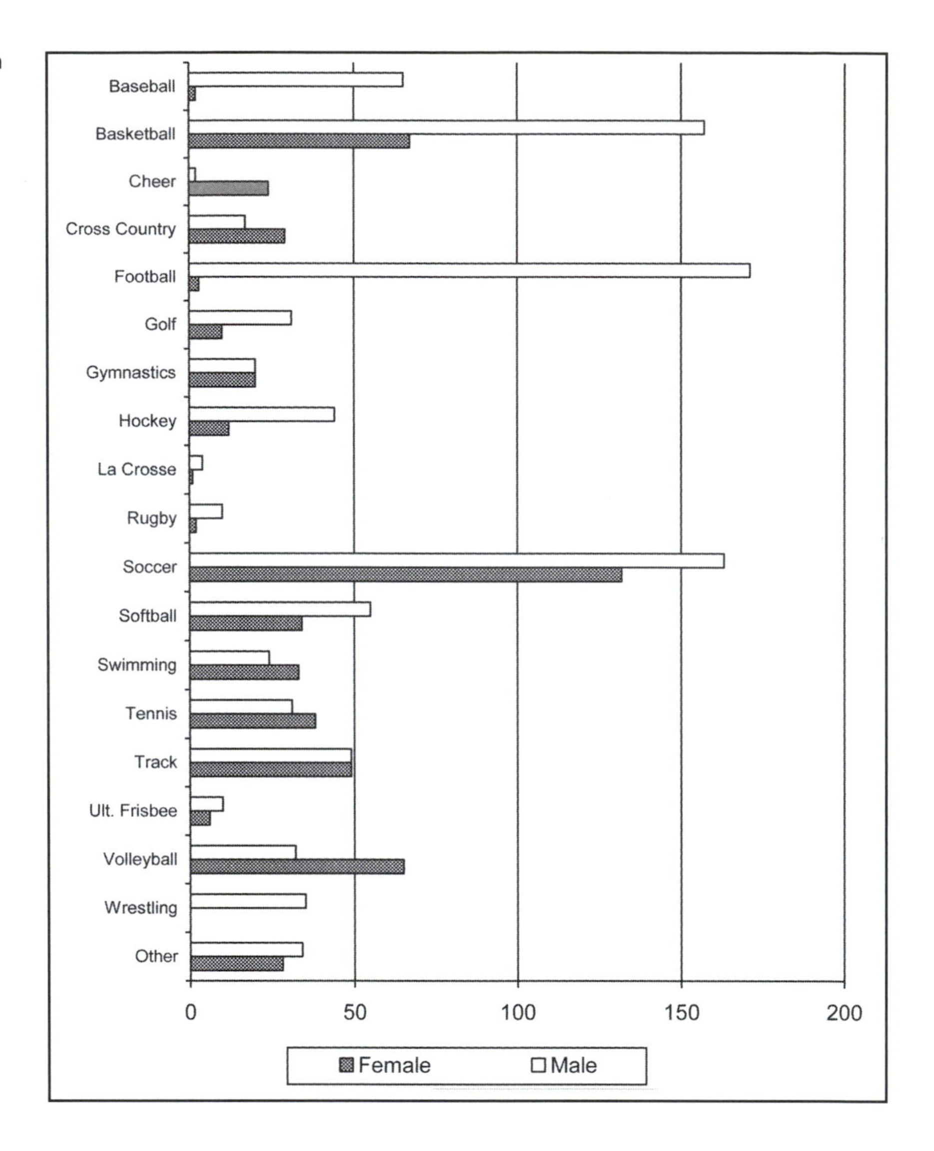

Figure 7-3. Sport/recreation activity when injured. Average age = 25.0 ± 13.5 yrs.

Performance enhancement programs are often designed to provide athletes of various ages and abilities an opportunity to take their performance to the next level through training plans customized specifically for their needs. Athletic trainers can provide programming on a daily or seasonal basis. One advantage to clinic-based sports performance programs is that they can provide their clients with easy access to other sports medicine professionals (such as physicians, physical therapists, dietitians, and exercise scientists). This type of access may not be available to individuals who enroll in classes/programs offered by self-employed strength/performance coaches.

Staff who work in these settings need to possess a thorough understanding of how to instruct individuals or teams to develop athletic skills needed for maximum athletic achievement while emphasizing techniques that decrease the risk of sports injuries. In addition, they must be able to recognize the different needs of clients participating in youth, high school, collegiate, elite, and master's level sports and activities.

The Athletic Trainer as Researcher in the Clinical Setting

Ongoing research is necessary for the athletic training profession to continue to evolve and grow. It is well recognized that the quantity of research produced by athletic trainers has grown considerably during the past 20 years. Most of this research, however, has been conducted by athletic trainers in the traditional collegiate laboratory setting or while interacting with collegiate athletic teams in practices and competitions. As a result, the athletes utilized as research subjects represent a very narrow demographic (college-aged [19 to 23 years old], healthy males and females) that do not represent athletes or active individuals who are high school, middle, or advanced ages. It is not clear, therefore, if the findings of research gained in the collegiate laboratory or on the collegiate athletic fields are always applicable to other active populations in noncollegiate settings.

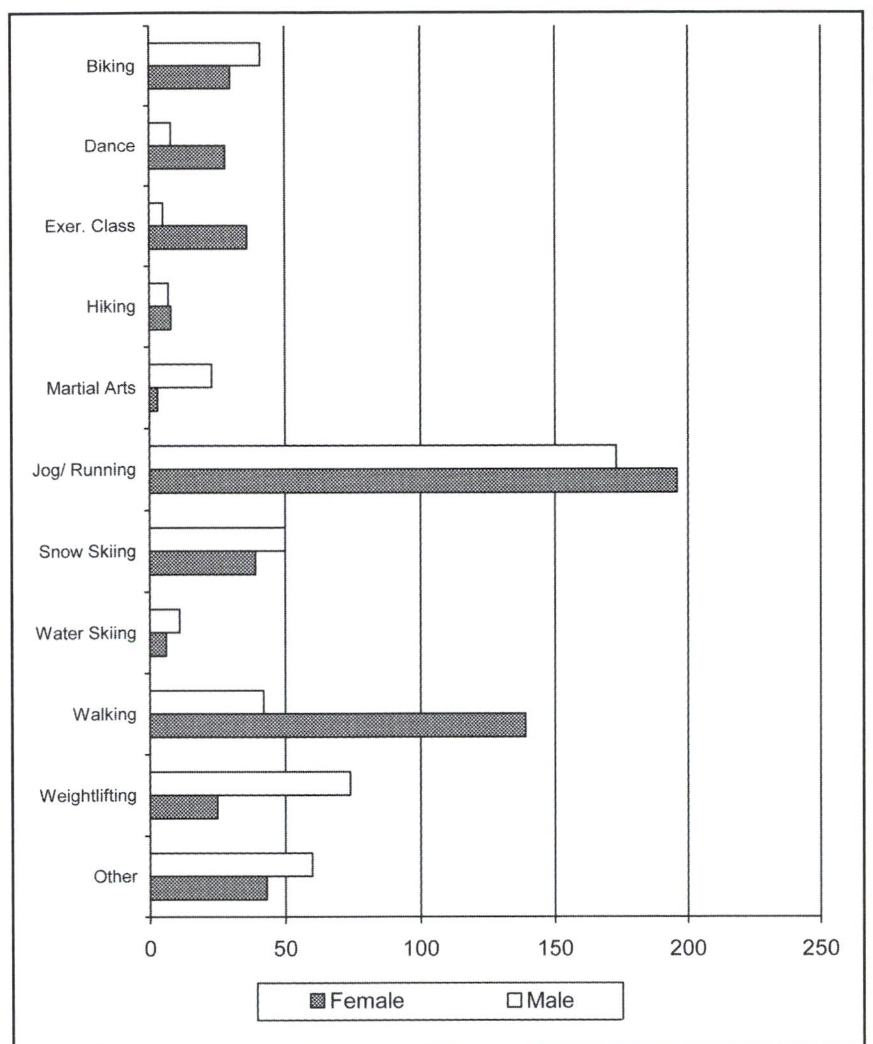

Figure 7-4. Fitness/exercise activity when injured for patients treated in sports medicine clinic. Average age = 40.1 ± 15.9 yrs.

There are several advantages for athletic trainers who conduct research in a clinical setting. First, athletic trainer researchers in the clinical setting have access to a more diverse patient population than athletic trainers in the university/collegiate setting. As a result, they can utilize a wider variety of individuals as research subjects in clinical outcome and intervention research. Second, clinical athletic trainers often provide medical coverage for a wide variety of athletic events so they have access to a variety of field research opportunities that include but are not limited to studying youth and high school-aged athletes, recreational athletes, or master's level athletes. Access to these noncollegiate populations is often desired because they represent a much larger number of individuals who can benefit from injury prevention or injury treatment research.

One disadvantage to conducting research in the clinical setting is that clinic administrators often mandate that their staff take part in only activities that can directly enhance revenue generation for their clinic. As a result, these administrators are reluctant to allow time for interested athletic trainers to conduct clinical sports medicine research. Another drawback is that few sports medicine clinics can provide the necessary research infrastructure and oversight commonly found at mid and large level universities. This lack of research infrastructure may make it difficult for athletic trainer researchers to access grant funding or conduct collaborative research studies with other researchers in related fields. Table 7-1 presents a typical timeline for a clinic-based research project.

Athletic trainers who conduct research alone or as part of larger multi-site research efforts have duties similar to other researchers, including the following:

- Supervising or assisting with screening of potential study participants
- Recruiting and retaining participants
- Discussing research protocol with potential research subjects, including potential risks and benefits
- Collecting data on study participants

Table 7-1

Procedures and Timeline for Starting a Clinic-Based Research Project

Date	Procedures
Oct 2008	Come up with a clinically relevant research question.
Nov to Dec 2008	Meet with other interested clinicians to discuss collaboration, identify clinic and staff resources, identify funding sources, and conduct a literature review. Meet with a biostatistician to discuss the research plan, obtain sample size estimates, and determine randomization procedures (if any). Write the initial research protocol.
Jan 2009	Submit the research grant applications to various funding agencies. Meet with hospital/clinic, academic, and secondary school administrators to discuss the study and obtain letters of support. Submit a review application to the Institutional Review Boards (IRBs) for Human Subjects. Often, IRB reviews may be required from the academic (college/university), clinic (hospital/clinic), and secondary school (school district) research committees.
March to June 2009	Revise and resubmit the research protocol to address concerns from the IRBs and funding agencies. Note: Special attention must be provided at this stage to work out compromises to meet the needs of multiple funding agencies and IRBs. Obtain final IRB approvals.
July 2009	Initial grant funds released by the funding agencies.
Aug 2009	Purchase research equipment, supplies, and subject incentives. Produce and distribute subject recruitment brochures and posters. Meet with clinic and school staff to discuss the research protocol. Provide subject inclusion/exclusion criteria and train them on subject recruitment and data collection procedures.
Sept 2009	Begin to enroll subjects.

- Following all required study procedures and protocol follow-up
- Assisting with the research data analysis and interpretation

MARKETING AND PUBLIC RELATIONS

Marketing services is a goal for athletic trainers in the clinical setting. Unlike their collegiate counterparts, athletic trainers in the clinical setting need to make various entities aware that an athletic trainer is available and the types of services they provide. There are 3 primary objectives for this type of marketing. The first objective is to make administrators, school officials, parents, civic groups, and sports associations aware of the services athletic trainers provide as a health care professional. The second objective is to make these same individuals aware that Anytown Sports Medicine Clinic can provide the needed services. The third objective is that the athletic trainers in Anytown Sports Medicine Clinic can provide these services on an efficient and cost-effective basis.

Nearly all hospitals and large multi-specialty clinics employ a public relations/marketing staff. Athletic trainers can utilize these professionals to help promote the athletic training services of the clinic. In addition, these staff may contact the athletic trainers to provide comments with regards to a news event. The public relations staff will then coordinate an interview with the athletic trainer and the media for broadcast.

On the other hand, if the clinic is small, the athletic trainer will not have the benefit of working with full-time marketing professionals. Athletic trainers in these smaller settings will need to develop their own marketing and public relations strategies and initiatives. While the marketing objectives remain the same, the methods used to get the marketing messages to interested stakeholders fall to the athletic trainer. This can be quite problematic unless the athletic trainers initiate media and public contacts on their own. These contacts can be established in a variety of ways, including:

- Introducing yourself to media personnel covering school and community athletic events
- Public speaking at school, booster/parent, or coaching organizations. Athletic trainers should also expand their target audience and ask to speak to local civic organizations that do not deal directly with athletes or sports medicine.
- Writing newspaper columns. Newspapers, especially those with smaller circulations, usually welcome advice/informational columns from many individuals. Athletic trainers can provide advice and information on a wide range of issues from sports nutrition to injury recognition and prevention. When possible, the column should be accompanied by a photo of the contributor and the clinic logo.
- Offering to provide interviews or commentary on talk radio programming
- Offering to provide television interviews

In addition, athletic trainers in the clinical setting need to realize that most if not all media welcome the opportunity to provide a local angle to a national sports medicine story. Interviewing "a local sports medicine expert" allows local media to provide greater depth and context to these stories. Using events in the national, regional, and local news is a very effective method to let people know what services certified athletic trainers perform in their clinic.

Contacting the Media to Market Your Expertise

Do not be afraid to reach out. Athletic trainers should also contact their media outlets when a significant event or situation occurs, but the importance is unrecognized by the local media. One example of effective use of a local event follows. During the second week of August, just as the preseason practices began for high school football players, the weather changed significantly to an extended period of high heat and humidity. One of the athletic trainers from the local sports medicine clinic contacted several television outlets and reminded them this would be a good time to do stories for their viewers reminding them of the danger heat injury posed and provide strategies high school athletes could use to prevent heat illness and injury. Within an hour, one of the local TV stations contacted the athletic trainer and immediately set up a live broadcast with the athletic trainer at the area school during the local news hour. The athletic trainer provided information that parents/coaches could use to recognize signs of heat illness. More importantly, however, the athletic trainer was able to provide tips for preventing injuries that included the necessity for fluid replacement, sound nutrition, and rest. At the end of the interview, viewers were encouraged to call the athletic trainer if they had any questions relating to the topic of heat injuries.

Other Clinic-Based Programming Initiatives

Special event programming is an effective method to make the public aware of the services and expertise of an athletic trainer and provide services that coincide with the mission (providing medical service, educating the public, etc) of the clinic. An example of a typical sports medicine clinic mission is found in Appendix B. Some examples of effective clinical programming include health fairs; sports physicals; and educational programs for parents, coaches, and athletes. When clinicians carry out programming, they need to make sure they contact all of the local media to make them aware of the event and cover it with an interview or story if they have time.

Health Fairs

Health fairs can be sponsored by corporate, educational, governmental, or community groups or health care providers and can be open to employees or the public in general. Athletic trainers can educate the public and increase the awareness of their work roles by providing services that include the following:

- Screening attendees for a variety of conditions that include blood pressure, body composition (% fat), and upper/lower extremity flexibility
- Handing out literature on injuries, medical conditions, performance enhancement, and preventing injuries
- Speaking with attendees one-on-one to address specific questions they have regarding their injuries
- Answering questions regarding appropriate injury prevention, treatment, or rehabilitation techniques

Sport Pre-Participation Physicals

Athletic trainers can play an important role in conducting pre-participation athletic physical exams, often called a "sports physical." In general, these physicals do not have the same benefits as a physical exam

Using the Media to Spread the Word

Media outlets (television, radio, newspapers) often cover the same stories within the same limited timeframe. Athletic trainers also need to remember that stories covered by one media source may be duplicated by other sources as well. These media outlets are constantly looking for stories, especially those with a local flavor.

As an example, look at the situation that occurred when a marathon was scheduled for the first time in a community. A month prior to the marathon, a local newspaper asked one of the athletic trainers at a local sports medicine clinic if he could write a column that would provide information that marathoners could use to help them recover in the days/weeks after the race. Even though he indicated he was not an expert in this area, the athletic trainer reluctantly agreed to gather research and talk to experts to put the column together. One week before the marathon, the column appeared in the local newspaper. The next day, a local television producer read the story and requested the AT to do a live broadcast reiterating similar information for their television audience. Finally, the day before the marathon, a radio reporter saw the television broadcast and set up a radio interview with the AT that discussed the same information (how to recover from a marathon) as the newspaper column and television broadcast. The radio station interviewed the AT and sound bites from this interview were played on the day of and immediately after the race.

conducted by the athlete's pediatrician. However, they are convenient, with many schools bringing physicians and other health professionals to the school to do the exams. The athletic trainer in the clinical setting can play an important role in these exams by screening the athletes for conditions not normally covered in the physician exam such as orthopedic screenings. These screenings can include the following:

- Recording the athlete's history of previous serious athletic injuries such as concussions, fractures, or severe sprains/strains
- Measuring
  - Joint range of motion
  - Ligament laxity
  - Upper and lower body flexibility
  - Body composition (% fat)

Another effective variation of this type of program is to have the clinic offer free sport physicals for low income athletes with low or no insurance coverage (See sidebar on p. 127 detailing the clinic mission statement).

Educational Programs

A very effective method of programming consists of providing educational seminars, conferences, meetings, and in-services for athletes, coaches, parents, and exercise enthusiasts. These type of educational programs often last 2 to 4 hours and are conducted in the evening or weekend. To be successful, these programs should target a specific audience and focus on a specific topic. The conference planners also need to realize that they need to involve the media to help spread the word that a specific program is being offered. Media personnel should be contacted early once the date, topics, and speakers have been identified. In addition to enhancing program enrollment, stories in the media will make the public who did not attend the program aware of the types of services/skills provided by the clinic personnel.

SUMMARY

- Understand the differences between the education and training for employment in the traditional collegiate and clinical settings.

  While some duties are similar for athletic trainers in the traditional and clinical settings, there are significant differences in the work environment and patient demographics in these two settings.
- Explain the rationale for employing athletic trainers in the clinical setting.

  Athletic trainers can fill a unique role in enhancing the quality of health care provided to individuals seen in sports medicine clinics. Athletic trainers employed in clinics often have specific duties for working as a physician extender, an outreach provider, a rehabilitation specialist, or in performance enhancement.
- Understand the importance of marketing and public relations and describe common techniques utilized in clinical settings to market their services.

  Clinicians must understand the importance of an effective public relations marketing plan. This plan should include active solicitation of the print, radio, and television media to make them aware of the services provided by the clinic.
- Identify programming initiatives.

  There are several effective programming techniques such as health fairs, sports physicals, and education programs that can enhance the perception of the services provided by athletic trainers in the clinical setting.

- Describe the advantages and disadvantages of conducting research in the clinical setting.

  Conducting sports medicine research in the clinical setting allows researchers to access research subjects not commonly represented in traditional sports medicine research. However, conducting this research may be more difficult than performing research in the traditional collegiate setting.

- Summarize contract language necessary to provide athletic training outreach services to schools, institutions, and organizations.

  All outreach services can only be provided after a specific contract has been signed by the school/institution/organization and the sports medicine clinic.

- Summarize the position description for a typical clinical/outreach setting.

  All outreach services can only be provided after a specific contract has been signed by the school/institution/organization and the sports medicine clinic.

ACTIVITIES

The following activities can be used to generate discussion among students and instructors. These cases are based on actual scenarios derived from the clinical employment setting.

Case Studies

Case Study 1: Athletic Training Outreach Coverage

Robert is an administrator at the Anytown Sports Medicine Clinic and also serves as a board member for the local Anytown Youth Soccer League. The soccer league has an upcoming youth soccer tournament with 32 teams scheduled to take place the next Sunday at the Anytown recreation facility. The Anytown Youth Soccer League relies on dozens of volunteers to run the tournament and uses the money raised on this day to fund the league for the rest of the year.

Robert has agreed to volunteer the members of the athletic training staff at the Anytown Sports Medicine Clinic to cover all of the tournament games throughout the day and waive the usual fees associated with covering weekend athletic events. As a result, the athletic training staff members will not be paid directly for their work. Instead Robert has offered each staff member "comp time" for the hours that staff members can use during a regular work week later in the year. (Note: "Comp time" is short for compensatory time. This is overtime that an employee is not paid for but may be able to use in place of vacation days in the future. It can be easily abused by both management and staff if not well documented.)

Several athletic training staff members have discussed covering the event among themselves and have some concerns. They feel that it is not fair to have area high schools pay for the athletic training outreach services of the Anytown Sports Medicine Clinic and allow the Anytown Youth Soccer League to receive the same services for free. In addition, the staff is concerned that they are being forced to volunteer to work this Sunday and do not feel providing "comp time" justifies the time away from their families.

Discussion Questions

- Is it acceptable for the Anytown Sports Medicine Clinic to charge fees to some schools or organizations for athletic training outreach services and not charge fees to other schools or organizations?
- Should the athletic training staff be required to "volunteer" to work the tournament?
- How should individuals of the athletic training staff approach Robert with their concerns?
- Is "comp time later this year" an equitable payment to the athletic trainers who work the tournament?

Case Study 2: Duties in Conflict—When Clinic and School Duties Collide

Cindy works as an athletic trainer at the Anytown Sports Medicine Clinic. During the week, her duties include working as a physician extender until 2:00 pm then traveling to Anytown High School at 3:00 pm to provide athletic training outreach services.

On this day, the clinic is especially busy since there were several patients over-booked on the schedule. In addition, a nursing staff member went home sick. As a result, the physician and staff are seeing patients 1 to 1.5 hours behind schedule. As Cindy prepares to finish her clinic work and head for the school, the physician approaches her and states that "she needs to stay in clinic to help out for a few more hours."

Cindy is concerned because she knows that several coaches and athletes expect her to be at the training room by 3:00 pm for treatments. In addition, the contract between the clinic and the school states that the athletic trainer must be at the school by 3:00 pm each day.

Discussion Questions

- What should Cindy do in this situation?
- How should Cindy deal with the physician making this request?
- If she stays and works in the clinic, should Cindy be responsible for contacting the athletic director and telling him she will not be at school on time?

REFERENCES

1. National Athletic Trainers Association. January 2007 NATA Total Membership by Job Setting. Available at http://www.nata.org/membership/MembStats/2007_1.htm. Accessed February 11, 2007.
2. Greene J. Athletic Trainers in an orthopaedic practice. *Athletic Therapy Today.* 2004;9(5):55.
3. American Medical Association. Certified athletic trainers in secondary schools (Resolution 431, A-97). Available at http://www.nata.org/statements/index.htm. Accessed October 10, 2006.
4. American Academy of Family Physicians. Athletic trainers for high school athletes. Available at http://www.aafp.org/online/en/home/policy/policies/sports.html. Accessed October 9, 2006.

Chapter 8

MEDICAL RECORDS AND DOCUMENTATION

Jill H. Murphy, MPT, LAT, ATC, CSCS

OBJECTIVES

At the end of this chapter, the reader will be able to:

- Identify the contents of the medical record
- Understand the implications of the Health Insurance Portability and Accountability Act (HIPAA) and explain the importance of maintaining patient confidentiality.
- Recall the purposes of documentation
- Summarize the standards of practice related to documentation in the athletic training field
- Compose the subjective, objective, assessment, and plan of care components of an initial evaluation
- Write specific impairment-related, functional, and measurable goals for a variety of patient diagnoses
- Explain how to avoid common documentation errors in the initial evaluation and daily and progress notes
- Demonstrate the ability to document evidence of skilled feedback when providing therapeutic exercise
- Summarize the importance of frequent reassessments of each patient's functional status using quantifiable tests and measures to demonstrate progress toward specific goals

From the professional athletics setting to the high school athletic training room, the importance of the medical record and the appropriate documentation it contains cannot be overemphasized. No matter the specific setting of practice, whether billing a third party or simply providing in-house athletic training services, without a thorough and detailed record of what problems are found, what the plan will be, what was done to address the problems, and the outcome of the interventions, there is no ability to communicate with other health professionals throughout the course of the patient's care, diminishing continuity of care and impacting the potential effectiveness of any future interventions throughout a patient's lifetime. Society has become increasingly dependent on technology for maintenance of medical records; however, the demand for immediate access for all potential health care providers to a patient's complete medical record must be balanced with fully effective security measures to maintain the confidentiality and privacy of the patient and his or her medical record. The administrative demands of athletic training record keeping have moved far beyond simply maintaining a medical record on each athlete; the information and organization system utilized within the medical record is a high priority for the athletic trainer. The health care provider must develop an exceptional ability to document in a way that effectively meets the needs of the patient, treating provider, referring provider, employer, insurance or other third-party provider, and potential legal and liability interests spanning a time frame from initial date of service delivery throughout the lifetime of the patient and beyond.

This chapter explains the role and importance of documentation in the medical record, as well as provides the necessary tools for documenting according to the standards of practice within the athletic training profession. The necessity of confidentiality and the implications of HIPAA for athletic trainers across a variety of settings will also be addressed.

MEDICAL RECORDS

The medical record contains all of the information about the patient's history, current problems, and interventions utilized to address those problems, as well as a documented record of any other forms of communication exchanged related to the patient's care, along with billing records and ICD-9 coding and physician orders that complete the medical record for each date of service. This medical record may be written or entered in a database through a variety of available software applications. The advantages of the electronic medical record are many, from easy, immediate access for all care providers, reduction of paper waste, legibility and clarity of documentation, and real-time availability of adjunct reports such as imaging and test results. In 1993, President Bill Clinton began calling for widespread use of a national electronic database of health care records by year 2014. In response to this call, membership for the American Health Information Community, National Provider Identity Numbers, e-signing and e-prescribing, and many other initiatives have begun to address the issues involved with this far-reaching goal, including protecting the security and privacy of such information.

PROTECTING PATIENT PRIVACY

CONFIDENTIALITY

As portability of and access to medical records improves, the most critical hazard is the potential for inappropriate use of confidential medical records. This presents a renewed challenge to health care providers to strictly maintain the privacy of patients' records not just for the paper medical and billing records but also for secured digital systems.

HISTORY OF HIPAA

In 1996, HIPAA was signed into law, and the finalized, modified federal privacy standards went into effect on April 14, 2003. The HIPAA guidelines create a standard for privacy protection of health information for health care providers, health plans, and health clearinghouses that maintain and transmit medical records in an electronic format. Because this electronic format included electronic billing, most health care providers were affected by this legislation. The only health care providers not included are those who do not electronically bill for services, which may exempt some collegiate and professional athletic trainers from falling under this law. Some high school providers may also be excluded from HIPAA regulations because they are covered by the privacy provisions of the Family Education Rights and Privacy Act (FERPA), which governs educational records in elementary, middle, and secondary schools. Many athletic trainers are part of a "hybrid entity," meaning they are employed by a facility that is subject to HIPAA guidelines but are employees who work in a noncovered setting such as a high school. Employers may require "hybrid entity" employees to follow the HIPAA privacy guidelines even though it is not required depending on the opinion of legal advisors. Athletic trainers in traditionally noncovered entity collegiate and professional settings may choose to follow the privacy guidelines of HIPAA in an effort to better protect the privacy of the athletes they serve. Newly hired athletic trainers are encouraged to investigate whether their employer is a covered entity under HIPAA, whether any additional, stricter state privacy regulations apply, and whether their employer has policies in existence to protect private health care information in their particular setting.

HIPAA IN PRACTICE

HIPAA privacy standards do not require covered entities to receive a patient's written consent before disclosing private health information for the purposes of treatment, billing, and other routine health care operations, such as audits, case management, and utilization reviews. Other important HIPAA guidelines include the following:

- Protected health information includes both personal health information and individually identifiable health information; past and present information that falls in these categories is protected under HIPAA.
- Each organization must designate a privacy officer to ensure that HIPAA privacy policies and procedures are being followed.
- Patients are provided authorizations before any health information is released from one entity to another. This includes the disclosure of any health information on a specific athlete to a coach. Once an authorization is signed, this information can be released as needed

depending on the wording of the specific authorization. For example, most authorizations in a high school and collegiate setting will authorize the disclosure of information to protect the health and safety of the athlete, indicating disclosure is allowed to coaches and game officials such as referees but not to the media.

- If an athlete or patient refuses to sign an authorization, treatment cannot be denied. However, in a collegiate setting, a signed authorization to release private health information can be a prerequisite to participation in the athletic program.
- Patients have the right to request their medical records; they may be required to make the request in writing and pay a small copy fee.
- Patients are provided a notice about privacy practices from each health entity they visit; the notice includes such information as a clear explanation of how their health information may be disclosed, their right to limit the disclosure of their information, and their right to request an accounting of how their health information was used.
- Information left on a patient's voicemail should be generic and kept to a minimum to not disclose details of the patient's diagnosis and/or treatment.
- Patients may request that only a certain phone number or address be utilized as contact information.
- Patients should be given the option of a private treatment area to keep conversations with patients and health care providers as private as possible.
- Medical files and schedules should not be left face up with patient identifying information visible to other patients in any health care setting.
- Covered entities must ensure that the disclosure of health information is completed to the minimum amount necessary to accomplish the intended purpose. Access to a patient's medical information is allowed only to those who need to know. An internal monitoring system is encouraged to be certain this rule is being followed.
- Covered entities are required to obtain the patient's written authorization to use or disclose information for research purposes. Such information is typically encoded to disguise the actual identity of the patient in the study.
- Patient information utilized for educational purposes must either be altered so that the actual patient cannot be identified in any way, or the patient may sign a release authorizing the specific use on a specific date and in a specific context for educational purposes. Examples of this might be a professor utilizing a patient's radiological scan for educational purposes or students who may attend a patient's surgery.

The Department of Health and Human Services also issued a Security Rule in 2005 creating a national standard to protect health information maintained or transmitted in electronic formats, including the internet, intranet, dial-up or leased lines, private networks, and any magnetic tape, disk, or compact disk media used to physically move data from one location to another. The Security Rule requires health plans to adopt a data security plan that is in writing with administrative, physical, and technical safeguards. Covered entities also must adopt "incident" reporting strategies, with no formal means specified by which internal incidents need to be reported to outside entities. Entities that have only paper records stored in filing cabinets are not covered entities.

HIPAA Penalties

There are serious penalties in place for violating HIPAA; the Privacy Rule is enforced by the Department of Health and Human Services Office of Civil Rights. A patient may file a complaint within 180 days of the violation (the time can be extended) with the Office of Civil Rights, and then the department investigates the claim and tries to resolve the issue informally. A person who violates HIPAA may be fined up to $25,000, or face up to 10 years in jail and a fine of $250,000 for serious offenses that involve a criminal investigation with the Department of Justice.

DOCUMENTATION FUNDAMENTALS

Effective documentation in any athletic training setting must thoroughly and adequately demonstrate the patient's need for skilled rehabilitation services by identifying and relating specific impairments to the patient's specific functional limitations. Impairments are losses or abnormalities of the musculoskeletal or other systems that are identified and measured by the clinician during the initial evaluation and in future reassessments; examples of impairments are range of motion deficits, weak muscles, edema, and muscle contractures. Functional limitations are restrictions or losses of ability to perform certain tasks that might ordinarily be expected as a result of a healthy organ or organ system; an example of functional limitation is the inability to or difficulty with walking, sleeping, jumping, prolonged sitting, or throwing. A part of the evaluation process is the determination that not only is the patient in need of skilled services to restore full function but also that the patient has a good, predictable likelihood of improving from the interventions provided. One benefit of good documentation is that it can then serve as a guide directing the natural progression of interventions as the patient attains goals throughout the course of treatment. The outcomes of effective documentation are clearly demonstrating the medical necessity of rehabilitation services for the patient that, when applicable, will result in gaining reimbursement from workman's compensation, third-party insurance, motor vehicle insurance medical payment funds, and/or from the individual patient on a self-pay basis. Skillful and artful communication of the needs of the patient is the clinician's means by which he or she differentiates him- or herself as a health care provider versus a personal trainer, which is also a key to gaining recognition from a variety of payer sources.

Documentation is a reflection of the quality of care that the athletic trainer provides each patient. It is the most common means by which determinations of potential fraud, abuse, and over-utilization of services are made. A well-designed plan of care in the initial evaluation and updates to that plan of care each visit encourage maximum utilization of time and provision of exceptionally skilled care with each patient, in addition to demonstrating the quality of and necessity for the rehabilitation services provided. In essence, good documentation practices are another way in which athletic trainers can improve their patient care.

Purposes of Documentation

The purposes of documentation can be summarized as follows:

- Provision of an accurate, thorough medical record. As a medical provider, an athletic trainer may be subpoenaed to appear in court as a witness to comment on an athlete or patient seen many years previous. Without a thorough record of all evaluation and intervention procedures; telephone conversations; and communication with the patient, case workers, coaches, doctors, and parents/family, it would be very difficult to testify as a credible and knowledgeable professional in a court of law. Any billing that may have been performed is also an important part of the medical record and may be utilized to support the services described in the actual treatment notes.
- Communication with referral source (physician). Upon completion, the initial evaluation is sent to the referring physician or other referring provider for approval of the plan of care, and this becomes the new prescription for rehabilitation services. More than one physician or health care provider is frequently involved with the patient's care, in which case the athletic trainer must provide other physicians or health care providers with progress notes in addition to providing these to the referring provider on a regular basis to inform the health care team of the patient's rehabilitation progress.
- Communication with coworkers. There have been several court cases in which allied health professionals did not document specific precautions and/or physician protocol information, and as a result, those precautions were not followed by coworkers assisting the patient, setting up a potential case for negligence for all professionals involved in the patient's care. Again, thorough communication with everyone involved in the patient's care is critical for the purposes of promoting continuity of care in addition to avoiding liability issues.
- Communication with others involved with the patient. The health care team does not just extend to medical professionals. In the case of a high school, collegiate, or professional elite athlete, the health care team extends to position coaches, head coaches, strength and conditioning coaches, emergency professionals, and any other professionals interacting in a way with the patient that might impair his or her ability to rehabilitate from injury successfully. Coaches and physical education professionals involved with the patient should be updated as often as needed in writing regarding the playing and participation status of the athlete; a copy of this also becomes a part of the medical record. For the patient who is rehabilitating from a work injury, written communication or written details of telephone and/or electronic communications with the patient and/or family, employer, case manager, and physician(s) must be documented, in addition to communicating with the referring physician if any changes in work restrictions might be appropriate.
- Protection from liability litigation. If the patient does not improve or respond to postsurgical or injury rehabilitation as expected, the medical record becomes critical to prove that the clinician did his or her duty versus providing negligent care. This is especially a concern if the patient is an athlete with high expectations of returning fully to his or her sport and is very disappointed with any remaining unresolved functional limitations impairing athletic performance, and perhaps limiting future potential scholarship and/or professional opportunities.

Common Documentation Terminology

In 1993, the National Center for Medical Rehabilitation Research (NCMRR) developed specific terminology for disability classification to assist in uniform communication for research in the area of rehabilitation. The second purpose of this classification system is to demonstrate the balance required between functional opportunities and functional demands with self-actualization as the final goal of rehabilitation. In general, the goal of rehabilitation is to remove barriers for patients. Athletic trainers treat patients at the impairment and functional limitation levels. In this way, they have a direct impact on patients' medical diagnoses and influence any remaining disabilities and societal limitations.

Pathophysiology is an interference with normal physiological and developmental processes. This is the medical diagnosis (ie, rotator cuff tear, multiple sclerosis, diabetes, hamstring strain).

An impairment is the loss or abnormality of cognitive, emotional, physiological, or anatomical structures or function, including all losses or abnormalities, not just those attributable to the initial pathophysiology. For example, if the patient has multiple sclerosis, the actual location of the problem is the build-up of plaque in the brain; however, a clinician would treat the impairments of decreased range of motion, decreased flexibility, muscle contractures, decreased strength, impaired endurance, and any other impairment. Impairments are measured or quantified during the initial evaluation.

A functional limitation is a restriction or inability to perform an action in the manner consistent with the purpose of an organ or organ system. What function can the patient with the humerus fracture no longer do with that arm that he or she should be able to do or was previously able to do? The existence of functional limitations is the reason why the patient is seeking rehabilitation services. Examples of functional limitations are the inability to throw, reach overhead, squat to the floor, and vacuum a floor.

A disability is the limitation or inability to perform activities and roles to the levels expected within physical and social contexts. On a global level, this is how functional limitations affect particular tasks at home or work that any adult or child would normally be expected to do. For example, cleaning the house, driving a car, sitting in class as a student, or caring for children are all examples of potential disabilities if the patient is unable to perform those tasks.

A societal limitation is a restriction attributable to social policy and/or barriers that limit the fulfillment of roles or deny access to services and opportunities that are associated with full participation in society. Examples of societal limitations are inadequate curb cut-outs or availability of handicapped parking. Generally, certified athletic trainers do not routinely work at this level of the rehabilitation process.

Source: U.S. Department of Health and Human Services, Research Plan for the National Center for Medical Rehabilitation Research, NIH Pub. No. 93-3509, March, 1993, National Institutes of Health, National Institute of Child Health and Human Development, Bethesda, Maryland.

Initial Evaluations

The initial evaluation is a record of the initial visit by the patient to the athletic trainer. The purpose of the initial evaluation is to introduce, describe, identify, and address the patient problem. Also, the athletic trainer must recognize the importance of this initial visit in introducing the patient to the arena of rehabilitation and to the unique role and skills of the athletic trainer. Serving as more than just a physical examination and revelation of impairments and functional limitations, the initial evaluation becomes an important opportunity to establish rapport and gain the patient's trust to improve the patient's compliance with the rehabilitation program. Improving the patient's confidence in his or her provider reaps significant gains in patient function.

The initial evaluation documentation includes the plan and prognosis for the episode of care just begun and provides the basis for all treatments and documentation to follow. The documentation should be thorough and consistent across all practice settings, with very few variations to the following format based on patient type, referral source, and/or specific additional requirements of any third-party reimbursement (see Appendix C for a sample athletic training initial evaluation form). Note that any treatment performed during the initial evaluation and an assessment of that treatment should also be documented in a daily note format.

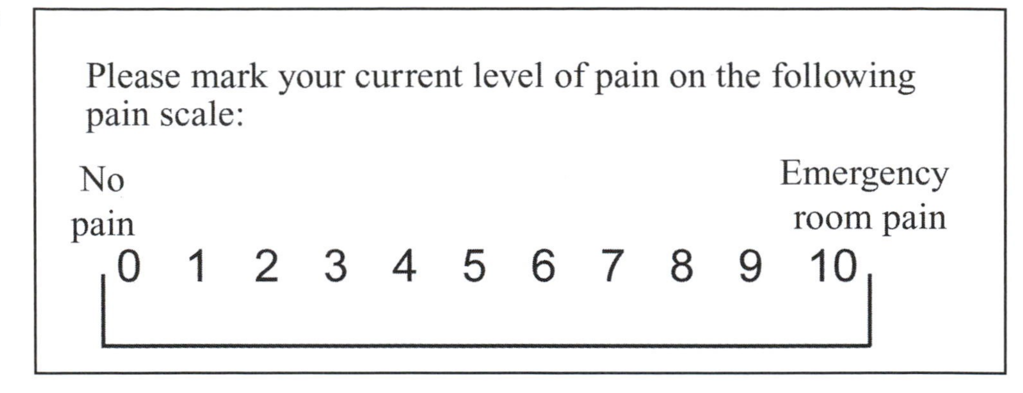

Figure 8-1. Visual analog pain scale.

Subjective

The subjective portion of the initial evaluation begins with the patient interview. It includes the following items reported by the patient and/or the patient's family:

- The current pain level and chief concern or symptoms can be documented using a visual analog pain scale (Figure 8-1), along with the pain scale number linked to specific activities or postures that make the symptoms better or worse. Also inquire if the patient feels most of his or her pain at night (red flag), whether pain fluctuates with or without movement (red flag), what the patient has already tried to relieve the pain and symptoms and symptom response to those pain-relieving attempts, and the initial and current location of pain and symptoms, including any neurological and circulatory signs or symptoms.
- The date of onset of the condition for which the patient is being treated is an important marker for any third-party payers separating this incident of care from any previous bouts of rehabilitation for any previous injuries. The date of onset must be a specific calendar date (month, day, year) (eg, mm/dd/yyyy). If the patient is unable to determine the precise date of injury, use the patient's assistance to estimate the date at the beginning, middle, or end of the month when the symptoms first appeared or became suddenly worse (eg, early May would then be 5/01/yyyy). If the patient has just had surgery for which he or she is in rehabilitation, the date of surgery (or manipulation) serves as the date of onset.
- The mechanism of injury describes the particular way in which the injury occurred, including the speed, direction, and angle of impact with object, person, or ground. The patient may have no recollection of any type of impact, in which case the mechanism will be listed as insidious. Also provide the location of the activity during which the patient was injured (at home, at work, motor vehicle accident, etc).
- The current functional limitations are any activities that the patient must modify or avoid doing altogether as a result of the injury. These range from changes and/or interruptions in sleeping due to pain or discomfort and difficulties with positioning for sleeping up to performing sprinting and jumping activities.
- The complete medical history includes any previous diagnoses, whether directly related to the current injury or condition or not. This information may raise red flags that the current symptoms may be nonorganic in nature or may indicate the need to modify the interventions selected if there are any contraindications to treatment, such as the use of electrical stimulation or diathermy on a patient with a pacemaker, or the use of ultrasound in a patient with a history of cancer. This information is typically solicited from the patient during the registration process by asking the patient to fill out a medical history questionnaire, which can then be reviewed by the athletic trainer and the patient during the subjective portion of the initial evaluation (Case Study 8-1).
- The complete surgical history along with the dates of the procedures will provide additional information regarding the extent of any previous injuries.
- Any previous injuries to the same location, including the dates of injury and severity of each injury, gives the athletic trainer an idea of the prior condition of the anatomical structures involved in the current injury.
- It is very important to clarify the current medications the patient is taking, along with the frequency of taking pain medications and nonsteroidal anti-inflammatories (NSAIDs). There are many potential drug interactions and side effects

Case Study 8-1

When Medical History is Key

Case. A high school soccer coach in his mid-thirties enters a high school athletic training room to be evaluated for calf pain that would not go away. The coach had participated in soccer clinics for coaches on 2 consecutive weekends and believed he had incurred a mild calf strain the first weekend, and then had made it worse the next, despite stretching and icing. He indicated there had been an unusual amount of swelling with the injury, along with redness. Inspection by the athletic trainer determined a large area of redness with significant swelling in a broad area extending throughout the posterior lower leg. The coach reported that the swelling had been getting worse in the past 3 days, even though he had been resting his leg. The patient was unable to perform a single leg heel raise due to pain but did not have a particular area of point tenderness upon palpation. Due to the redness and unusual swelling, the athletic trainer recommended the coach report to an emergency room as soon as possible and recommended to the physician that the patient may need a Doppler ultrasound to rule out the presence of a deep venous thrombosis (DVT). Before the coach left the athletic training room, he mentioned that he had a heart transplant several years earlier, reinforcing the athletic trainer's decision to call ahead and send the patient to the ER immediately. The patient returned to the athletic training room several days later, reporting that the Doppler ultrasound was negative but that he did have a bacterial infection that arose from his initial mild calf strain due to the immune-suppressing medications he had been taking for years to protect his heart transplant. The prescribed treatment was bed rest for 3 days and a course of oral antibiotics followed by a follow-up with his physician. The importance of taking into consideration the patient's complete medical history during an initial evaluation, no matter how healthy and young the patient may look, cannot be overestimated.

Debriefing Questions

- In the high school setting in which this incident took place, is was not customary at the time to ask a coach to complete a medical history form prior to being evaluated. Based on the information presented above, would you make this a requirement in your athletic training setting?
- What bearing did the patient's medical history have on the final diagnosis and treatment?

(eg, some cholesterol-lowering medications have the side effect of muscle pain) that the athletic trainer should take into consideration during the initial evaluation. Questions regarding frequency of dosing, especially for pain and anti-inflammatory medications, can help determine if the current pain level the patient describes is typical or atypical of how he or she may feel the rest of the day and whether pain is adequately under control. It is during this question the patient may relate difficulties or side effects of any prescribed medications, which may need to be addressed by either reassurance from the athletic trainer or by referring the patient back to the physician via patient phone call or appointment in order to clarify dosing or change any medications that are not adequately addressing the patient's pain control needs. Often patients will take medications on an as-needed basis, thinking the medication is intended for use only when they are in pain, when in fact NSAIDs need to be taken routinely as prescribed by the physician in order to have the desired effect. In this case, the athletic trainer should counsel the patient to take the medication strictly as directed by the physician.

- The social history of the patient may include many items critical to tell the story of the patient and his or her current problem. This could include the individual's race or descent if pertinent (eg, African Americans are more likely to suffer from sickle cell anemia), marital status, caregiver status, and in what type of dwelling he or she lives, especially with a description of any stairs or barriers that may be important to note or if any roommates or other members of the household are present and able to assist the patient at home if necessary. Also determine the societal role of the patient (eg, if the patient is a student, a mother, or a grandparent) and note if the patient has family members that require physical care from the patient and any other social responsibilities that may affect the rehabilitation prognosis.
- Previous limitations in function must be stated to clarify the patient's initial level of function and help determine the eventual level of function to

which the patient can be reasonably expected to return following rehabilitation. Simply document any activities that the patient was unable to do previously; if there are no previous limitations, this also must be documented with no exceptions.

- The particular requirements of workplace, school, sport, hobby, and any other pertinent activities and their associated movement patterns will be important to document and perhaps incorporate in future rehabilitation sessions and to consider as potential rehabilitation goals.
- Physician precautions for rehabilitation and restrictions on work or participation in recreational and/or athletic activities should also be noted and followed during the initial and subsequent visits.
- Each patient should be asked about his or her rehabilitation goal during the initial evaluation. A patient can simply be asked, "What would you like to be able to do at the end of your rehab sessions that you cannot do today?" The patient needs to take an active interest to gain the independence and self-motivation needed to successfully complete the rehabilitation process. The more input the patient has in his or her rehabilitation goals, the more motivated the patient becomes (Box 8-1).

Box 8-1

About the Patient's Goal

Some patients will have goals that seem unrealistic. Question the patient further regarding his or her level of function immediately prior to the injury he or she sustained. Then take into consideration the chronicity of the condition and any permanent damage incurred during the injury process. Be honest but tactful in discussing more achievable goals with the patient if his or her goals are likely not attainable. Also mention to the patient that should he or she respond very well to rehabilitation, new goals can be developed that may be closer to the final goal the patient had in mind.

Many patients that athletic trainers are likely to see have very high level, sports-related rehabilitation goals. It is good to document the patient's goal, but realizing the limitations of third-party reimbursement is an important consideration when setting the actual rehabilitation goals. Sources of third-party reimbursement may refuse to pay for any rehabilitation even if one goal is related to return to sport activities, as these insurers are not required to pay for a patient's return to sport but only for the patient's return to functional daily activities. The only exception might be a junior high or high school student's return to physical education class, which is considered necessary to fulfill the expected role of being a student.

Objective

The objective portion of the initial evaluation contains the quantified impairments measured and documented using a standardized, repeatable method in order to easily re-test to demonstrate progress in future visits. The impairments that are measured are those body system deficits that are preventing the patient from performing a specific task or activity. Table 8-1 lists common impairments that are assessed during an initial evaluation. Some of these items may not be tested if not applicable to the patient's problem as determined during the subjective portion of the initial evaluation.

In addition to measuring and documenting specific impairments, it is becoming increasingly more important to assess functional limitations in a quantifiable way. Functional limitations may be assessed by observing or timing the patient or by asking the reliable patient what he or she can and cannot do in very specific terms. Functional limitations that specifically relate to the patient's current injury or condition may include difficulties with the following tasks among others:

- Sleep is a very important goal for all patients, as sleep is imperative to the body's reparative ability. All patients should be asked about sleep quality and the ability to position themselves comfortably to fall asleep without delay. It can be quantified by asking the patient the average number of times pain awakes him or her at night, any delay in falling asleep due to pain in number of minutes, and the average number of hours of lost sleep per night due to pain.
- Bed mobility, basic transfers, and advanced transfers can be quantified by using the Functional Independence Measure (FIM) scale (Box 8-2), the number of seconds to perform the activity, the number of attempts successfully completed compared to the number attempted, and any modifications made from pre-injury performance, such as slower speed or use of assistive device. In addition, note any safety concerns if present.
- Activities of Daily Living (ADL) Scales measure the performance of the basic activities required for living, including indoor walking, bed-to-chair transfers, toilet transfers,

Table 8-1

Measurement Methods of Common Impairments

Impairment	*Measurement Method*	*Units/Description*
Edema	*Tape measure of girth	cm
	*Volumetric measurements	mL
	Visual estimation	trace, 1+, 2+, 3+
Range of motion (ROM)	*Goniometer	degrees
	*Tape measure	cm
	*Inclinometer	degrees
	% estimate in the spine	%
Strength	*MMT	Kendall scale of 0/5, 1/5, 2/5, 3/5, 4/5, 5/5, with + and – when appropriate
	*Grip strength-dynamometer	#
	*Isokinetic strength	Force/torque (# or N), % force: contralateral limb, % force:body wt
Flexibility/muscle length	*Goniometer	degrees
	Visual estimation	min, mod, or severely decreased
Special tests	Various specific tests	+ or -, laxity (1+, 2+, 3+)
Joint mobility	Paris Joint Mobility Scale	0 Anklylosed 1 Severely hypomobile 2 Hypomobile 3 Normal 4 Hypermobile 5 Very hypermobile 6 Unstable; subluxation or dislocation
	Capsular end feel	Empty, soft, firm, hard, bony
Nerve mobility	ULTTs, LE special nerve tests	+ or – for reproduction of Sxs
Point tenderness	Palpation Scale+	Grades I or 1+ Pain with palpation Grade II or 2+ Wince & c/o pain Grade III or 3+ Wince and withdraw Grade IV or 4+ Patient will not allow palpation
Balance/proprioception	*SLS eyes open and closed SLS knee bent/straight	sec
	*Balance Master	Balance Master Assessment
	*Berg Balance Scale (BBS) or other special scales	BBS results, compared to normative data in patient's age range
Skin integrity	Observation	Qualitative description of ecchymosis and/or wound appearance (smell, drainage color and amount, redness or other signs of infection present)
	*Tape measure diameter or length/height	cm

* = most accepted forms of measurement
MMT = manual muscle testing, ULTT = upper limb tension testing, LE = lower extremity, SLS = single limb stance, Sxs = symptoms

+Reprinted from Magee DJ. *Orthopedic Physical Assessment.* 4th ed. Philadelphia, PA: WB Saunders; 2002.

Box 8-2

Functional Independence Measure (FIM) Scale

Bed mobility, transfers, and ambulation are graded by the level of assistance needed. The Functional Independence Measure (FIM) Instrument is an extensive tool frequently used in hospital, skilled nursing, and sub-acute rehabilitation settings. The FIM contains a scale that helps quantify the patient's level of ability for a broad range of tasks; the full FIM Instrument can be quite lengthy. However, the FIM scale is an excellent way to quantify typical areas of functional limitation in the outpatient setting, including bed mobility, basic and advanced transfers, and ambulation.

7 Complete independence in timely and safe fashion

6 Modified independence; patient needs assistive device or more time to perform activity

5 Supervision; patient can complete the task but needs someone there for verbal cues or safety; no physical assistance needed

4 Min assist; patient performs at least 75% of physical work required by the activity

3 Mod assist; patient performs at least 50%, but less than 75% of the work required by the activity

2 Max assist; patient contributes only 25% to 50% of total work required

1 Total assist; patient requires total physical assistance for the activity

don/doffing socks, and don/doffing shoes. The Barthel Index and the Katz Index of ADL are examples of specific ADL scales.

- Instrumental Activities of Daily Living (IADL) Scales measure the performance of additional daily living activities that assist the patient in independent living, such as the ability to use a telephone, manage medications, prepare meals, perform housekeeping, do laundry, use transportation, and manage finances. Examples of IADL scales are the Rapid Disability Rating Scale, Arthritis Impact Measurement Scale, Klein-Bell Activities of Daily Living Scale, and the Functional Independence Measure (FIM) (see Box 8-2 for additional information).
- Driving can be assessed by noting the patient's ability to grip and turn the steering wheel with both hands, ability to manually shift if applicable, and can be quantified by asking the patient about the distance in time or miles the patient is able to drive safely and independently without modifications or breaks.
- Ambulation can be assessed by the need for assistive devices, the number of feet the patient is able to walk assisted or unassisted, the amount of assistance needed if applicable, the type of surface on which the patient is able to ambulate (uneven, slippery, carpeted or uncarpeted, ramps), modifications in gait speed from previous ambulatory abilities, and any qualitative deviations in gait quality about which the athletic trainer may wish to comment. For older populations, the Gait Speed and the Timed Up and Go (TUG) tests are just 2 of many ambulation tests that may be assessed during or subsequent to the initial evaluation and compared to available normative data for specific age ranges.
- The ability to ascend and descend stairs may be assessed by observing or by asking if the patient needs to hold onto the railing with one or both hands, needs an assistive device, utilizes a reciprocal (one foot on each step) or nonreciprocal (2 feet on each step) gait pattern, the number of stairs the patient can complete before needing to rest, and the seconds or minutes it takes the patient to ascend and descend a flight of stairs.
- Balance or limits of stability may be assessed utilizing a basic test of single leg balance with eyes open or closed, with knee bent or straight, tandem or Romberg stance, or more specific tests such as the Berg Balance Scale, Tinetti, and the Forward or Multi-directional Reach Tests.
- Reaching should be assessed utilizing the most common reaching maneuvers, heights, and directions performed by the patient in his or her home or work setting, including such common tasks as reaching into the back seat, reaching to get the mail out of the mailbox from a car, reaching for items from a high closet shelf, and lifting and reaching to place an infant or child in a car seat. The patient's ability to reach can be quantified by measuring standing reach or use of the more specific Forward or Multi-directional Reach Tests.
- Lifting, pivoting, squatting, and carrying should be assessed utilizing job or home specific lifting heights, weights, distances, and typically sized objects, along with the number of times lifted over a period of time, and demonstrated safety or lack of safety with current lifting mechanics.

- Kneeling can be assessed along with the patient's ability to transfer on and off the floor. This is especially important for a patient with a balance deficit who might fall to the floor and have difficulty getting up, or for a parent who frequently plays with children on the floor, in addition to the common tasks of kneeling to perform gardening, picking items up off the floor, and lifting heavy items from the floor.
- Climbing is a critical task for children to fully develop motor skills, but climbing ladders is also a very functional movement for adults to perform outdoor and indoor household and work-specific tasks.
- Running may be evaluated by distance, speed, gait deviations, form, efficiency, and safety.
- Jumping can be assessed by distance or height, seconds to perform repetitive jumps, single or bilateral jumps, number of jump attempts safely landed, and qualitative descriptions of the patient's landing pattern.
- Sustaining prolonged postures or repetitive activities may be quite difficult for the patient with an edematous joint or spine injury. This can be quantified by the number of minutes spent sitting, standing, walking, or performing repetitive work tasks before the patient needs a break, along with any modification in activity, assistive devices used, or safety issues noted.
- Assess any other functional tasks required at school, home, or work.

Assessment

The athletic training assessment contains the medical diagnosis, summarizes the information collected in a problem list format, and states the patient's prognosis. Every assessment should include the following items:

- Athletic training diagnosis
- Impairments
- Functional limitations
- Prognosis

> **What Questions Does the Assessment Answer?**
>
> Your assessment answers the following question: why does this patient require rehabilitation skills and services?

The athletic training diagnosis must be the same as the physician's diagnosis; however, this may vary by state practice act. In most states, if a specific diagnosis is not stated on the physician's script, the athletic trainer must contact the physician to get this information. The athletic trainer may provide an additional, even more specific diagnosis in addition to the physician's diagnosis if this better describes the patient's problem or injury. If the patient sustains a new injury over the course of rehabilitation, the physician must be consulted.

> **IMPORTANT!**
>
> Please refer to the exact rules and guidelines specific to your state's athletic training practice act regarding the requirement of a specific physician diagnosis and any additional requirements for athletic trainers practicing in your state. Certain third-party payers may require additional information as well. It is customary to contact the payer prior to seeing the patient to gain a prior authorization to treat the patient and to determine the patient's insurance coverage of rehabilitation services provided by an athletic trainer before any rehabilitation services are provided.

The impairments listed in the assessment are a highlighted version of the objective data collected during the initial evaluation (eg, 2+ right knee edema, decreased right knee ROM [3 to 77 degrees), decreased R LE strength [4/5]). The most pertinent functional limitations should also be included (eg, Pt wakes 4x/night due to knee pain, sit to stand transfers with bilateral UE support).

A large portion of the assessment section will consist of the impairments and the related functional limitations. This can be achieved in 2 different ways (Box 8-3). First, the highlighted impairment information may be listed and then related to the functional limitations by stating that the impairments are limiting the patient's ability to perform whatever functional limitations are listed. The second, more preferred method of stating the assessment is relating each impairment to a specific functional limitation. For example, the patient's knee edema is limiting the patient's ability to sleep without waking due to pain; the patient's decreased knee AROM is limiting the patient's ability to perform car transfers, etc. Either way, the assessment must clearly relate impairments to the patient's functional limitations in order to support the medical necessity of rehabilitation.

Box 8-3

Assessment Example

Dx: 2° R inversion ankle sprain

Separate list for impairments and functional limitations:

The patient presents with the following impairments: 2+ R ankle edema with moderate ecchymosis, decreased R ankle AROM (df: -8°, pf: 35°, inv: 10°, ever: 4°; all with pain), decreased R ankle strength (ant tibialis: 4+/5, post tibialis, soleus, peroneals: 4/5, gastroc: 2+/5), and impaired gait and proprioception (NWB R LE with 2 crutch assist). These impairments are limiting the patient's ability to sleep without pain interruption, ascend/descend stairs with WB on R LE, stand on tip-toes to reach into top closet shelves for items, ambulate for community and in-school to walk between classes, don/doff pants in standing, and participate in PE or recreational activities.

Prognosis: The patient's prognosis is good for attaining the following goals.

Relating impairments to each functional limitation:

1. 2+ R ankle edema with moderate ecchymosis is limiting Pt's ability to sleep through the night without waking due to pain.
2. Pt is unable to ascend/descend stairs with WB on R LE 2°decreased R ankle AROM (df: -8°, pf: 35°, inv: 10°, ever: 4°; all with pain).
3. Pt is unable to stand on tip-toes to reach into top closet shelves for items due to decreased R ankle strength (ant tibialis: 4+/5, post tibialis, soleus, peroneals: 4/5, gastroc: 2+/5).
4. Pt's NWB R LE status & need for 2 crutch assist is limiting Pt's endurance for community and school ambulation between classes.
5. Pt is unable to don/doff pants in standing due to decreased proprioception (unable to WB on R LE).
6. Pt is unable to participate in PE or recreational activities.

Prognosis

The final portion of the assessment is the prognosis, or statement regarding the patient's potential for successful rehabilitation. The prognosis may be excellent, good, guarded, or poor, depending on the individual patient and diagnosis. An excellent or good prognosis indicates that the patient is extremely likely to attain the stated goals in a timely and predictable fashion with no foreseeable barriers to improvement. A guarded prognosis may be appropriate for the patient who is attempting rehabilitation as a last ditch effort to try to avoid surgery for a rotator cuff or meniscus tear, for example. A poor prognosis is reserved for patients who will not benefit from any athletic training services due to the presentation of a problem that may not be in the athletic trainer's scope of practice, such as an athlete presenting with a previously undiagnosed ACL tear. If the athletic trainer perceives the patient's odds of succeeding in rehabilitation (and thus the prognosis) as poor, the plan of care should be a referral back to the physician or to another clinician if appropriate. The plan should not be an attempt at rehabilitation if the prognosis is truly poor. Sources of third-party reimbursement will not pay for rehabilitation for patients who have no chance of improving their functional limitations.

Athletic trainers must take into account the chronicity of the patient's condition, the patient's potential need for surgery, if any, and likely patient compliance when establishing the rehabilitation prognosis.

Keep in mind that the prognosis is intended to describe the likelihood of the patient attaining his or her realistic goals in his or her particular situation. This may not mean fully resolving all symptomatic complaints and regaining full range of motion, strength, and function, as some patients may attend rehabilitation sessions to strengthen prior to surgical procedures. Consider the following examples:

- When treating a patient who has an ACL tear and is attending rehabilitation preoperatively, the goals may focus on reducing edema and increasing range of motion and strength; however, full return to function is not likely (which is why the patient is planning to have surgery following rehabilitation). Therefore, the prognosis would be "good for attaining the following goals," with the following goals being realistic according to the expected progress of the patient over that time period with the understanding that the patient still has a deficient ACL.

- In cases in which the athletic trainer and physician may suspect the patient may have a rotator cuff tear, requiring surgery, the athletic trainer may document that the prognosis is "good, unless a complete tear is present."

The prognosis should be an honest portrayal of the patient's situation and should fully explain a less-than-excellent prognosis and why the patient may still benefit from rehabilitation despite a guarded prognosis. Finally, an athletic trainer may anticipate that a patient with a chronic pain problem may not fully regain all function at the end of the current bout of rehabilitation. In this case, the athletic trainer may state the prognosis as good but write goals that do not depend upon full relief of pain and symptoms and full return to function in order to meet the goals. Goals can be modified and new goals can be written should the patient exceed the athletic trainer's initial expectations for recovery.

Considerations must also be made for patients who have barriers to rehabilitation, such as cognitive deficits or learning disorders, motor learning difficulties, language barriers, or other organ system impairments such as low vision, poor hearing, or vestibular problems. When barriers to learning or other potential problems exist that may prolong the patient's anticipated treatment time, the concern should be stated along with a prognosis of guarded, if necessary. A guarded prognosis in this case indicates that it is doubtful the patient will meet all of his or her goals due to an identified barrier rather than the medical diagnosis. The chart then should contain the following statement, "The patient's prognosis is guarded due to limitations in the patient's ability to comprehend the athletic trainer's instructions for his or her home exercise program due to a previously diagnosed cognitive deficit." Or, "The patient's prognosis is guarded due to the patient's low vision, limiting his ability to remember his home exercise program due to difficulty seeing and reading his home exercise program hand-outs."

Plan of Care

The plan of care is a summary of the interventions needed to completely address the impairments and functional limitations listed in the assessment within a specific timeframe, along with goals that will assist in demonstrating progress throughout the course of rehabilitation. The plan of care consists of the following items:

- The duration of treatment is the total length of time over which the patient will need skilled rehabilitation services (eg, 6 weeks). The duration may also include the anticipated time (in minutes) the patient will need per visit.
- The frequency of treatment is the number of times the patient attends rehabilitation visits over a given period of time (eg, 2 times a week).
- The intervention list indicates the treatment techniques, modalities, exercise instruction, and any other treatments likely to be performed over the course of rehabilitation.
- The goals are the means by which progress is demonstrated during the rehabilitation process and serve as the criteria for discharge. At least one goal for every 2 weeks of treatment is recommended in order to adequately demonstrate progress. Goals must relate an impairment to a functional limitation, focus on a specific task, be quantifiable or measurable, and have a specific deadline for achievement.

Effective Goal Writing

Every goal should relate an impairment to a functional limitation. When writing a goal, the athletic trainer can choose either the impairment or the functional limitation as the standard to determine whether or not the patient has met the goal, but he or she still must mention the other component even if it is not the standard by which goal achievement is measured. Each goal should contain the following information (Box 8-4).

Box 8-4

Sample Goal

Increase R LE strength so the Pt can carry a grocery bag up and down 1 flight of 14 stairs safely (8 wks).

- Specific action: stairs
- Quantifiable activity: 14 stairs
- Duration/reps of activity: ascend/descend 1x
- Impairment addressed: decreased LE strength
- Functional limitation addressed: carrying grocery bag up/down stairs
- Timeline for achieving goal: 8 wks

- Specific action to be performed by the patient
- Quantifiable, measurable, repeatable activity
- Duration/reps of activity

- Impairment that, if addressed, will allow the patient to perform the above activities
- Functional limitation addressed (unless the activity is the actual functional limitation)
- Timeline for achieving the goal

In the goal (see Box 8-4), the standard by which goal achievement is determined is the patient's ability to ascend/descend 14 stairs while carrying a grocery bag, which is the functional limitation. The impairment, decreased lower extremity strength, is mentioned because it is very likely that the patient's inability to ascend/descend stairs is limited by the patient's lower extremity weakness. It is important to state this correlation, as most third-party payers specifically look for this statement in chart reviews of allied health professionals' goals.

There are several ways to correlate the impairment with the functional limitation in a goal. The most accepted practice of goal writing is to make the actual standard for goal achievement the functional limitation while mentioning the impairment addressed. Goal #1 (Box 8-5) is an example of this type of goal. Goal #2 is acceptable, but an impairment related to the patient's inability to don/doff his or her shoes would make this goal slightly better from a reimbursement standpoint. The third goal (impairment based, with functional limitation listed) is also acceptable. The preference of medical record reviewers is Goal #1, as the functional limitation is always the most important part of the goal to demonstrate that the patient's functional needs are being met in rehabilitation.

Box 8-5

Types of Goals

Goal #1: Functional limitation based, with impairment listed

- Increase R knee AROM, so Pt can return to tying and don/doff shoes independently for 2 consecutive days (3 wks).

Goal #2: Functional limitation based, with no impairment listed

- Pt will return to tying and don/doff shoes independently for 2 consecutive days (3 wks).

Goal #3: Impairment based, with functional limitation listed

- Increase R knee AROM = to L, so Pt can return to tying and don/doff shoes independently (3 wks).

Goal Presentation Options

Option #1: Preferred Method

Long-Term Goal #1 (to be met in 8 wks)

Increase R knee AROM, so Pt can squat to the floor to pick up a briefcase without knee pain on 3:3 attempts.

Short-Term Goals (to be met in 4 wks):

#1A: Decrease R knee edema, so Pt can sleep through 2 consecutive nights without waking due to pain without use of pain medications.

#1B: Increase R knee AROM, so Pt can perform a sit to stand transfer from a low seating surface on the first attempt on 2 consecutive days.

Long-Term Goal #2 (to be met in 8 wks):

2) Increase R LE strength, so Pt can ascend and descend 2 flights of stairs with reciprocal gait pattern and without UE assist while carrying a laundry basket safely.

Short-Term Goals (to be met in 4 wks):

#2A: Increase R LE strength, so Pt can return to safe driving to and from rehabilitation appointments (20 minutes) without increased knee pain.

#2B: Increase R LE strength, so Pt can ambulate for one full day as needed at home without an assistive device.

Option #2 Allowed Method

Goals are listed in chronological order based on when goals should be achieved.

Goals:

1. Decrease R knee edema, so Pt can sleep through 2 consecutive nights without waking due to pain without use of pain medications (2 wks).
2. Increase R knee AROM, so Pt can tie his R shoe independently on 2 consecutive days (4 wks).
3. Increase R knee AROM, so Pt can squat to the floor to pick up a briefcase without knee pain on 3:3 attempts (6 wks).
4. Increase R LE strength, so Pt can ascend and descend 2 flights of stairs with reciprocal gait pattern and without UE assist while carrying a laundry basket safely (8 wks).

Sources of third-party reimbursement value certain terms in goals because these terms help ensure the safety of consumers at home and in the community. The injuries related to falls are very expensive to treat and are related to increased mortality rates in elderly patients. Therefore, the terms *safely, without loss of balance,* and *independently* or *without supervision* are useful terms in goals applicable to many functional situations (landing from jumping, stepping off a curb, ascending/descending stairs, climbing ladders, etc). Using a certain number of successful attempts to total number of attempts ratio can help quantify a functional task that is otherwise difficult to measure and set a standard for goal achievement. For example, the patient can perform independent sit to stand transfers 2 out of 3 attempts without loss of balance. See Appendices D and E for additional examples of relating impairments to function for particular patient diagnoses and for additional goal writing tips.

Sources of third-party reimbursement may regard certain terms as red flags when found in a patient's medical record. These words can include any nonspecific terms, such as *proper, good, better,* and *improved,* because these terms really do not mean anything when added to a patient goal. There is no way to quantify the terms good, better, and improved, and therefore no ability to prove that the patient did meet that goal. Box 8-6 contains a summary of the most common errors in goal writing.

Box 8-6

Common Errors in Documentation: Goal Writing

- No relationship stated between impairments and functional limitations
- No measurable outcome
- Nonspecific task
- More than one measurable outcome
- Nonspecific activity (listing physical education class, but not what activity is being done)
- Use of nondescript words (ie, good, better, improved, proper)

Workman's Compensation Goal

For a patient with workman's compensation reimbursement, at least one of the final goals should relate to a specific workplace task that, if attained, will allow the patient to return to work with minimal or no work restrictions.

Goal Setting for Athletes and Highly Functional Patients

Highly functional patients and athletes are patients with real medical problems with associated impairments and functional limitations, but because the patients function at such a high level, sources of reimbursement may question their treatment goals and plan. It is often very challenging to write effective goals for these patients because there comes a time during their treatment that they can do most daily activities, just not their recreational activity or full return to their sport. The goals of any patient need to address impairments that directly affect functional limitations in areas of ADL, IADL, and daily living tasks, not inclusive of sporting or recreational activities, or even work activities unless the injury is a workman's compensation injury. This does not mean that this population should not be treated. Instead, this compels the athletic trainer to focus more on daily activities and the fulfillment of roles of societal expectations for each patient rather than specific sporting tasks. For example, a goal may be to return to full participation in physical education class, which is a normal expectation of a student to be able to fully participate without limitations and is a required part of any educational coursework from kindergarten through high school. A goal may be for a mother to return to climbing the stairs while holding her child instead of a goal returning the mother to running 5 miles without pain. Another example would be a football player returning to his prior activities of kneeling or running up and down stairs safely and efficiently instead of returning him to explosive movements out of his 3-point stance. This does not mean the patient's goal is not considered over the course of rehabilitation. It simply requires the athletic trainer to focus on athletic movement patterns that are common to everyday life and incorporate these in the functional assessments performed and goals established.

One method of assisting the athletic trainer in finding movement patterns in everyday life that may mimic the requirements of typical sporting activities is to take a moment to analyze the functions all humans perform on a daily basis for survival. The following represent the common categories of functions that an injury or illness may impact:

- ADL are basic activities required for everyday living, such as eating, bathing, dressing, toileting, grooming, mobility, basic transfers (sit to stand, stand to sit, supine to sit, sit to supine, and toilet), advanced transfers (bath/shower, car, floor), and ascending and descending stairs.
- IADL include daily activities that are a bit more advanced but still required for independent living, such as use of a telephone, shopping, food

preparation, housekeeping, laundry, driving a car, hailing a taxi, riding the bus, taking medications, and financial responsibility.

- Advanced daily activities are those activities that are not included in the ADL or IADL lists but still are negatively affected by illness or injury. Sleep is a very sensitive function interrupted early on by pain and swelling, including affecting the patient's ability to position comfortably to fall asleep without delay, and is critical to the healing process. Patients also frequently have advanced household indoor and outdoor chores to accomplish that may include bending, lifting, squatting, kneeling, scrubbing floors, climbing a ladder, and carrying substantial weight over a distance.
- Postural activities are those activities humans perform for prolonged periods of time as a result of changes in technology over the centuries and commonly as part of a vocation or tasks in the home. Common postural activities involve sitting, standing, walking, driving vehicles, and being passengers in vehicles for prolonged periods of time.
- Repetitive activities are those activities done for prolonged amounts of time with little deviation in the variety of muscles utilized over that period of time. For example, typing, searching the internet, playing video games, knitting, sewing, playing piano, craft projects. When performed over a period of time, all of these activities induce fatigue related to over-use of particular muscles and joints and may be limited by an injury.
- Community interaction includes both community mobility, such as ambulation endurance without a sitting break required for shopping in a mall and grocery and department stores; walking through an airport; and walking across parking lots to the doors of a restaurant, church, or school. This may also include using an escalator or a moving walkway, getting in and out of an elevator, and opening and closing heavy doors. Community interaction also assumes a human is moving safely through these community environments, including crossing the street at a controlled intersection in 17 seconds; crossing the street without stoplights; climbing stairs with or without railings; stepping up a curb; reacting to and avoiding obstacles; and timing the entrance and exit off an escalator, bus, or subway car.
- Societal roles vary widely among humans, and a patient's societal roles can change throughout the course of one day. Children are expected to be able to participate in playing and learning activities, including learning movement patterns or skills in physical education classes. Adults are expected to be able to care for their children and pets, and at times for older and disabled adults, in addition to participating in vocational and leisure activities. Adults and children are expected to participate in community activities, as socialization is a healthy human behavior that contributes to quality of life. For this reason, the above-listed activities are generally recognized by sources of third-party reimbursement as activities that normal individuals should be able to return to performing with as few limitations as possible following an illness or injury. Keep in mind that insurance companies do not reimburse for rehabilitation focused on returning a patient to work unless that patient is a workman's compensation patient.
- Sources of third-party reimbursement do not typically recognize the value of restoring a patient's general health and wellness; instead they tend to value only those basic activities that will help the patient live through the day in a relatively normal way. However, if the patient has a secondary diagnosis such as diabetes, depression, or morbid obesity, goals can be written to address returning to some activity level the patient previously had been performing to help control blood sugar levels and treat obesity and depression. For example, if the patient is obese, a goal could be written to get the patient back to walking 45 minutes a day to help decrease or maintain his or her current weight level. If the patient is diabetic or has high cholesterol, the patient's goal may be to return to 45 minutes of activity to help control blood sugar or cholesterol levels. If the patient has no secondary diagnoses, a goal could be written to return the patient to 60 minutes of exercise for cardiac fitness without pain or limitations. However, do not continue to treat a patient for the sole reason of meeting this goal when all other goals have been met, otherwise reimbursement for continued treatment is likely to be denied. Third-party payers are starting to recognize the role of exercise in the treatment and prevention of diseases; however, at this time, this recognition is limited to the treatment realm rather than the preventative benefits of returning to the previous high level of activity or exercise.

A second means by which athletic trainers can think of goal setting for athletes and other highly functional patients is by considering the following 4 levels of function and utilizing the goal-setting strategies provided for each.

1. Level One: The patient can perform basic daily activities without pain or symptoms, but cannot participate in recreational activities and has pain or symptoms with advanced daily activities. A patient example for this level is the football lineman with low back pain who can no longer practice or perform weight lifting due to his back pain. Further question this patient about his ability to sit through his night class, lift a suitcase into a vehicle, move furniture, and lift his backpack full of books off the floor and carry his backpack between classes. Even though the patient's goal of returning to football is not one of the actual goals utilized for rehabilitation, if the patient can return to the aforementioned activities, he will be ready and able to return to playing football and weight training. For patients in this category of function, consider goals that address endurance with daily and postural activities, household chores, community mobility and social interaction, community safety, societal roles, caring for children, and general health and wellness. Simply ask the patient what he or she cannot do in these categories and write a goal linking the appropriate impairment with that functional limitation.
2. Level Two: The patient can perform all daily activities but has pain or symptoms during recreational activities. The level two patient is a homemaker who can perform all of her household activities and care for her children, but she has iliotibial band tendonitis when she runs her typical 10 miles per day. For this patient, her goal may be to ascend and descend stairs after running because this might be painful for her. Another goal could be the ability to squat to the floor to pick up a toy or child, as squatting, after running, might be painful. A third goal could be the ability to run without pain to prevent her child from getting into danger in time. This patient may also be trying to lose baby fat or simply get back into shape. Returning to exercise for cardiac fitness is always a good goal, if accompanied by several other great goals linking impairments to reasonable functional limitations. With this patient level, consider higher level household chores and high-level daily activities requiring endurance, in addition to addressing societal roles, community safety, and general health and wellness.
3. Level Three: The patient can perform daily activities but has pain or symptoms after recreational activities. A patient example here is the lawyer who can do all of his activities and can even perform training for the upcoming marathon. However, he has nagging left hamstring pain when he is done running distance or interval training. This patient is certainly in the most difficult category of patients for which to create goals. Again, think of goals for activities that would be difficult when the pain is present (after running). The attorney who only has pain after he runs would likely find it difficult to bend to tie his shoes, bend to pick up a paper off the floor, or carry groceries up and down a flight of stairs. Question the patient thoroughly to discover what home activities bother the patient after he returns from his run, and use these activities as standards or the focus of the goals. Consider the categories of common functions in relation to how the patient can function once he is in pain after running. Keep in mind that a patient initiating rehabilitation at this level is not likely to need a large number of rehabilitation visits, so only a limited number of goals are needed.
4. Level Four: The patient can perform daily activities and recreational activities without complaints. The level four patient can do all activities but may have had pain last week at the doctor's visit, or the patient is concerned about the painless clicking in his knee when he ascends and descends stairs about once a week. Some patients are sent for rehabilitation even though they do not truly need it. This occurs rarely but does happen in a clinical setting. Often, the doctor writes a script for rehab 1 week prior to the patient coming to rehab, and often doctors prescribe anti-inflammatories that seem to take the problem away. In these cases, it is the job of the clinician to determine if the biomechanical problems likely causing the pain are still present and worth treating to prevent reoccurrence of the injury once the patient completes the medication. When obvious biomechanical deficiencies are present and function is likely to be hampered in the near future, consider seeing the patient for 1 or 2 visits to introduce a home exercise program to address those deficiencies. If the clinician finds nothing abnormal during the evaluation and no pain complaints or functional deficiencies are present, communicate this to the physician in your plan of care in the initial evaluation and explain to the patient that no additional treatment will be necessary.

Initial Evaluation Summary

- During the subjective part of the initial evaluation, ask the patient what he or she cannot do in detailed, measurable terms. Include the patient's inability to fulfill a societal role, such as a student walking to class, a mom lifting a child into a car seat, or an individual's ability to ascend/descend stairs to an upstairs bedroom. Remember to document a specific date of onset and include a statement about the patient's prior level of function.

- The objective section should contain all objective measurements, including quantification of functional limitations when possible.
- The assessment should describe how the objective data are impacting the patient's functional ability.
- The plan of care should correlate the goals to the interventions that will be performed. Goals must be measurable and functional and contain a deadline for achievement.

ICD-9

Along with the initial evaluation, the athletic trainer also must complete the billing and ICD-9 coding to identify the patient diagnosis(es). The ICD-9 is based on the World Health Organization's Ninth Revision of the *International Classification of Diseases*. This is the official system of assigning codes to diagnoses and procedures common to all hospitals and clinics in the United States.

Daily Notes

Every patient encounter is thoroughly documented in a daily note (Appendix F). The daily note contains subjective, objective, assessment, and plan of care data in a more limited and updated format than contained in the initial evaluation. Many sources of reimbursement are analyzing daily notes to determine if skilled services were actually provided throughout the treatment and using this analysis to decide if the services will be reimbursed. The clinician must use the daily note to demonstrate his or her unique clinical skills and decision-making process by documenting why that particular treatment or modality was used, not just how it was utilized during the treatment. It will help the clinician if at least one impairment is reassessed every visit, so quantified data can be documented and compared to previous data to determine if progress has been made and to help decide if the overall treatment plan needs to be modified. This brief data collection in addition to subjective information gained from the patient helps to focus the treatment session on the most pressing needs of the patient, improving the quality of care given during that treatment session. Goals should also be reassessed at least one visit per week to determine the level of overall progress so that if necessary, modifications to the current treatment plan can be made if little progress has been made toward goal achievement.

- The subjective portion of the daily note should contain the information the patient provides in response to questions such as, "How are you doing today? What is bothering you the most today? What functions are you now able to perform that you were not previously able to perform prior to starting rehabilitation?" Pain should be assessed during every visit, whether or not a pain scale is utilized. Any changes in function should be noted. The subjective portion of the daily note may be written in the first or third person.
- The daily note objective section should contain the data reassessed each visit and also contains the information regarding the treatment provided on that date of service unless a separate treatment section is used. Specifics should be provided on any modalities performed (including settings, the clinical reasoning behind making that modality selection for this particular patient, and the patient's response to the modality treatment, if any), and a description of the skilled treatment performed by the athletic trainer such as manual therapy, therapeutic exercise, instructions in posture or body mechanics training, functional activity training, recommendations on activity modifications, and any other instruction and/or treatment performed. Any exercises that have specific names that do not clearly identify the purpose of the exercise and do not adequately describe the exercise should be further clarified. For example, if the clam exercise is performed, it is important to note that the clam exercise is performed for gluteus medius strengthening, as a medical reviewer may not be familiar with the name and purpose of each exercise commonly known within rehabilitation circles.
- The daily note assessment should state the patient's response to the skilled intervention just received in specific and meaningful terms. Assessments detail the patient's response to treatment, along with progress made during the treatment session, why problems were encountered with any techniques, overall progress made (or not made as expected) toward goal achievement, and/or the patient's subjective response to treatment with clinician explanation of why such a response was elicited. The

patient's response to a new home exercise also qualifies as a professional assessment. This is the area of the daily note that gives the clinician the best opportunity to demonstrate his or her professional judgment and decision-making skills. Do not squander this opportunity!

- The plan can be a list of specific interventions for the next treatment, or any adjustments to the current plan of care based on the patient's status. A specific plan developed in advance for the next visit for any new exercises or modalities to try saves time during the next visit so you can simply begin precisely where you left off in the previous treatment session. Assess goals on a weekly basis and identify which goals have been met, which the patient has made progress toward achieving, and which the patient still has not yet achieved. Modify goals when appropriate for the patient. This may include a goal upgrade (making the standard more difficult to achieve), downgrade (making the standard easier to achieve), extension of the deadline for achievement, modification of the standard/task, or the establishment of entirely new goals if the old goals have been achieved. Use good judgment when deciding to modify goals. With more experience, the initial evaluation goals will be more on target regarding tasks the patient will be able to perform in a given timeframe, making the need for rewriting or modifying goals unnecessary and rare occurrences for patients who do either far better or worse than expected. Box 8-7 highlights some of the common pitfalls in the daily notes aspect of documentation.

Box 8-7

Common Errors in Documentation: Daily Notes

- Failure to include the visit number (visits actually attended)
- Failure to list the treatment time listed in minutes
- Failure to sign and date all entries
- Failure to document all treatment modalities and procedures used
- Failure to reassess objective data and goals
- Lack of skilled assessment every visit
- Evidence of nondiagnostic, nontherapeutic, routine, repetitive, and reinforcing procedures without evidence of skilled feedback

The daily note is also the place to document any and all other patient contact and any communication related to the patient, such as phone calls to and from the physician, patient, case manager, employers, and the patient's family. Education of the patient and the family (if applicable) must be documented each visit, including the topic of education, format (verbal, written, demonstration, video, etc), and how the patient responded to the education (demonstrates exercise, indicates understanding, etc), and whether any barriers to education exist. Any changes in work status or work restrictions should be noted, as well as any cancelled or no show appointments.

Workman's Compensation Updates

Documenting changes in work status is particularly critical for workman's compensation patients. Workman's compensation case managers often require weekly or bi-weekly updates on patients, including work status, response to treatment, physician work restrictions, and the next physician visit.

Progress Notes

The progress note is a specialized daily note that contains an abbreviated, complete reassessment of subjective and objective information, with appropriate updates to the plan of care regarding frequency and duration of future rehabilitation, as well as updated goals (Appendix G). Progress notes are the means by which clinicians update the physician on the progress of the patient and communicate any other needs or concerns regarding the patient. The progress note refocuses future treatment sessions and serves as a script for continued treatment. The athletic trainer may also recommend to the physician that other evaluation/diagnostic tests be performed and/or other interventions be considered if the patient is not progressing as well as anticipated.

- In the subjective portion of the progress note, document what the patient perceives has been the percentage of improvement in pain and/or function since initiation of rehabilitation. Also ask the patient about pain level (can utilize pain scale), any functional abilities regained, and any functional abilities that the patient is unable to perform or needs to modify in order to perform.
- In the objective section, the athletic trainer should document the results of the re-evaluation, including any range of motion,

strength, edema, special tests, flexibility, and any other test items that would help measure progress and determine if a particular goal has been met. Functional tests to reassess the standards written for the goals are also helpful, especially in the later stages of rehabilitation.

- The progress note assessment should address changes in impairments and functional limitations, refer back to the previous months' treatments and progress if applicable, and highlight improvements in the patient's overall status as well as limitations yet to be overcome.
- The plan of care in the progress note can be established first by deciding which goals have been met, partially met, and not met, and then by providing updated deadlines for completion for goals during the next bout of rehabilitation if the patient is continuing rehabilitation. If any goals have not been met that were expected to be met in the current time frame, include an explanation as to why the goal(s) were not met and modify and add new goals if necessary. Based on the patient's improvements and further needs, the frequency and duration of future sessions should be requested for the physician's approval, as well as listing any new or modified treatment modalities or techniques and stating any new focus of treatment for the current bout of care.

Box 8-8 contains some of the common errors in writing progress notes as a part of the documentation process.

Discharge Notes

Once the patient has met all of his or her rehabilitation goals, or the patient has reached a plateau in progress despite the utilization of a variety of treatment approaches, the patient is ready to be discharged from rehabilitation. The discharge note contains the same information and format as the progress note and can replace the daily note for the patient's last visit in rehabilitation along with the details of the treatment provided that day. It serves as a summary of the patient's subjective and objective status, what treatments were performed, along with the patient's overall response, and the focus of the patient's home exercise program to address any remaining functional limitations independently. The discharge note contains objective data (impairments and functional limitations) reassessed on the final day of rehabilitation, a statement of goal achievement or lack of achievement and why, and further treatment recommendations, in the same format as the progress note.

Box 8-8

Common Errors in Documentation: Progress Notes

Failure to:

- Refer back to the previous month's treatments
- Show objective comparisons reflecting progress or lack thereof
- Show clinical decision-making related to continuing or discontinuing rehabilitation
- Address modification/update of goals and list any new goals
- List new interventions to be added
- Comment on any interventions eliminated and why
- Show functional application of goals related to impairments
- State current/new focus of treatment
- State changes in frequency or visit number in treatment

STANDARDS OF PRACTICE IN DOCUMENTATION

Variations by Setting

The standards of practice in documentation should not vary by individual practice setting, despite some variations that may currently exist, especially in colleges, universities, and professional athletic training settings. The goal of documentation is to improve patient care, which is the goal of every rehabilitation setting, regardless of the need for proving medical necessity for the purpose of gaining reimbursement for the services provided. Often medical facilities complete an internal chart audit as a means to improve documentation (see Appendix H for a sample chart review format). There are a few settings that may necessitate additional paperwork for a variety of reasons and needs, such as military, industrial, and clinical settings when treating particular caseloads, such as patients with workman's compensation. In these cases, additional work-related information and updates on a routine basis may be required in addition to typical documentation expectations. For these patients, incorporating work or other relevant tasks very similar to those the patient will be returning to will be of utmost importance, in addition to including return to work or return to specific relevant task goals included in the plan of care.

Relating Standards of Documentation to Standards of Practice

Heightened documentation standards required by sources of reimbursement have forced rehabilitation professionals to evaluate the means by which rehabilitation treatments are delivered in daily practice. This has happened in the past when insurance companies no longer reimbursed for the application of hot packs and ice in rehabilitation settings. This forced allied health professionals to change the way they practiced by either choosing modalities that were reimbursable or by providing more skilled techniques or services instead. Sometimes patients were asked to come in before or stay after treatments to undergo heating or cooling treatments free of charge. Change is a constant in the health care field, and although change can be threatening, in the end it is always beneficial if the result is improvement in patient outcomes and the quality of services provided.

Some relatively recent modifications in the practice patterns of athletic trainers in response to the expectations of source of reimbursement include the following areas:

- All treatment time that is billed requires skilled intervention. The use of a treatment log, complete with today's date, sets and reps, and weight lifted can be easily misconstrued as routine, repetitive exercise without evidence of skilled feedback, which would not gain reimbursement. Instead, the athletic trainer needs to spend the treatment time perfecting exercise technique, form, and progression of the exercises and encouraging the patient to perform the exercise program at home. The patient may also be encouraged to come in early or stay late after the appointment time to complete exercises that require specialized equipment but do not need skilled intervention. If at any time during the treatment session the athletic trainer is merely supervising exercise (with the exception of monitoring vitals or attempting a new exercise), there is no skilled intervention being provided, so no skilled intervention codes can be billed for those minutes. If the patient could do the same exercises at home or in a pool supervised by a lifeguard, then the patient should not be billed for doing these exercises in the clinic. If the patient is independent with the home exercise program, he or she should be discharged from rehabilitation. If the patient needs to work on technique with a few of the exercises he or she is doing at home, document not only the exercise performed but also the technique or advice given to the patient.
- Functional testing utilizing gold standard tests is highly recommended when available to assess functional limitations. These gold standard tests have research-proven reliability and validity. Such tests may include the FIM, the Berg Balance Scale, the Timed Up and Go, and single limb or tandem stance balance tests.
- The athletic trainer must be very careful when treating more than one patient at a time. If 2 or more patients are being treated at one time, the group therapy charge, not a therapeutic exercise charge, must be used to appropriately describe and bill the intervention being provided. The exception to this rule is when skilled assessment or intervention is taking place in a one-on-one basis, and only the time of this one-on-one skilled intervention is billed as such for each patient.
- Modalities are classified and billed according to those that require supervision and those that are unsupervised. Supervised modalities include ultrasound and iontophoresis, while electrical stimulation is considered an unsupervised modality. A supervised modality requires the clinician to supervise the actual treatment (eye contact of the treatment being performed). Remember to include the clinical rationale for using the modality for the particular patient problem every visit during which the modality is being performed.
- Reimbursement based on the quality of care provided, which is determined by the efficiency and effectiveness of the treatment given to assist the patient in meeting his or her functional goals, is the next major trend in reimbursement for rehabilitation services. Reimbursement will be based on the quality and efficiency of the services provided in order to give incentives for the appropriate provision of high quality services and to reduce unneeded or inappropriate care performed to increase revenue.

Box 8-9 lists the common errors that occur in general documentation.

Patient Advocacy

If a source of third-party reimbursement denies payment on a rehabilitation claim or on a medical device recommended by the allied health professional and the physician (such as a home traction unit), the athletic trainer needs to determine if all the required documentation was completed and forwarded to the payer, assess the reason for the denial, and forward any additional information to the payer if requested. A claim may be denied for a variety of reasons, so

Box 8-9

Common Errors in General Documentation

- Inadequate documentation to prove services were rendered
- Notes do not have the correct date of service
- Notes sent do not reflect the actual services billed
- Someone other than the billing provider performed the services
- Total of billed treatment exceeds total treatment time
- Care continued even when the patient is no longer functionally improving and is not expected to improve
- Patient is performing a maintenance program
- Procedures are billed that could have been effectively carried out with the patient by a nonprofessional after instruction is completed
- Failure to document that the physical condition or function of the patient was sufficiently impaired to require treatment
- Failure to state the patient's level of function prior to the injury
- Treatment not applicable to meaningful daily living needs
- Treatment progressed beyond the patient's prior level of function
- Modalities performed for an extended period of time without clear documentation of the continued benefit of each specific modality or treatment
- Focus of treatment is on higher level activities (advanced balance exercises, recreational or social activities, work activities, general fitness, endurance, etc)

Documentation Red Flags for Reimbursement Audit

The federal Medicare program is administered by the Center for Medicare and Medicaid Services, which is the entity that determines which rehabilitation services are covered and publicizes documentation requirements for reimbursement by Medicare. Because Medicare is the only nation-wide health care program, individual insurance companies typically follow Medicare guidelines for documentation, which is why the following list of red flags for a Medicare audit are presented here.

- Daily intervention beyond 1 week
- Lack of frequency of treatment tapering over the course of rehabilitation
- Performing the same modalities throughout the course of treatment
- Lack of active, restorative, and functional based treatment (modality-only treatment)
- Large gaps in treatment without re-evaluation, change in diagnosis, and change in interventions
- Claims submitted for more than 12 to 15 visits per episode of care
- Use of unlisted modalities such as laser or anodyne
- Documenting only impairments without relation to function; justifying interventions based solely on range of motion and strength
- Basing care decision on nonmeasurable terminology (increased/decreased, minimal/moderate/maximal, etc)
- Treatment based solely on patient's pain complaints

discovering why the claim was denied is the first step to resolving the issue. If all of the required information was sent and the denial is not reversed, the athletic trainer must determine if the patient does (or did) need additional skilled rehabilitation and what evidence can demonstrate that need. Then, include this information in a letter to the provider, clearly demonstrating why further rehabilitation is medically necessary for the patient. Do not give up after the first try, as many sources of reimbursement may routinely deny the first and second claim. If the patient does require additional rehabilitation, and appeals and reauthorizations are allowed according to the patient's specific policy, a few thoughtfully persuasive phone calls and letters are likely to succeed in gaining reimbursement on the patient's behalf. See Appendix I for a sample patient advocacy letter.

SUMMARY

- Identify the contents of the medical record.

  The complete medical record contains all of the patient's medical information, including history, physician orders, daily and initial evaluation documentation including progress and discharge notes, billing records and ICD-9 codes, and any other communication from and about the patient that is pertinent to his or her care.

- Understand the implications of HIPAA and explain the importance of maintaining patient confidentiality.

  The introduction of HIPAA further underlined the necessity for maintaining patient confidentiality in all settings at all times.

- Recall the purposes of documentation.

  The purposes of documentation are to provide an accurate medical record and prove the medical necessity for the patient, in addition to creating a record that can be used at future dates for previous treatment history, litigation purposes, and for communication with colleagues, including physicians.

- Summarize the standards of practice related to documentation in the athletic training field.

  The standards of practice in documentation should not vary by individual practice setting, despite some variations that may currently exist, especially in colleges, universities, and professional athletic training settings. The goal of documentation is to improve patient care, which is the goal of every rehabilitation setting, regardless of the need for proving medical necessity for the purpose of gaining reimbursement for the services provided.

- Compose the subjective, objective, assessment, and plan of care components of an initial evaluation.

  Documentation by athletic trainers can be recorded in a SOAP note format or any other format that includes the subjective, objective, assessment, and plan (including goals), as well as treatment information.

- Write specific impairment-related, functional, and measurable goals for a variety of patient diagnoses.

  Patient goals should relate an impairment to a functional limitation. When writing a goal, the athletic trainer can choose either the impairment or the functional limitation as the standard to determine whether or not the patient has met the goal but still must mention the other component even if it is not the standard by which goal achievement is measured.

- Explain how to avoid common documentation errors in the initial evaluation and daily and progress note.

  Documenting the specifics of each treatment, including not only what was done, but why each exercise or modality was completed, as well as writing goals that link impairments to functional limitations and include a specific action to be performed and a deadline for completion are several ways to avoid documentation errors.

- Demonstrate the ability to document evidence of skilled feedback when providing therapeutic exercise.

  One means by which athletic trainers can demonstrate their skill as health care practitioners is by performing and documenting brief assessments on a daily basis, as well as providing and documenting one-on-one care and feedback to each patient throughout the rehabilitation process.

- Summarize the importance of frequent reassessments of each patient's functional status using quantifiable tests and measures to demonstrate progress toward specific goals.

  Frequent re-evaluation over the course of treatment and updating the goals and plan of care help guide the treatment process and improve quality of care.

ACTIVITIES

The following activities and cases are designed to reinforce material presented in the chapter and to allow for discussion among students and instructors. Many of these examples are drawn from actual patient cases.

Objective Scramble

Take the following objective information, and match the data to the following headings: (Note: not all answers will be used, and some may be used more than once.)

Pain scale	ROM	Distal joint screen
Special tests	Skin integrity	Neurological system
Strength	Proprioception	Proximal joint screen
Posture	Joint mobility	Functional tests
Point tenderness	Edema	Flexibility

Right shoulder initial evaluation data:

__________ 1. Light touch sensation intact B UEs

__________ 2. R shoulder abduction PROM: 124°

__________ 3. B elbow, hand, wrist AROM WFL

__________ 4. R G-H jt capsular end feel: empty

__________ 5. + Hawkins-Kennedy test for impingement

__________ 6. Pt able to tuck in the back of her shirt

__________ 7. R supraspinatus MMT: 4+/5

__________ 8. C-spine AROM WFL and pain-free

__________ 9. Pt's pain is 2/10 at rest; 6/10 with mvmt

__________ 10. B mod decreased pec minor length

__________ 11. Pt has FHP & B mod fwd shoulders

__________ 12. Pt able to reposition R shoulder at 90-90 with ~ 80% accuracy

__________ 13. Pt's inf capsule has mod decreased mobility

__________ 14. Pt able to lift R hand to head to wash her hair

__________ 15. R shoulder flexion AROM: 145°

__________ 16. R shoulder edema: trace at ant and lat G-H jt

__________ 17. + Neer impingement test

__________ 18. 2+ pt tender R supraspinatus tendon

Goal Rewrite

You have a patient who has been diagnosed with a second-degree moderate inversion ankle sprain. Using the guidelines provided in the chapter, rewrite the following goals. See Box 8-5 to review.

1. Decrease pain and swelling by 50% (3 days)
2. Increase AROM by 50% (1 wk)
3. Attain FWB (1 wk)
4. Increase strength by 50% (3 wks)
5. Improve agility and function by 50% (1 wk)
6. Return to unlimited stair ambulation (10 days)
7. Return to full competition with protective taping (2 wks)

Case Study

Review the case study provided below; students are encouraged to develop appropriate goals for this case.

Diagnosis: s/p R ACL reconstruction

Subjective: 16 y.o. female high school basketball player presents to rehab 2 days post-op; she injured the knee when doing a jump stop in the 3rd quarter of a varsity basketball game 1 mo ago; athlete denies any previous knee injuries. Reports 4/10 R ant knee pain at rest; no increase in pain with amb. Is avoiding 2 flights of stairs at home, has 3 step entry into house. Finds car transfers difficult and is unable to drive until released by MD.

Past Med Hx: None

Medication: Vicodin

Job tasks: High school student; in P.E. class—currently playing volleyball; part-time summer job as a lifeguard

MD restrictions: No P.E., running, jumping, or driving until further notice

Objective: Edema: 3+ R knee with moderate ecchymosis post and medial knee

Incisions: Healing with very minimal drainage; no signs of infection

ROM: R knee PROM: flex: 2-56° ext: -2° L knee PROM: flex: 0-148° ext: 4°

Patellar mobility: Severely decreased glides x 4 & tilts

Strength: 30% R quad activation with quad set
L quad & ham MMT: 5/5
12° extensor lag with R flexion SLR
Mod decreased R VMO:VL ratio

Palpation: Min pt tenderness medial joint line

Neurological: Intact B LE's

Foot/ankle screen: AROM WFL

Function: Unable to tie or don/doff shoes I
Uncomfortable in sitting due to dependent position & limited R knee flex
Squat to ~25° knee flexion with B UE support; PWB on R LE
Gait: R knee immobilizer with 2 crutches IPt not able to FWB for single limb stance R LE

Special tests: Lachman's & ant drawer (-)

Assessment: 16 y.o. female presents to rehab 2 days s/p R ACL reconstruction with 3+ R knee edema, decreased R knee PROM (2-56°), decreased L LE strength (12° extensor lag), and impaired gait and proprioception. These impairments are limiting the Pt's ability to perform ADL's such as tying her shoes I, driving a car, sitting in dependent positions, prolonged ambulation, stair ambulation, kneeling, running, and jumping.

Prognosis/Rehab Potential: Good for attaining the following goals.

P: Goals:

Plan of Care: rehab 2-3x/wk x 10 wks for ROM, edema control, scar and patellar mobs, strengthening, gait/proprioception training, functional activity training, and HEP.

Documenting Initial Evaluations: Subjective Findings

Use the outline below to guide you through an injury evaluation with one of your classmates. Write a thorough subjective portion of an initial evaluation using a scenario provided from the instructor or simply make one up for this exercise. Be accurate and concise, writing only pertinent information within the following format. Use of standard medical abbreviations is encouraged.

Patient: ______________________ MD: ______________________

DX: ______________________

MD precautions: ______________________

____

W/C: ______________________

Today's date: ______________ Date of surgery: ______________

Date of onset/mechanism of injury/previous Rx:

Social Hx:

Chief complaint/functional limitations:

Medical/surgical Hx:

Medications:

Work/school/recreational tasks/activities:

MD work/school/recreational restrictions:

Writing Daily Notes

Using a scenario similar to the one above, interview one of your classmates and simulate an injury and potential treatment session for that injury. Fill out all appropriate blanks for your single treatment session. If a blank does not apply to your patient, write N/A for not applicable.

Patient:______________________ MD:______________________

DX:______________________

MD Precautions:______________________ Date of surgery:______________________

Visits approved:______________________

Date: Visit #:___/___
Units billed/time: Date: Visit #:___/___
Units billed/time:
S:

O:

Modalities:

HEP/Pt/family education:

Education format:

Pt/family response:

A:

P:

LAT:

Writing Progress/Discharge Notes

Interview the same classmate you interviewed for your daily note and base this progress note on his or her responses for the subjective portion (including change in functional limitations). In the objective portion, include some information on the patient's ROM, strength, point tenderness, special tests, and any other information that would be appropriate. Remember to keep this section somewhat abbreviated. Complete the assessment portion, making up the patient's progress and items that still need more intervention. Finally, initial goals #1 and #2 have been met. Please write goals #3 to #5, to be attained over the next 4 weeks. Also include appropriate interventions to complete the plan of care.

____ Progress Note ____ Discharge Note

Patient:____ MD:____
DX:____
Today's Date:___________________________________ Date of surgery:______________________________
Date of 1st visit:________________________________ Date of last visit:_____________________________
Patient compliance: Visits attended:________
Visits scheduled:_______

Athletic Training Interventions:
Subjective (chief complaint; functional limitations):

Objective:

Assessment:

Plan of Care:
Goals (met, modified, continued):
#1-2) Met.

#3)

#4)

#5)
Frequency and duration of additional rehab:
Athletic Training Interventions:

Licensed Athletic Trainer:______________________ Date:____
Cont athletic training:______ D/C:________
MD comments:________________________________ MD signature:________________________________
Date:____

ADDITIONAL INFORMATION

The following information related to this chapter can be found in the appendices.
Appendix C Athletic Training Initial Evaluation
Appendix D Examples of Function and Impairment-Based Goals
Appendix E Goal Writing Tips
Appendix F Daily Notes
Appendix G Athletic Training Progress/Discharge Note
Appendix H Athletic Training Chart Review
Appendix I Sample Insurance Appeal Letter
Appendix J Standard Medical Abbreviations

BIBLIOGRAPHY

Department of Health and Human Resources, Office of Inspector General (2005, March). Results of the Medical Review Performed on Selected Medicare Claims for Physical and Occupation Therapy Services Provided During Calendar Year 2002 in the State of Texas. http://oig.hhs.gov.

Dittmar S, Gresham G. *Functional Assessment and Outcome Measures for the Rehabilitation Health Professional.* Gaithersburg, MD: Aspen; 1997.

Downie W, Leatham PA, Rhind VM, et al. Studies with pain rating scales. *Ann Rheum Dis.* 1978;37:378-388.

Fearon H, Levine S. APTA Reimbursement for Rehab in the Out-Patient Setting: Rules for Engagement [Workshop]. (1/8/05).

HIPAA Basics: Medical Privacy in the Electronic Age. www.privacyrights.org/fs/fs8a-hipaa.htm.

Hunt V. Meeting clarifies HIPAA restrictions. *NATA News,* 10-12.

Issues and Insights: CPT Coding: Winning at the Numbers Game [Online chat]. (12/9/2003). www.apta.org/rt.cfm/reimb/codingchat.

Magee DJ. *Orthopedic Physical Assessment.* 4th ed. Philadelphia, PA: Saunders; 2002.

Manual System. Pub 100-02 Medicare Benefit Policy; Transmittal 88; May 7, 2008

Mason D. Congress, Medicare, and pay for performance. *PT Magazine.* 2005;26-28.

Moore RJ, Mandelbaum BR, Watanabe DS. Evaluation of neuromusculoskeletal injuries. In: Schenk RC, ed. *Athletic Training & Sports Medicine.* 3rd ed. Rosemont, IL: American Academy of Orthopedic Surgeons; 1999:80.

Simon Ravitz K. The HIPAA privacy final modified rule. *PT Magazine.* 2002;21-25.

US Department of Health and Human Services. Improper Medicare Fees-for-Service Report—Fiscal Year 2004. Available at http://www.cms.hhs.gov/CERT/downloads/FY2004LongReport.pdf. Accessed March 3, 2009.

United Government Services, LLC. *Medicare Memo.* 2004;12:8.

United Government Services, LLC. *Medicare Memo.* 2004;6:10.

United Government Services, LLC. *Medicare Memo.* 2004;5:10-11.

United Government Services, LLC. *Medicare Memo.* 2000;11:35-37.

ADDITIONAL READINGS

Berg KO, Wood-Dauphinee SL, Williams JI, Maki B. Measuring balance in the elderly: validation of an instrument. *Can J Public Health.* 1992;83(Suppl 2):S7-S11.

Gnella C, Paris SV, Kutner M. Reliability in evaluating passive intervertebral motion. *Phys Ther.* 1982;62(4):436-444.

Granger CV, Hamilton BB, Dieth RA, Zielezny M, Sherwin FS. Advances in functional assessment for medical rehabilitation. *Topics in Geriatric Rehabilitation.* 1986;1:59-74.

Kendall FP, McCreary EK, Provance PG. *Muscles, Testing and Function.* 4th ed. Baltimore: Williams and Wilkins; 1993.

Chapter

INSURANCE AND REIMBURSEMENT
ADDRESSING THE BOTTOM LINE

Brian Anderson, ATC and Elizabeth Swann, PhD, ATC

OBJECTIVES

At the end of this chapter, the reader will be able to:

- Recognize and define key terms associated with insurance and reimbursement
- Explain the associated components of insurance policies
- Summarize the different types of insurance plans or programs
- List several ways to contain health care costs
- Explain the purpose of CPT codes for reimbursement
- Discuss the requirements for athletic trainers to be reimbursed for their services

The role of insurance and reimbursement for athletic trainers varies by setting and mission of the clinic, hospital, or school that employs them. The 2 main purposes that athletic trainers would utilize for insurance would be either for cost-containment or revenue and reimbursement. The goal of the organization, either as a cost-containment or a revenue and reimbursement entity, would determine how athletic trainers view and utilize insurances. For those employed in secondary schools, colleges and universities, and even industrial settings, their primary purpose in understanding insurance is for the coordination and access to additional medical services such as diagnostics, specialists, and various health care facilities. The main focus for insurance of those employed in clinics or treatment facilities is for the reimbursement for the services they are providing. However, an increasing number of settings, including secondary school and university-based athletic trainers, are beginning to pursue reimbursement for services as a means to show monetary value for items traditionally provided for free. In order to accomplish either a cost-containment model or revenue and reimbursement model, one must understand the insurance industry and how the various parties and components work together in providing the patient with the best access to health care. Today the insurance industry is composed of a variety of individuals, entities, and components that provide a complex and intricate network of systems in an effort to provide for the health care of the patients and compensate the providers for the services that are provided.

Did You Know?

Historically, access to health care was provided in full or in part by one's employer in an effort to keep individuals on the jobsite.

UNDERSTANDING THE PERSONNEL

There are many people or entities involved in determining an insurance program. The 3 most significant are the subscriber, provider, and the insurance carrier.

Table 9-1

Components of Insurance Policies

Components	Definition
Premium	Amount paid by the subscriber for the policy.
Deductible	Amount which the subscriber is responsible for paying prior to the insurance company taking responsibility for the claim or bill.
Co-pay	Amount paid by the subscriber upon visit to the provider prior to receiving services.
Co-insurance	Applied after the deductible amount has been met by the subscriber in which a percentage of the remaining balance would be distributed between the insurance company and the subscriber.
In-network benefits	Those services provided by preapproved providers with whom the insurance company negotiates a fee for that service.
Out-of-network benefits	Those services that are provided outside of the established network of providers; the insurance company will still provide payment, although the portion payable by the subscriber may be greater.

The subscriber is the individual or group of individuals being insured, typically a family or an individual. The provider is the entity that is providing the service to the subscriber, typically a physician's office, diagnostic facility, hospital, treatment center, or anyone deemed appropriate by the insurance carrier/company. The insurance carrier/company is an entity responsible for setting fee structures with providers, paying bills for the subscriber, and determining the benefits to be paid. It is important to remember that the insurance company is a for-profit corporation with responsibilities to employees and stockholders as well as the subscriber and health care provider. Insurance companies must then rely on the premium paid by the subscriber (individual and/or corporation) to fund the insurance programs, pay operational expenses, as well as ensure profits. An insurance company does not simply pay bills/claims on behalf of the subscriber/patient—they negotiate a set fee for each service to be provided with the health care provider. That provider agrees to that particular fee structure in exchange for providing service to the subscribers within that plan.

Another individual or entity that is important in the insurance industry is the primary care physician, commonly referred to as the PCP.[1] This is especially prevalent for those in health maintenance organizations (HMOs) (to be discussed later). The PCP is most often an internal medicine/family care physician who is responsible for coordinating the care of his or her patients to specialists, diagnostics, and treatment facilities in a financially responsible manner, essentially serving as the gatekeeper to health care for those on such plans.

Role of the Primary Care Physician

A primary care physician (PCP) is a physician, such as a general practitioner or internist, chosen by an individual to serve as his or her health care professional and who is capable of handling a variety of health-related problems, of keeping a medical history and medical records on the individual, and of referring the person to specialists as needed.

In some health care plans, particularly managed care plans, the subscriber must designate a PCP who then becomes the gatekeeper for his or her medical care, and all referrals to specialists must first come through the PCP before the subscriber can see a specialist for his or her illness in order for full benefits to be paid by the insurance company. In this case scenario, the PCP coordinates all health care for the person.

COMPONENTS OF INSURANCE POLICIES

One must understand the components that distinguish one insurance plan from another in an effort to understand insurance policies (Table 9-1). The 2 components that are most obvious are deductibles and premiums. The premium is the amount paid by the subscriber (patient or consumer) for the policy.[2] In many cases, this cost will be paid in part by the subscriber's employer as a benefit. There will be an associated deductible amount in addition to the premium. The deductible is the amount for which the subscriber is responsible for paying prior to the insurance company taking responsibility for the claim or bill. The premium and deductible have an inverse relationship to each other. Typically, the higher the deductible amount, the lower the premium and visa versa. For instance, a subscriber or patient with a deductible of $1000 would be responsible for the first $1000 of a claim prior to the insurance company paying for the remainder of the claim.

The next components to assess would be co-pays and co-insurance. These further complicate how the payment of claim is divided among the parties (subscriber or insurance company). A co-pay is the amount paid by the subscriber upon visit to the provider prior to receiving services. As a typical example, the subscriber would need to pay $20 prior to seeing the physician. Following the payment, the claim or bill would be submitted to the insurance company for payment according to the parameters of the policy. An example of another typical case where a co-pay would exist would be for prescription medications, where the subscriber would pay an amount ($10, $20, etc) prior to receiving medications. Some policies will limit the amount a subscriber will pay for co-pays on an annual basis. For example, a policy may include a maximum of $3000 in co-pay amounts for an annual benefit period. In addition to co-pays, another method in which an insurance company will share the cost of the services with the provider is by utilizing a co-insurance. Co-insurance is applied after the deductible amount has been met by the subscriber in which a percentage of the remaining balance would be distributed between the insurance company and the subscriber.[1,2] Traditionally, this percentage would be 50%, 70%, 80%, or 100%. The higher the percentage amount, the more favorable it is for the subscriber. A 80% co-insurance would be applied after the deductible has been meet at which point the subscriber would be responsible for 20% of the bill and the insurance company would pay the 80%. This can become complicated when there is a co-pay combined with a deductible amount as well as a co-insurance.

All of these components essentially divide the responsibility of paying for health care among different parties in an effort to share the burden of potentially large expenses. All of these components have an effect on the premium or cost the subscriber initially pays whether or not he or she ever seeks medical attention. A relatively healthy individual would elect to have a lower premium with a higher deductible combined with co-pays and co-insurance such as 70/30 (subscriber responsibility of 30% with insurance company responsible for 70%) because they will not utilize medical services. The individual needing significant amounts of medical services would likely choose a higher premium and lower deductible amounts combined with lower or no co-pays and a more favorable co-insurance of 80/20 or 100% (20% payable by the subscriber and 80% by the insurance company or 100% paid by insurance company). This will be more costly upfront with the premium but save the subscriber money if he or she frequently seeks medical services. This combination of premium, deductibles, co-pays, and co-insurance makes it difficult for subscribers to choose an insurance plan because it is not easy to compare one policy to another.

Another concept to understand is in-network versus out-of-network benefits. In-network benefits are those services provided by preapproved providers with whom the insurance company negotiates a fee for that service. This is financially favorable to the subscriber as well as the insurance company in that it helps to control costs. Out-of-network benefits are those services that are provided outside of the established network of providers; however, the insurance company will still provide payment although the portion payable by the subscriber may be greater.[1] For example, a plan may have an 80/20 co-insurance for in-network services but a 50/50 co-insurance for out-of-network services. The subscriber has the ability to choose a physician or service provider but will have to pay out of pocket for a larger percentage of the total bill. Not all plans have out-of-network benefits, therefore if the subscriber wishes to see that service provider, he or she will be responsible for the entire bill.

The relationship between included versus excluded coverage must also be understood. A subscriber's policy may limit some services based upon the medical necessity of the service toward his or her health care. When a service is excluded, the insurance company is not going to compensate the provider. The following are examples of services that may be excluded on various plans:

- Military service injury/illness
- Health prevention programs
- Dental care
- Massage treatments
- Injuries sustained during a suicidal act
- International services

The following are examples of unique inclusions to many health care policies:

- Mental health
- Chiropractic care
- Transportation/lodging expenses for distant treatment services
- Medical evacuation

Table 9-2

Common Types of Indemnity Payments

Type	Description
Reimbursement—actual charges	Under this type of plan, the insurer will reimburse you for the actual cost of specified procedures or services, regardless of how much that cost might be.
Reimbursement—percentage of actual charges	Under this type of plan, the insurer pays a percentage of the actual charges for covered procedures and services, regardless of how much those procedures and services cost. A common reimbursement percentage is 80%. This has the same effect as a 20% co-payment.
Indemnity	Under this type of plan, the insurer pays a specified amount per day for a specified maximum number of days. Although your reimbursement amount does not depend on the actual cost of your care, your reimbursement will never exceed your expenses.

Adapted from Health Insurance. Indemnity vs. Managed Care. Available at http://www.agencyinfo.net/iv/medical/types/indemnity-managed.htm. Accessed August 8, 2008

TYPES OF INSURANCE PLANS/PROGRAMS

All of the previous mentioned components make up the way health insurance plans are structured, funded, and managed. Housed within an insurance company are a variety of plans, which also vary from one company to another. Health insurance plans can be broadly divided into 2 large categories: 1) indemnity plans (also referred to as "reimbursement plans") and 2) managed care plans.[3]

Indemnity Plans

An indemnity plan reimburses the subscriber for his or her medical expenses regardless of who provides the service; although in some cases the reimbursement amount may be limited. The coverage offered by most traditional insurers is in the form of an indemnity plan.[3] Different plans use different methods for determining how much a subscriber will receive for his or her medical expenses. Table 9-2 explains reimbursement for the 3 most common methods.

Managed Care Plans

There are several types of managed care plans but only preferred provider organizations (PPOs) and HMOs will be addressed in this chapter. Although there are important differences between the different types of managed care plans, there are similarities as well.[4] All managed care plans involve an arrangement between the insurer and a selected network of health care providers (doctors, hospitals, etc). All offer policyholders significant financial incentives to use the providers in that network. There are usually specific standards for selecting providers and formal steps to ensure that quality care is delivered.[3] PPOs and HMOs are described in more detail below and their advantages and disadvantages are listed in Table 9-3.

The PPO has a system that allows the subscriber the most flexibility in his or her choice of providers. For example, a PPO network may identify 50 orthopedic surgeons within a geographical area that the patient may elect to utilize for services and receive those services with the more favorable pricing, such as a $20 co-pay with a 100% co-insurance, meaning the cost for the visit for the patient was a maximum of $20. If the patient were to choose an out-of-network physician, he or she may receive that service with an expense such as a $20 co-pay with an 80/20 co-insurance. The patient would pay the $20 plus 20% of the remaining charges. Patients have the right to choose which services they elect to receive and by whom. Another convenience traditionally offered by a PPO plan is the ability to access care directly or without going through a PCP or gatekeeper. They can also be referred from physician to physician without having to obtain permission/authorization from the PCP. Additionally, more physicians will accept or be contracted with these types of plan as it affords them greater payment for services in a less complicated manner. A PPO plan typically will cost the subscriber more money in premium than other plans but allows for more coverage and convenience as well as less monies paid out at the time of service.

Table 9-3

Advantages and Disadvantages of PPOs and HMOs

Plan	Advantages	Disadvantages
Preferred provider organizations (PPOs)	Free choice of health care provider Out-of-pocket cost generally limited	Less coverage for treatment provided by non-PPO physicians More paperwork and expenses than HMOs
Health maintenance organizations (HMOs)	Low out-of-pocket costs Focus on wellness and preventative care Typically no lifetime maximum payout	Tight controls can make it more difficult to get specialized care Care from non-HMO providers generally not covered

Adapted from Health Insurance. HMOs, PPO & POS Plans. Available at http://www.agencyinfo.net/iv/medical/types/hmo-ppo-pos.htm. Accessed August 8, 2008.

HMOs offer another option for subscribers that typically has a less costly premium. HMOs traditionally utilize the PCP as the organizer of services for the subscriber. Prior to receiving nonemergency services, the subscriber must obtain a referral from the PCP for a prescribed health care service that is usually limited to a particular time frame (eg, 60 days) or patient encounters (eg, 15 visits). This in part is orchestrated through a very tight network of service providers. The insurance company will develop relationships with a variety of service providers in a geographical area (typically fewer than the PPO network) to provide the subscriber with options that he or she can discuss with his or her PCP. Typically, there are no out-of-network benefits as it is cost prohibitive for the HMO to allow subscribers to utilize providers outside the contracted network of providers. In addition to the inconvenience of fewer providers and coordination through the PCP, the cost for services is traditionally higher at the time the service is provided and may include a $20 co-pay with an 80/20 co-insurance after a deductible is met.

Health Savings Account

Another type of insurance program is the health savings account (HAS). These fluctuate in popularity and are uniquely arranged from one company to the next, but generally speaking they function like a PPO in that the subscriber has wide access to service providers but costs are self-funded by individuals or employer groups. Typically, an employer group would have a fund dedicated to the payment of claims and then contract with an insurance company for their payment and negotiating power with the providers. The managing agents of the account determine the services provided with a HSA. For instance, the HSA could determine that preventive medicine would have a positive influence on the cost of long-term care for disease and sickness and provide the subscriber with access to fitness classes or gym memberships. Essentially, the managing group is weighing the benefits of healthy activity versus the long-term cost of treating cardiovascular disease. Granted, this type of thought process could take place within any of the other health plans, but the flexibility lends itself to the HSA plan because the monies are controlled by the managing group, which has representation from the subscriber. The managing group would then pay a fee to the insurance company in order to have access to their provider discounts as well as infrastructure to pay claims.

Medicare and Medicaid

Medicare is a federal program that provides health insurance to retired individuals, regardless of their medical conditions.[5] Medicaid is a health insurance program for people with low income and is a joint federal-state program to provide medical assistance to aged, disabled, or blind individuals (or to needy dependent children) who could not otherwise afford the necessary medical care.[6]

Most people become eligible for Medicare upon reaching age 65 and becoming eligible for Social Security retirement benefits, although there are criteria that would enable a person to become eligible for Medicare before the age of 65.[5] There are 3 parts to Medicaid that are outlined in Table 9-4. Obviously, Medicare is an insurance coverage plan that does not generally apply to high school or college/university athletes but is relevant to clinic settings.

Table 9-4

Parts of Medicare Coverage

Coverage	*Description*
Medicare Part A (Hospital insurance)	Generally known as hospital insurance, Part A covers services associated with inpatient hospital care (ie, the costs associated with an overnight stay in a hospital, skilled nursing facility, or psychiatric hospital, such as charges for the hospital room, meals, and nursing services). Part A also covers hospice care and home health care.
Medicare Part B (Medical insurance)	Generally known as medical insurance, Part B covers other medical care. Physician care—whether it was received while you were an inpatient at a hospital, at a doctor's office, or as an outpatient at a hospital or other health care facility—is covered under Part B. Also covered are laboratory tests, physical therapy or rehabilitation services, and ambulance service.
Medicare Part C (Medicare + Choice)	The 1997 Balanced Budget Act expanded the kinds of private health care plans that may offer Medicare benefits to include managed care plans, medical savings accounts, and private fee-for-service plans. The new Medicare Part C programs are in addition to the fee-for-service options available under Medicare Parts A and B.

Adapted from Health Insurance. Medicare. Available at http://www.agencyinfo.net/iv/medical/types/medicare.htm. Accessed August 8, 2008.

Each state administers its own Medicaid program based on broad federal guidelines and regulations. Within these guidelines, each state 1) determines its own eligibility requirements; 2) prescribes the amount, duration, and types of services; 3) chooses the rate of reimbursement for services; and 4) oversees its own program.[7]

To qualify for Medicaid, you must meet 2 basic eligibility requirements. First, you must be considered categorically needy because you are blind, disabled, or elderly. Second, you must be financially needy.[6] This means that your income and your assets must fall under a certain limit set by the state in which you live.[6]

Medicaid pays for a number of medical costs, including hospital bills, physician services, home health care, and long-term nursing home care.[6] States may elect to provide other services for which federal matching funds are available. Some of the most frequently covered optional services are clinic services, medical transportation, services for the mentally disabled in intermediate care facilities, prescribed drugs, optometrist services and eyeglasses, occupational therapy, prosthetic devices, and speech therapy.[6] It is important to check with the insured's state Medicaid office to determine what coverage is offered. Unlike Medicare, it is possible for high school and intercollegiate athletes to have Medicaid as their form of insurance coverage.

COST-CONTAINMENT CONSIDERATIONS

As mentioned earlier in the chapter, one of the roles athletic trainers play in dealing with insurance is having access to referral services (specialists, diagnostic, treatment) in an effort to provide expedited access to care for their patient population. This process is utilized in the secondary school settings but predominately utilized in the college and university environment. Essentially, many athletic trainers are coordinating the insurance coverage of the school with that of the student-athlete in an effort to provide cost-effective and timely care. This is sometimes not easy to accomplish due to the timing of the injury, the area of the country the student-athlete is from, type of insurance plan the student-athlete's parents have, etc.

Typically, a secondary school or university athletic department will obtain an excess or secondary policy to cover student-athletes when they are injured as a part of their participation in sport. An excess or secondary insurance is a method of payment for services under the plan that takes effect after any and all primary (student-athlete/student-athlete's parents) insurance has been exhausted. This type of insurance has its own unique set of concepts that make up how it is structured and delivered. Typically, these plans are associated with university (especially National Collegiate Athletics Association [NCAA] institutions) policies and have a medical maximum limit of

$75,000, which meets the NCAA's catastrophic deductible limit.[7] Essentially, the university athletic trainer is coordinating 3 insurances: 1) student-athlete's primary (if such exists), 2) school's secondary (excess) policy, and 3) the NCAA's catastrophic policy.[7]

As one would think, in the event of an athletic-related injury while the student-athlete is participating in school activities, the student-athlete's primary insurance typically provided via the parent is utilized for any services provided (specialists, diagnostics, surgery, etc). Any cost not covered, which could include co-pays, deductibles, co-insurance, or uncovered procedures, would then be the responsibility of the school's secondary insurance program. Once the overall cost reaches the threshold of $75,000, the NCAA's (for NCAA schools only) catastrophic plan would take responsibility.[7] Most schools in recent years have elected to utilize the student-athlete's primary insurance in an attempt to control costs to their secondary program. In addition, many schools mandate that student-athletes have primary insurance and furthermore have insurance that covers athletic-related injuries because many of the insurance plans offered through student health exclude injuries sustained during athletic participation.

Secondary Insurance Concepts

A school's secondary insurance program can be just as complicated as the insurance structure mentioned in the first half of this chapter. Excess plans have varying deductibles, plan structures, and inclusions and exclusions. Some traditional inclusions/exclusions to consider for a secondary/excess policy for a school are listed in Box 9-1.[3]

Box 9-1

Inclusions/Exclusions for Secondary Insurance Policies

- Heart and circulatory benefit: If this benefit is included, then coverage would be extended to pay for those conditions arising from athletic-related arrhythmias or cardiac episodes that can be attributed to participation in athletics.
- Pre-existing conditions: This benefit is payable when an athlete is cleared to participate in athletics but then sustains an injury to the same body part that was previously injured. An example of this would be an athlete that has a past medical history of a right ACL tear in high school and then sustains the same injury in college. If the school has a pre-existing condition inclusion in their policy, their service would be covered by their plan. It does not mean the school has to utilize this practice for all types of injuries. This also does not suggest that the university's insurance would provide coverage to an athlete that sustained an ACL tear in high school and the school's insurance would pay for its repair.
- HMO/PPO denial clause: The benefit is important for the school's secondary insurance in that if the provider gets denied for payment by the student-athlete's primary insurance for whatever reason (no out-of-network benefits, failure to obtain a proper referral/pre-authorization, etc) the school's insurance would be responsible for the claim. If this benefit is not included, the responsibility would become the student-athlete's or in many cases the school would pay for this service out-of-pocket. This would need to be explained in the school's policies related to financial responsibility for athletic injuries.

TYPES OF EXCESS/ SECONDARY PROGRAMS

Most excess/secondary insurance programs for student-athletes are centered upon the deductible amount and type. There are typically 2 types of deductible amounts: 1) traditional disappearing and 2) aggregate.[9]

Traditional Disappearing

Traditional disappearing deductibles range in size from $0 to $10,000 or more per injury. The purpose of the "disappearing" deductible is to have the insurance company pay any remaining balances after a certain pre-set deductible figure had been paid by the individual or school. Because of this, a school with a $0 deductible will naturally pay more for the premium than what they would expect to pay for a higher deductible. It is also important to note that the premium is experience related, which means the more the claims paid out by the insurance company the higher the premium will be for subsequent years.

If a school purchased a policy with a $0 deductible, the school's insurance company would be responsible for any bills ranging from $0 to $75,000 after the student-athlete's primary insurance has paid any amount it is going to pay. For example, a student-athlete obtains a magnetic resonance image (MRI) for a knee injury she sustained during soccer practice. The bill for the MRI is $1900, which is submitted to the student-athlete's primary insurance for payment (she has a $1000 deductible with a $50 co-pay and an 80-20 co-insurance). Based on negotiated rates by her primary insurance company, they adjust the bill to $1400. In this example, the first $1000 due to the student-athlete's deductible would be the responsibility of the school's insurance, thus leaving $400 to be divided 80/20 with 80% or $320 the responsibility of the student-athlete's insurance and the remaining 20% of $80 again the responsibility of the school's insurance. In summary, this $1900 claim was reduced by $500 of which the student-athlete's insurance paid $320 and the school's insurance paid a total of $1080, which would then become a part of their claim history to determine future premiums.

Another consideration that schools utilize to reduce the cost of their premium is a higher deductible such as $2500. This becomes effective if the student-athlete's insurance meets the first $2500. Utilizing the example above with the $1900 MRI bill and the same student-athlete primary insurance, the situation would have worked out as follows: instead of the $1000 in primary deductible and $80 in co-insurance going to the secondary insurance for payment, the school would have paid the $1080 "out-of-pocket," meaning the school (in most cases) would have paid that portion of the bill, thus having no impact on the school's claim history. In this case, if the student-athlete was to need surgical intervention and incurred an additional $10,000 in bills the situation would continue to build. Since the student-athlete's primary insurance deductible has been met, the $10,000 may be distributed as such. Let us assume that there is a $50 co-pay for surgery of which the same 80/20 co-insurance would still exist. The soccer player's primary insurance adjusted the billable charges to $7500 based on negotiated fee structures. The remaining balance is $7450 after the $50 co-pay deduction of which 80% or $5920 is the responsibility of the student-athlete's insurance and 20% or $1490 is the remaining balance. Based upon the additional expenses, the student-athlete's primary insurance meets the deductible for the secondary plan and thus the school was not accountable for any out-of-pocket expenses. However, there is now an increased expense in claim history on the school's secondary insurance. Due to the fact that the student-athlete had primary insurance, the school saved a significant amount of money and claims activity versus the student-athlete without any primary insurance. The same case for a student without any primary insurance would look as follows: $10,000 in surgical fees plus the initial $1900 in diagnostic charges for a total of $11,900. Of this the school would be responsible for $2500 in out-of-pocket expenses and the school's secondary policy would be responsible for the $9400. This has a significantly larger impact on current as well as future insurance cost versus the insured student-athlete.

Aggregate Deductible

Some schools have considered and are utilizing aggregate deductible plans for their secondary insurance. An aggregate deductible acts similar to a family deductible. Instead of utilizing a deductible amount as in the case above of $2500 per person per injury, the school's insurance utilizes an aggregate deductible for all of their student-athletes. Once they collectively reach a set amount, typically $50,000 or higher, then the insurance company would be responsible for the remainder of the bill versus when the individual reaches the amount such as in the example of $2500. As an example, a school may elect to have a $100,000 aggregate deductible with a management fee of $35,000. The $100,000 or aggregate amount is placed into a claims fund that essentially pays for claims as they occur. The $35,000 is considered the premium of management fee for processing claims and managing the account. It is still the goal of the university to utilize primary insurance to the extent possible. Sticking with the female soccer player example, the $1080 that was paid by the school's insurance company in the $0 deductible example in this case would have been deducted from the $100,000 aggregate amount. It would be in the school's best interest to keep the claim activity below the $100,000 amount as any monies not utilized would be rolled into the following year's amount, thus saving the school money. If the claims activity was to exceed the $100,000 aggregate amount, the subsequent year's program would reflect any additional cost either in a higher premium/management fee and/or a higher aggregate amount.

In an effort to minimize the time and expenses associated with coordinating all of these insurance processes, many schools elect to become "self-insured," essentially assuming the financial risk of a student-athlete's health care from $0 to $75,000 (NCAA schools)[7] or whatever the medical maximum amount for that organizing body. In such cases, it is critical that the school utilize the student-athlete's primary insurance to its maximum in an effort to decrease the cost to the university.

As you can tell, this process can become complicated with having to coordinate all the necessary primary insurance to best serve the school's interest in controlling cost but at the same time have access to quality medical care.

STRATEGIES TO MINIMIZE COST TO SCHOOL OR SCHOOL'S INSURANCE

Many of the strategies to reduce costs of the school's athletic health care center on primary insurance and the concepts discussed in the first part of this chapter. Substantial effort should be directed toward coordinating and maximizing the insurance policies student-athletes have to lessen the burden incurred by the school and/or the school's insurance. This requires a great deal of understanding pertaining to how all these processes work.

Mandating Primary Insurance Prior to Participation

This is becoming a more accepted practice as a school's medical costs are directly affected by the percentage of student-athletes with or without insurance. In the event that the student-athlete does not have insurance, the school's secondary policy becomes the primary and thus contributes to the amount of claims filed against that policy, which increases the school's premium for years to come. This is sometimes a hard practice to mandate in universities where students are receiving scholarships as many students simply do not have the financial means to purchase primary insurance. Some schools require primary insurance for those volunteering/walking-on prior to participation.

Adjusting Primary Care Physician for In-Network Benefits

If a school mandates insurance, it does not guarantee that the student-athlete will have coverage where services are likely to be provided. Such is the case if a student-athlete is from out of state and on an HMO that does not provide benefits to the geographical area where the student-athlete is attending school. In many cases, there can be an exemption filed with the primary insurance for visiting or guest privileges. One strategy would be to have the student-athlete's primary care physician changed to the school's team internist or physician in the area so that those services (specialist, diagnostics, surgery, etc) would then be considered in-network and thus drastically reduce the impact on the school or the school's secondary insurance plan. An example of this would be the student-athlete that needed surgery and diagnostics totaling $15,000. Although the student-athlete had primary insurance, the provider that performed the surgery may not have been contracted with the student-athlete's insurance program, thus the $15,000 would be the sole responsibility of the school or school's insurance. If the student-athlete could have been switched to a physician in the local area as his or her PCP and then referred to in-network providers, the student-athlete's primary insurance would have been accountable for a large portion of the $15,000 and the school's secondary insurance would only be responsible for co-pays, deductibles, and any co-insurances. If adjusting the PCP is not an option, the student-athlete could always be sent home to have the services provided with his or her family physician, which would then be an in-network service. This is an inconvenience to the athlete as well as the school, but it would be fiscally responsible.

Negotiating Fees With Providers

It is a common practice for schools to negotiate fees with providers that they routinely utilize.[10,11] This would come into play when you have athletes that are uninsured or out-of-network where the schools in agreement with the provider would establish a set fee for a particular service. Common services include MRI, x-ray, office visits, common procedures, etc. This practice could also be applied to services provided to student-athletes with high deductible plans in an effort to reduce the amount of money filed against the school's secondary insurance or self-insurance fund.

Timely and Accurate Claim Filing

Most school secondary insurance programs require a series of items in order to process the claim for payment. First and foremost, the school representative, usually the athletic trainer, would need to complete a "Notification of Injury Form" that would identify the injury as athletically related and needing medical attention. The provider would need to file a CMS 1500/UB-92 claim form (explained in the reimbursement portion of this chapter), essentially the bill, with the student-athlete's primary insurance for processing and payment.[1,2,9] Upon payment from the primary insurance to the provider, the subscriber (student-athlete or his or her guardian) will receive an explanation of benefits, commonly referred to as an EOB. In order for the school's secondary insurance to provide payment for the balance of the unpaid claim, they are going to need to receive the Notification of Injury, CMS 1500 Claim Form as well as the EOB from the student-athlete's primary insurance company. Upon receiving that information, the secondary insurance or their third-party administer (TPA) will process and make payable any amount due to the provider. The TPA simply is the claims processing arm of the insurance company. This process typically falls within the duties of the athletic trainer and can become quite time consuming due to the number of individuals involved with processing a secondary insurance claim.

COST OF SECONDARY/ EXCESS SCHOOL INSURANCE

There are a lot of factors that go into determining a school's cost for secondary insurance. The first, as alluded to earlier, is the deductible amount the school wishes to carry. However, one of the most significant influences in determining the cost of secondary insurance is the school's claims loss history. A loss history is the amount of money spent by the insurance company to pay for the claims that were submitted. Typically, an insurance company will need a 3-year history plus the current year's loss runs in order to make a prediction of the cost to provide insurance for that particular school. Thus it is in the best interest of the school to contain cost or expenses filed against the schools' insurance as much as possible in an attempt to provide the best possible financial situation. What is not taken into consideration in working with these high deductibles is the amount of out-of-pocket expenses needed to make up that $10,000, which could be as high as an additional $250,000 in some cases, making their total cost for health care equal to $600,000. A current display of school premium and deductible plans can be found on the Collegiate Sports Medicine Foundation Web site (www.csmfoundation.org) within the Center for Cost-Containment and Insurance.

REIMBURSEMENT FOR SERVICES PROVIDED

Outside of cost-containment considerations, revenue and reimbursement is the most attractive reason to understand how the health care insurance industry operates. Athletic trainers in all settings are seeking and receiving reimbursement for services being provided as certified and licensed athletic trainers. This process has been more traditionally focused around the clinical/industrial athletic trainers, but recently all settings, including secondary schools, have been involved in some form of reimbursement process. It is important to keep in mind that the insurance industry is much like a moving target and one must constantly keep up with the environment, legislation, and issues affecting this process. Athletic trainers pursuing reimbursement for services first should address their state practice acts as well as any other state legislative issues affecting the reimbursement for services provided by athletic trainers.[10] A strong practice act without limitations in services provided or restrictions as to reimbursement opportunities will lend itself favorably to obtaining third-party reimbursement.

Typically when one speaks of reimbursement, he or she is referring to third-party reimbursement or the act of being compensated for a service from someone other than the patient/client/athlete (eg, an insurance company). However, one should not limit one's options for payment from a third-party source. The easiest, quickest, and least restrictive form is direct or cash-based compensation for services. Many individuals will elect to go beyond what their insurance plan provides them as it relates to rehabilitative services either in the duration of treatment or in the initial treatment itself. This simply involves marketing one's self to the public and establishing fees for services or groups of services on a cash payment system. This is permissible as long as the clinician is practicing within his or her scope and practice act in which he or she is providing services. This would also allow the patient the ability to seek reimbursement for the money he or she spent on athletic training services through his or her insurance if his or her insurance will reimburse him or her for those services.

In large scale, compensation for athletic training services is dependent upon the recognition of insurance carriers for those services. Regardless of the provider (athletic trainer, physical therapist, diagnostic facility, etc), there are a certain number of steps that need to be established in order for insurance carriers to reimburse that entity or individual for services provided to their patients. First, the patient would need to have "medical necessity" established for the types and frequency of care to be delivered. Typically, this comes in the form of a physician's letter establishing the medical necessity for a prescribed test, treatment, or service. Second, the facility and provider must be recognized by the insurance company as "capable" of providing services covered within their plan as well as establishing a fee structure for payment. This is the most difficult step in athletic training reimbursement efforts because insurance companies are not recognizing the athletic trainer as an approved provider of physical medicine both locally and nationally. Effective May 23, 2007, as a mandate under the Health Insurance Portability and Accountability Act (HIPAA), it will be necessary to obtain a National Provider Identifier (NPI) number in order to bill for health care services recognized by the Center for Medicaid and Medicare Services (CMS). Whether the athletic trainer is billing under Medicare or not, it will be necessary to receive this identifier as other insurance companies will look to standards established by Medicare as a benchmark for services that they will provide to their subscribers. One can obtain an NPI number by visiting the Department of Health and Human Services Web site at www.cms.hhs.gov/NationalProvIdentStand. It is important to note that having an NPI number does not guarantee reimbursement, although it is conceivable that in the near future the absence of an NPI will preclude the possibility of reimbursement. In addition to medical necessity and approval of insurance carriers in many cases, especially with HMOs, it will be necessary to obtain a referral for "athletic training services," not "physical therapy" from the prescribing physician. This distinction should also be noted in the establishment of medical necessity as well. Once medical necessity, referral, and approval from the insurance company is obtained, one must establish the parameters or limitations the patient will participate in the services provided. This can consist of co-pays that will need to be collected, deductible limits, and co-insurance as well as filing instructions for the provider. All of this must happen before the patient enters the facility for services to be rendered. During the initial visit, it is necessary for an initial evaluation to determine the patient's current limitations to activity as well as establish both short- and long-term goals of the treatment process. As with occupational therapists and physical therapists, athletic trainers have been provided a clinician-specific code for evaluation and re-evaluation (97005 and 97006) as identified by the Current Procedural Terminology or CPT codes.[12] Following an evaluation, the athletic trainer/clinician establishes a plan to accomplish the goals laid out by the physician and patient throughout the course of therapy. Additional CPT codes are utilized for the course of rehabilitation. Some of the more common procedures are listed in Table 9-5 and an example of CPT codes for a daily treatment appear in Box 9-2.[12]

What Are CPT Codes?

Current procedural terminology (CPT) codes define the specific therapeutic procedures (or services) that a provider has done for a patient. They are 5-number codes and are published annually in the CPT manual by the American Medical Association (AMA). The purpose of the coding system is to provide uniform language that accurately describes medical, surgical, and diagnostic services. Physicians, hospitals, and other health care providers use CPT codes to report medical services to private and public health insurance systems for purposes of reimbursement. A standard system of coding also allows for reliable nationwide data collection. CPT is trademarked by the AMA, which first published the codes in 1966.

Box 9-2

An Example of a Daily Treatment

- 97110 (therapeutic exercise)—2 units
- 97112 (neuromuscular re-education)—1 unit
- 97140 (manual therapy)—1 unit

In addition to the CPT codes being submitted to the insurance company for payment, a detailed accounting with goals and objectives needs to be established in the documentation for the patient encounter. Essentially, progress is going to need to be established, with complete evaluation, re-evaluation, treatment notes as well as discharge notes provided for payment.[3-6,9,11] Documentation for record keeping and reimbursement is covered in Chapter 8.

SUMMARY

- Recognize and define key terms associated with insurance and reimbursement.

  Like all entities, insurance companies have a unique vocabulary to help support their business functions. In order to interact with insurance companies it is important that you learn their jargon and what it means. Some basic terminology includes provider, subscriber, primary care physician (PCP), deductible, co-insurance, co-pay, in-network benefits, out-of-network benefits, PPO, HMO, managed care, indemnity plans, and CPT codes.

- Explain the associated components of insurance policies.

  Health insurance policies help defray the cost of medical expenses incurred as a result of injury or illness. The person(s) that are covered under the policy are referred to as subscribers, while the entity providing the service to the patient is called the provider. Generally, the insurance company is responsible for setting fee structures with providers, paying bills for the subscriber, and determining the benefits to be paid. Insurance companies are "for-profit" companies and are therefore in the business to make money.

  A premium is the amount paid by the subscriber for the insurance policy and the deductible is the amount that the subscriber is responsible for paying before the insurance company begins paying the claim. One way to control the cost of

Table 9-5

Common Rehabilitation Common Procedural Terminology Codes

CPT Code	Description
97110 (each 15 minutes)	Therapeutic exercise; used when performing therapeutic exercises to develop strength and endurance, ROM, and flexibility to one or more areas. One-on-one interaction with patient.
97112 (each 15 minutes)	Neuromuscular education; used when performing neuromuscular re-education of movement, balance coordination, kinesthetic sense, posture, and proprioception.
97140 (each 15 minutes)	Manual therapy; used when joint mobilization, manual lymphatic drainage, manual traction, myofascial release, craniosacral, soft tissue mobilization, or desensitization techniques are utilized.
97113 (each 15 minutes)	This charge is used for aquatic therapy when using the pool for therapeutic exercise, NOT conditioning activities.
97504	Orthotic fitting and training; used for orthotic training for upper and lower extremities. This charge should not be used in addition to a gait training charge.
Each of the following are based on 15-minute increments:	
97035	Ultrasound
97035	Phonophoresis
97032	Electrical stimulation
97033	Iontophoresis
97034	Contrast baths
97022	Whirlpool
97010	Hot packs
97010	Cold packs/ice massage
97016	Compression pump
Note: The rule of 15: Most physical medicine codes as above are in 15-minute increments. Any procedure provided from 7 to 22 minutes would be one (1) billable unit, 23 to 37 would be two (2) billable units, and so on.	

insurance coverage is to select a higher deductible, thus reducing the premiums. A co-pay is the amount the subscriber pays to a provider before receiving services. Co-insurance is applied after the deductible amount has been met by the subscriber and the remaining balance is distributed between the insurance company and subscriber as determined by the policy. Although there are some commonalities about co-insurance payments, it is policy specific.

Finally, some policies will require the insured to see a provider who is "in-network," which means the provider has been preapproved by the insurance company and a fee has been previously negotiated for his or her service. Out-of-network benefits are incurred when a provider is used with whom a prearranged fee has not been negotiated. While the insurance company will generally provide some payment, the amount the insured is responsible for is greater than if an in-network provider been used.

- Summarize the different types of insurance plans or programs.

Insurance plans fit into 2 broad categories: indemnity plans and managed care plans. Indemnity plans reimburse the subscriber for his or her medical expenses regardless of who provides the services. There can be several payment arrangements depending on how the indemnity plan is structured (see Table 9-2). Managed care plans generally involve a selected network of health care providers that the insured must see in order to maximize his or her insurance payment benefits (in-network benefits). Two common types of managed care plans include PPO and HMO. Additional insurance coverage options include HSA, Medicare, and Medicaid. The latter two are both federally and state funded and are available only to people who meet certain eligibility criteria.

- List several ways to contain health care costs.

  Several ways to contain health care costs were addressed in the chapter, including mandate primary insurance prior to participation, higher deductible on policies, adjusting the PCP to a local physician for in-network benefits (or having the athlete go home to his or her PCP if adjusting the PCP is not an option) negotiate fees with providers, and accurately file claims

- Explain the purpose of CPT codes for reimbursement.

  CPT codes define the specific therapeutic procedures (or services) that a provider has done for a patient. CPT codes provide a standard nomenclature that accurately describes medical, surgical, and diagnostic services. Physicians, hospitals, and other health care providers use CPT codes to report medical services to private and public health insurance systems for purposes of reimbursement.

- Discuss the requirements for athletic trainers to be reimbursed for their services.

  Foremost, compensation for athletic training is dependent upon the recognition of insurance carriers for those services. All claims for athletic training services will be denied without this recognition. Regardless of the provider, there are certain steps that need to be followed for insurance to reimburse for services rendered to a patient. Medical necessity has to be established, which generally comes from a physician; the facility and provider must be recognized by the insurance company as "capable" of providing services covered within their plan as well as establishing a fee structure for payment; obtain physician referral for "athletic training services," use the correct CTP codes; and document the patient's treatment regimen and progress appropriately.

REFERENCES

1. Ray R. *Management Strategies in Athletic Training*. Champaign, IL: Human Kinetics; 2005.
2. Rankin J, Ingersoll C. *Athletic Training Management*. New York, NY: McGraw Hill; 2001.
3. Health Insurance. Indemnity vs. managed care. Available at http://www.agencyinfo.net/iv/medical/types/indemnity-managed.htm. Accessed August 8, 2008.
4. Health Insurance. HMOs, PPO & POS plans. Available at http://www.agencyinfo.net/iv/medical/types/hmo-ppo-pos.htm. Accessed August 8, 2008.
5. Health Insurance. Medicare. Available at http://www.agencyinfo.net/iv/medical/types/medicare.htm. Accessed August 8, 2008.
6. Health Insurance. Medicaid. Available at http://www.agencyinfo.net/iv/medical/types/medicaid.htm. Accessed August 8, 2008.
7. National Collegiate Athletic Association. The Legislation & Governance Page. Available at http://www.ncaa.org/wps/ncaa?ContentID=18. Accessed July 14, 2008.
8. CIGNA Health Insurance. The Customer Care Page. Available at http://www.cigna.com/customer_care/index.html. Accessed July 14, 2008.
9. Konin, J, Frederick M. *Documentation for Athletic Training*. Thorofare, NJ: SLACK Incorporated; 2005.
10. Albohm M, Konin J, Campbell D. *Reimbursement for Athletic Trainers*. Thorofare, NJ: SLACK Incorporated; 2001.
11. Finkam S. *Athletic Training in Occupational Settings*. Thorofare, NJ: SLACK Incorporated; 2004.
12. American Medical Association. The Professional Resources Page. Available at http://www.ama-assn.org/ama/pub/category/3113.html. Accessed July 14, 2008.

IMPROVING PERSONAL EFFECTIVENESS

OBJECTIVES

At the end of this chapter, the reader will be able to:

- Differentiate between assertive, aggressive, and passive behaviors
- Describe the communication process
- Identify some barriers to effective listening and develop strategies to overcome these barriers
- Use verbal and nonverbal skills to actively listen
- Explain the Thomas-Kilmann Conflict Model
- Describe the SBI model for giving positive feedback and feedback for improvement and the skills necessary for this to be effective
- Describe what a difficult conversation is and why some conversations are considered difficult

As described in Chapter 1, effective leaders (and employees) has a heightened awareness about their behaviors and the impact they have on others. This occurs through giving, receiving, and seeking feedback and acting on the feedback they believe will make them a better leader—a willingness to change. Another model to consider in this change process is moving from a stimulus→response (S→R) model (Figure 10-1A) to a stimulus→conscious thought (pause)→responsible choice model (Figure 10-1B). The S→R would reflect one's unconscious habitual pattern of behaving. The shift occurs when we can pause between the stimulus and the response and as a result consider another way of responding or behaving. This results in a shift from spontaneous behavior to considered behavior (Figure 10-1C). The skills described in this chapter are critical to successful leadership and are embedded in all of the leadership qualities enumerated in Chapter 1. These skills are also paramount in shifting from spontaneous behavior to considered behavior. The purpose of this chapter is to address several specific skill sets that are necessary to be a successful leader and/or employee and to provide specific techniques where appropriate.

ASSERTIVENESS

Assertiveness is the ability to express one's self honestly without denying the rights of others.[1] This definition holds the notion of appropriateness in that there are limits to self-expression; those limits are the boundaries of others' rights to be treated decently, without demands, coercion, or judgment.[1] In my experience of teaching countless assertiveness workshops, I have observed that many times being assertive is confused with aggressiveness, when in fact they are 2 different sets of behaviors. This section will provide an overview of the differences between assertiveness, aggressiveness, and passivity as well as a model to explain how these behaviors are demonstrated.

Assertive, Aggressive and Passive Behaviors

Table 10-1 compares and contrasts these 3 types of behavior. The primary delineation between assertive and aggressive behaviors is taking into

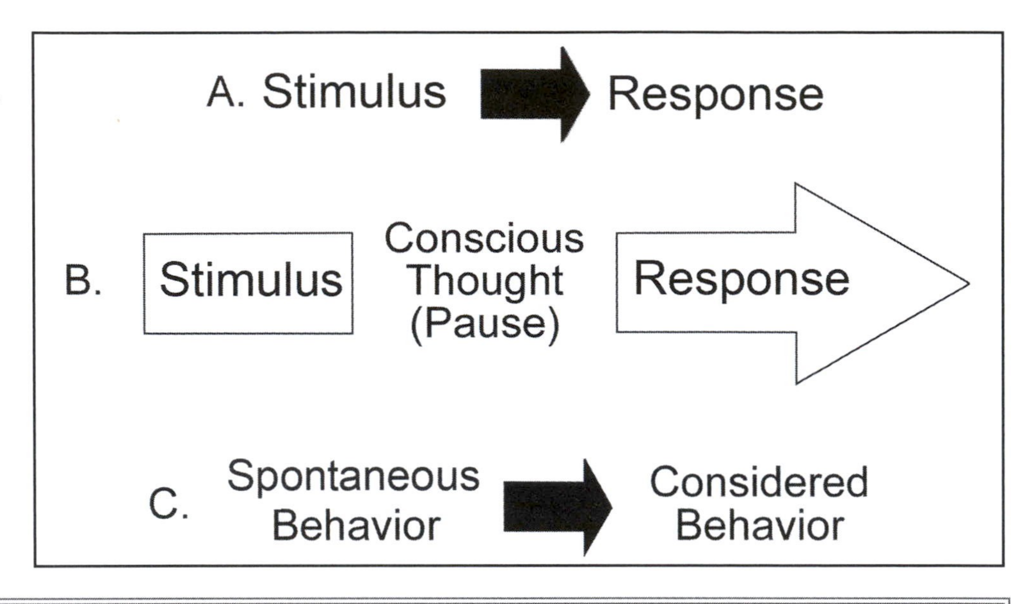

Figure 10-1. Movement from a stimulus-response model of behavior to considered behavior.

Table 10-1

Comparison of Three Types of Influence Behaviors

Passive Behaviors	*Assertive Behaviors*	*Aggressive Behaviors*
Demonstrates a lack of respect for his or her own needs and rights	Protects own rights and respects the rights of others	Violates rights, takes advantage of others
Does not express his or her honest feelings, needs, values, and con cerns	Achieves goals without hurting others	Expresses feelings, needs, and ideas at the expense of others
Allows others to violate his or her space, deny his or her rights, and ignore his or her needs	Assumes ownership of his or her thoughts, feelings, desires, needs, as well as ownership of the consequences of his or her actions	May achieve goals at the expense of others
Rarely states his or her desires when often that is all it would take to have them met	Socially and emotionally expressive	Defensive, belligerent; humiliates others
Nonverbals, may undercut their expression of a need or position	Feels good about self and has appropriate confidence in self	Explosive, unpredictably hostile and angry
Allows others to choose	Chooses for self	Intrudes on others' choices

account the rights of others. People demonstrating aggressive behavior are only concerned about their rights, wants, and desires at the expense of someone else's. People demonstrating assertive behavior are not only concerned about their rights, but also the rights and needs of others. Passive behavior on the other hand demonstrates a lack of respect for one's own needs and rights, as well as the rights and needs of others taking precedence over theirs.[2] Passive behavior is also characterized by not disagreeing with others, keeping feelings hidden from others, and not speaking out in regards to what is on their mind.[2] There is a further type of behavior referred to as concealed aggressiveness[2] or passive-aggressive behavior, which is when one subtly makes sure that his or her rights and needs prevail. The behavior is very subversive to others.

Assertiveness Model

The Interpersonal Influence Model[2] is an assertiveness model that takes into account the 4 assertiveness behaviors described in Figure 10-2. The 4 quadrants in the model are formed by the amount of openness (low to high) and the amount of consideration for others (low to high) a person engages in. Openness is an individual's willingness to disclose to another his or her thoughts, feelings, past experiences, reasons, etc.[2] Consideration for others is an individual's willingness

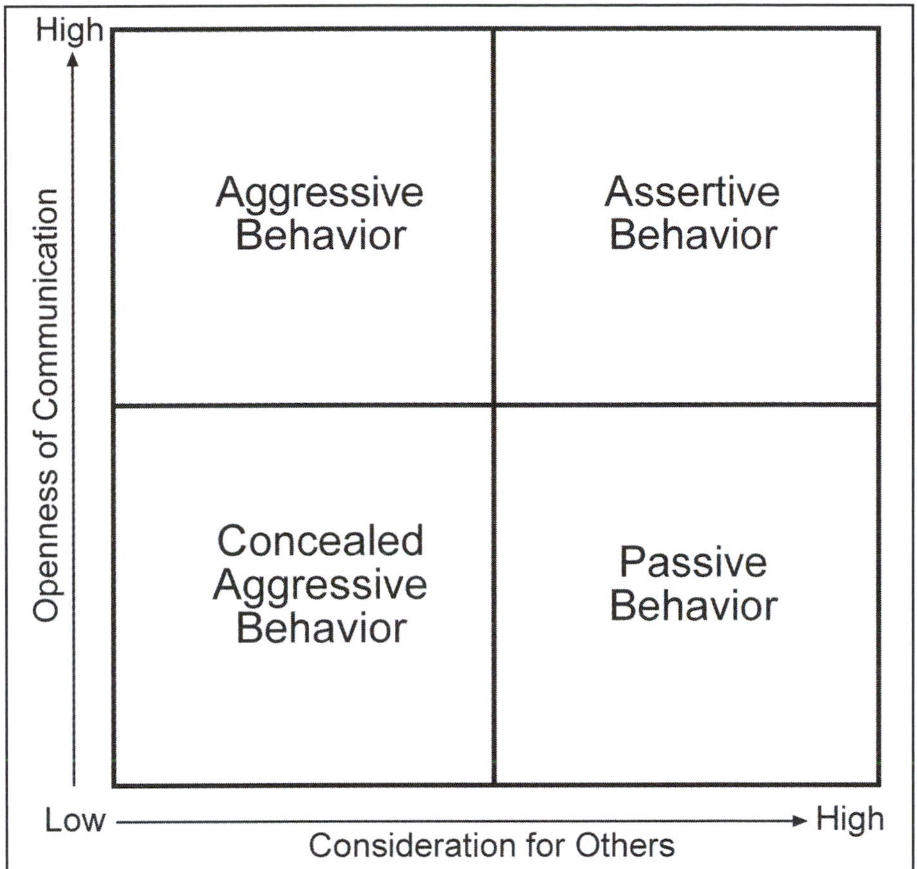

Figure 10-2. Assertiveness behavior model. (Adapted from *Interpersonal Influence Inventory*. 4th ed. King of Prussia, PA: HRDQ; 2004.)

to accord others the same rights he or she accords him- or herself. The influence pattern is determined depending on the relative use of each of these sets of behaviors. Based on human nature, we all have a primary pattern that we engage in. The Interpersonal Influence Inventory[2] (HRDQ; King of Prussia, PA, www.hrdq.com) is a self-assessment that can be used to determine your primary influence pattern.

While there may be times that all of these behaviors might be warranted, the assertive pattern of behavior is preferred. There are many times when an athletic trainer needs to be assertive, particularly when the well-being of an athlete is at stake and you are intervening on his or her behalf with coaches, administrators, or others.

LISTENING

Listening is a core interpersonal skill and one which we probably do not do very well. Yet, given that it is a cornerstone skill in the communication process, I find it interesting that if you ask virtually any group of professionals or nonprofessionals if they have had any formal academic training to improve their listening skills you will get only a few hands raised. We teach math, reading, and writing skills in the formal school system and maybe a speech class, yet we rarely teach the skill set associated with listening. While there are some people who are inherently good listeners (as with other behavioral skills) without formal training, for the vast majority of people listening does not come naturally. Fortunately, like many of these behavioral skills, listening can be learned. The purpose of this section is to describe the communication process, heighten your awareness of the barriers to listening and the associated strategies to overcome them, and use verbal and nonverbal skills to improve your ability to listen.

Effective Listening

Box 10-1 lists some interesting communication facts; the results of which show that on the whole people are poor listeners. Of particular interest is the fact that we are capable of mentally handling 400 to 500 words/minute while only speaking at an average rate of 125 words/minute. This is one reason that listening is difficult.[3] It is virtually impossible to stay connected to another person and listen to him or her 100% of the time. Your brain quickly fills in those "down times" it has in other ways. Sometimes words remind another person of his or her own experiences

Box 10-1

Interesting Communication Facts

- Most workers spend roughly half of their business hours listening. Research studies show that, on average, individuals listen at a 25% level of efficiency.
- If each of the 100 million workers in this country made a simple $10 listening mistake each year, the cost would be a billion dollars per year.
- After a 10-minute talk:
  - 20 minutes later—listener forgets 42%
  - 60 minutes later—listener forgets 56%
  - 8 hours later—listener forgets 64%
  - 6 days later—listener forgets 75%
- Average rate of speech for most Americans is 125 words/minute while the brain can handle 400 to 500 words/minute.

Adapted from Fisher S. *Effective Listening*. Amherst, MA: HRD Press, Inc, 1996.

(referred to as a trigger) and mentally result in the person taking a "mental trip" to that past memory/experience, unknown to the other person in the conversation. Thus, the use of the skills described later is helpful with maintaining that connection to another person, although not 100% foolproof.

Insight: Remember that in a conversation you are not capable of listening (staying connected) to the other person 100% of the time, thus do not expect them to do the same for you.

How many times have you been asked, "Did you hear me?" and you responded, "Yes, I heard you." This is probably a true statement in that you heard words coming from a person's mouth, but really made no meaning of the words; you heard something, but you were not listening. Hearing and listening are different phenomena. Hearing is done with the ears. It is the sense by which noises and tones are received as stimuli. Hearing is a sensory experience in which sound waves are gathered indiscriminately. Conversely, listening is an intellectual and emotional process that integrates physical, emotional, and intellectual inputs in search for meaning and understanding.[3] Thus, we probably hear a lot of things, but really only listen to a fraction of what we hear. An effective listener is characterized by the following:

- Discerning and understanding the sender's meaning
- Listening not only to the words, but to the meanings behind the words
- Hearing what is said between sentences, the nonverbal cues (ie, what the speaker thinks and feels)
- Participating actively (not passively)
- Interacting with the speaker in developing meaning and reaching understanding

Some speech communication specialists have found that when you are listening your heart speeds up, your blood circulates faster, and your body temperature rises.[3] In other words, it takes energy to listen and is thus referred to as active listening.

Communication Process

Figure 10-3 depicts a simple illustration of how the communication process occurs. Step 1 in Figure 10-3 illustrates the process where one person, the sender, transfers what is referred to as a "mind picture" as accurately as possible from his or her head into the head of another person, the receiver. However, the receiver never knows exactly what "mind picture" the sender has in his or her head because it is impossible to read another person's mind. All the receiver can do is guess, relying on interpretation of the message he or she hears—whether verbal or nonverbal. In step 2, the sender codes his or her verbal message. The receiver cannot possibly know what "mind picture" is in the head of the sender. If the sender wants to share it, he or she must select an appropriate verbal code that will accurately represent his or her picture. The sender transmits that verbal message (code) in step 3 and must be decoded (step 4) by the receiver. In this step, the receiver guesses or makes an inference about the meaning of the words. Real understanding of another happens only when the receiver's mind picture (the results of decoding) closely matches what the sender intended in his or her expression (step 5). To be sure that the receiver's impression matches the sender's expression, the receiver must listen and then respond (feedback—step 6). From this feedback, the sender gets tangible evidence of how the receiver decoded the message.[4]

If each party engaged in conversation will be 100% responsible for the success or failure of the communication and uses the skills associated with active listening, the communication will be richer, fuller, and more meaningful and will reduce the likelihood of miscommunication.

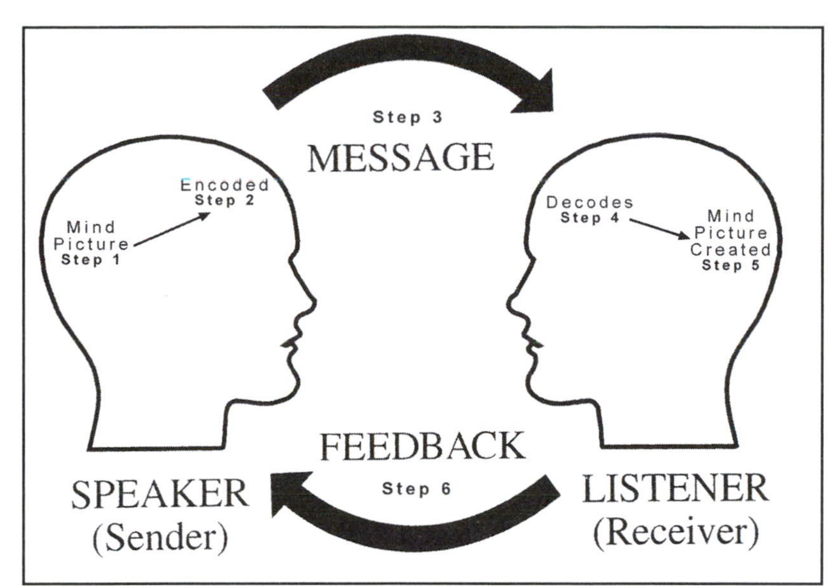

Figure 10-3. Communication process. (Adapted from Fisher S. *Effective Listening*. Amherst, MA: HRD Press, Inc.; 1996.)

Communication Barriers

Barriers to successful communication can be classified as physical, emotional, and/or intellectual. These 3 barriers can be further segmented into internal or external barriers, creating a matrix that appears in Table 10-2. Most of the communication barriers found in the external-physical quadrant are easily resolved, such as moving the conversation to another area if there is loud noise or visual distractions or asking someone to speak louder or slow down his or her rate of speech. The barriers that fall in the other 5 quadrants can be more difficult to manage, such as health problems, distracted by personal problems, unfamiliar with the content, or having biases about the person who is speaking. However, many of the others can be managed, such as asking people to clarify language you do not understand or words that are unfamiliar to you, not multitasking, and/or suspending your innate desire to respond. Many times when someone is talking to us we are not actively listening, rather we are mentally crafting our response, particularly if we feel verbally attacked. Covey's[4] fifth habit in his book, *7 Habits of Highly Successful People*, states, "Seek First to Understand, Then to be Understood." This requires one to suspend his or her judgment and to be genuinely curious in what the other person has to say and how he or she says it (the emotion behind it). While at best this is difficult to do for many people, the 4 core verbal skills discussed later in the chapter will help.

Receiver and Sender Blocks

There are many reasons it can be difficult to listen to somebody; some are a result of the sender's difficulty in putting what he or she wants to say into words, doing all of the talking, a "know it all" attitude of the sender, not feeling free to say what he or she really means, etc (Box 10-2). Additionally, there can be blocks present for the receiver of the message that make it difficult to stay connected to the sender and listen to what he or she has to say (Table 10-3). I believe several of the receiver blocks listed in Table 10-3 are more prevalent than others, including words that have different meanings, preoccupation, triggers, thinking about how to respond, spare time, uninterested, and judgmental.

Box 10-2

Sender Blocks to Communication

- May not be in touch with his or her real feelings (a fuzzy "mind picture")
- May not feel free to say what he or she really means
- May have difficulty putting his or her "mind picture" into words
- May not know (or care) whether receiver has decoded correctly
- Uses too much jargon
- Sender uses speech pattern and tone that is annoying
- "Know it all" attitude on part of sender
- Prefaces own messages—devalues self (eg, starts off messages with the phrase "Maybe it's just my opinion, but ...")
- Does all the talking and very little listening

Table 10-2

Communication Barrier Matrix

	Physical	*Emotional*	*Intellectual*
External	Noise Visual distractions Behavior of coworkers Climate of workplace Speaker not speaking loudly or clearly enough	Lack of feedback from your supervisor Faulty feedback from the speaker Negative incentives for listening Being a target for speakers emotions	Being unfamiliar with the content of the message Being unfamiliar with the speaker's word usage Having problems with the speaker's language or speech Receiving an incorrect message
Internal	Fatigue Health problems Pain/discomfort Hearing loss	Being distracted by personal problems Reacting emotionally Hearing what you want to hear Being biased in your listening Jumping to conclusions or making assumptions	Having difficulty remembering information Having trouble applying what you have learned to the situation Having difficulty understanding or processing the message Trying to do two things at once

Adapted from Fisher S. *Effective Listening*. Amherst, MA: HRD Press, Inc, 1996.

Table 10-3

Receiver Blocks: Explanations and Examples

Receiver Blocks	*Explanations and Examples*
Words have different meanings	Example: If you say "Hi, how are you?" to a number of subordinates, there will be many interpretations: "Well, here's old snoopy again, trying to check up on us." "It certainly is wonderful that he is really interested in my progress." "What does he mean by that?" "All right already, I know we are behind, so get out of here and let us catch up." "Now that's something to remember when I get up there in management. You can't run an operation sitting behind a desk in some isolated office. You have to roam the ship to get a first-hand feel for what is going on." "Uh oh he knows how I messed up yesterday." "That is what I like about him, always ready with a helping hand when you need it."
Pre-set ideas	The receiver may have pre-set ideas about the value of what will be said (ie, unimportant, boring, old news)
Difficult to understand	The receiver may have difficulty understanding and rather than telling the sender it is difficult, the receiver just nods as if understanding.
Redundant	The receiver may feel the sender is redundant
Preoccupation	The receiver may be preoccupied. For example: A New York columnist reported that a socialite was so preoccupied with making a good impression, she did not hear her guests. To test this theory, he came late to the next party and was greeted by her at the door. "I'm sorry I'm late, but I murdered my wife this evening and had the hardest time stuffing her body in my trunk." The socialite beamed, "Well, darling, the important thing is that you have arrived—now the party can begin."

(continued)

Table 10-3 (continued)

Receiver Blocks: Explanations and Examples

Receiver Blocks	*Explanations and Examples*
Triggers	The sender says something that is a "trigger" for the receiver. We all have words or phrases that serve as triggers and provoke emotional responses that cause us to disconnect from the sender.
Filters	Due to past experiences, the receiver may filter out what the sender is saying. For example: "That person has never had an original idea in her life." or "That person has never made a relevant point in his life."
Thinking	The receiver may be busy thinking about what he or she will say next and does not decode what the receiver is sending.
Charisma	The charisma of the sender may block the communication.
Nonobservant	The receiver may not carefully observe the nonverbal message.
Decodes selectively	The receiver hears only what he or she wants to.
Spare time	The receiver is capable of thinking many times faster than the sender can talk. Average rate of speech for most Americans is 125 words per minute. Brain can handle many times this amount. Results in "spare time" for the listener.
Authority	The receiver may choose to listen only to authority.
Uninterested	The receiver is not interested in the topic and does not bother to clarify.
Judgmental	The receiver may be highly judgmental of the sender or topic.

Words do have different meanings for different people, and we typically define a word not necessarily by the dictionary's definition, but rather by experience. I would venture to say we all have had experiences when something was miscommunicated because a word was defined differently. To compound this problem, receivers of a message typically do not inquire into vague language, such as "I understand," "I am not respected around here," and "We need to communicate better." The words *understand*, *respected*, and *communicate* are all vague words, and if we were to ask 10 people what they mean we would get several different answers. For example, what translates to respect to one person can be different for another since his or her operational definitions of respect are different. In my experience, I have seen many people say they do not feel respected by another person, yet the other person believes the behaviors they are engaging in do show respect. When the 2 people can share their definition of respect and feel listened to by the other, the relationship can move from a point of common ground, not difference.

We have already mentioned that different words can serve as a trigger for others (receivers) of which the sender is totally unaware. The trigger will mentally transport the receiver to the experience that the trigger evokes. For example, the word "fine" served as a trigger for a client of mine. When he heard someone use the word fine, particularly in a conflictual situation, it translated for him as "bad." While that is generally not true for most individuals, based on his past experiences when he heard the word fine it generally meant bad. Not only did this serve as a trigger for him, but it also is an example of using experiences to define a word.

Often we are preoccupied with many of the events, issues, and problems that are going on in our life and at any given moment we are just unable to compartmentalize these struggles. If that is the case, I suggest simply asking the other person if the conversation can occur at a different time. Granted, there are some things that cannot wait but my experience is that people understand that there are times that are better than others to have a conversation. If a person knows that you will be in a better state of mind in a couple of hours or the next day, he or she is generally willing to wait, knowing that you will be able to listen to him or her instead of just hear what he or she has to say.

Finally, being uninterested in a topic is a little tougher, particularly if that is compounded by being highly judgmental of the person sending the message. Just because you care about a topic and want to talk about it does not necessarily mean the other person cares about it or is even remotely interested in the topic. Often when someone is interested in something the expectation is held that we should all be interested in it. The true synergy arises when we find ourselves in dialogue around a topic that all parties have an interest in and energy to support the conversation.

How Do You Know When Someone Is Listening?

The list below provides a few behaviors that people will exhibit when they believe that the other person is listening to them.

- Responds with empathy
- Makes eye contact
- Avoids distractions
- Paraphrases what you have said
- Leans forward
- Nods
- Asks appropriate questions
- Receptive body language
- Probes for missing information
- Takes notes

Nonverbal Language

Body language is the message the body tells. Generally, your behavior speaks louder than words. Body language can support or refute what you are saying or at the very least send a mixed message. While your words may be saying "Yes" to something, your real stance is "No" and this "No" can come out in your body language and can carry a bigger impact on the other person than your words. Such behaviors as your arms crossed across your chest versus by your side or leaning forward in a chair versus sitting back can all send messages to another person as to your interest in what he or she has to say or your response to it.

However, just as words can be misinterpreted, so can body language. Body language is data that we "take in" as part of our meaning-making process, and when body language is not congruent with the spoken message, it generally creates confusion since one is not exactly sure what is being communicated (ie, a mixed message). As mentioned earlier, if both parties are 100% responsible for the communication, then one would inquire as to the mixed message he or she is receiving. For instance, "I hear you saying that you have no concerns about your surgery and the tremor in your voice and wrinkled forehead tell me otherwise." At least by heightening the athlete's awareness of the mixed message being received, an opportunity is provided to explore any reservations the athlete has about his or her surgery.

Our natural human pattern is to see something, make meaning of it for ourselves based on our point of view, and to then perceive it as fact; all of this is done in a split second. We rarely inquire about what we saw and the meaning we made of it. If we chose to "check out" our observations, it can: 1) heighten a person's awareness about his or her behavior and/or 2) give him or her the opportunity to provide another meaning to you for the behavior. A global example of multiple meanings for a specific body language or mannerisms is that in one country it can have one meaning and have a different connotation in another country.

Table 10-4 provides a list of some of the more common body behaviors with explanations that people can use to improve communication as well as being used as a "test" for perceiving if someone is listening to them or at least interested in what they have to say. Of the behaviors listed in Table 10-4, pay attention to the use of silence. I believe silence can be a very powerful technique during a conversation. I find it remarkable that when a question is asked, a response is expected almost immediately. Another great use of silence is when we give feedback to someone that he or she is not aware of or expecting. To sit in silence for several seconds or more gives the person time to process the message and make meaning of it for him- or herself. Many times the reason silence is not used is simply that the person is not comfortable in silence and needs to fill the space. Sometimes we just want a difficult conversation to be over.

Verbal Techniques

Verbal techniques are used as a part of your speech pattern to improve communication through enhancing understanding. These skills can help minimize some of the communication barriers discussed earlier in this section. Four verbal techniques will be described here: 1) paraphrasing, 2) perception checking, 3) asking questions, and 4) probing.

Paraphrasing

Paraphrasing is the act of restating, in your own words, what a person has said. Your restatement tries to capture both the cognitive (content/facts) and the affective (feelings) components of the message. It is a way of checking whether you and the sender are

Table 10-4

Nonverbal Techniques

<table>
<tr><th>Attribute</th><th colspan="2">Explanation</th></tr>
<tr><td rowspan="5">Voice</td><td colspan="2">The chart below may help you become aware of the impact your voice has on others.</td></tr>
<tr><td>Voice Attribute</td><td>Definition</td></tr>
<tr><td>Tone</td><td>Tone of voice involves the pitch of the voice (high or low) and the emotional overtones (enthusiastic, sad, bored, anticipatory, fearful).
A higher-pitched voice usually elicits excitement or tension in listeners.
A lower-pitched voice is generally calming and helps people slow down or relax.</td></tr>
<tr><td>Inflection</td><td>Inflection is the way a person varies the tone of voice when speaking. In any sentence, a person will raise and lower his or her voice to convey meaning.
A person who uses little or no inflection speaks in a monotone.</td></tr>
<tr><td>Pace</td><td>The pace with which you speak affects the group as well.
Too fast a pace may make the group hyperactive or tire them out.
Too slow a pace may put them to sleep.
Vary the pace of your speaking to fit the task.</td></tr>
<tr><td>Eye contact</td><td colspan="2">The listener must maintain eye contact with the person(s) he or she is speaking to, which shows that he or she is actively listening. If the listener looks away, the speaker loses a sense of focus as well. Eye contact shows that the listener is really paying attention. Use eye contact frequently as the person speaks and feel free to record ideas as well.
Recording the speaker's ideas is just as powerful as eye contact. It proves that you are listening and validates the person's contribution. Turn back to the speaker when you are finished recording and, if he or she is still speaking, continue to listen actively.</td></tr>
<tr><td>Attentiveness</td><td colspan="2">When you listen actively and maintain eye contact, you are being attentive. Not only does it involve all aspects of active listening and maintaining eye contact, but it means listening with all of the senses.
Be attentive to what the speaker is saying, how he or she is saying it, what the underlying mood of the message is, what is not being said, the atmosphere in the room, the reaction of others in the room, and so on.</td></tr>
<tr><td>Facial expressions</td><td colspan="2">Most people:
Do not always realize facial expressions affect whether or not people believe you are listening to them.
Generally take-in the expressions of another person but may not be aware that they are frowning, scowling, smiling, or even appear expressionless or "deadpan."</td></tr>
<tr><td>Silence</td><td colspan="2">Being okay with silence is a core skill for a good listener, particularly after asking a question. For some people, it takes time to process the question and formulate an answer. Some people have a tendency to:
Ask a question and then answer it
Pose a question and when it is not immediately answered, ask it again
Note: Be ready to give someone 30 seconds or more to formulate his or her answer.</td></tr>
<tr><td>Distracting habits</td><td colspan="2">Some common, distracting habits include:
Rattling coins/keys in pockets
Fiddling with clothes, jewelry, or hair
Clicking the top of a pen on and off
Scratching arm, ear, or nose
Pacing
Moving papers, charts, or other materials without purpose
Squinting or frowning
Habits become part of your demeanor unconsciously, and they are sometimes hard for you to notice. Many distracting mannerisms are the result of not knowing what to do with your hands while other people are talking.</td></tr>
</table>

hearing the same message. In my years of teaching paraphrasing, there are 2 areas that I have found to be pitfalls with this skill. First, to use this skill effectively you must be willing to interrupt the other person. One intent of paraphrasing is to help you stay connected to the other person and if the sender is into a 5-minute monologue, this can be difficult. The reason interrupting is difficult is because a prevalent societal norm is that this is considered rude. However, I urge you to consider that if you are into a long monologue, would you rather be interrupted by someone who says he or she needs to see if he or she understands what you are saying or allow you to go, then after 5 minutes tell you he or she did not understand what you were saying? Generally, people would prefer to be interrupted so you can both be on the same page.

Secondly, notice that there are 2 parts to this skill. You must capture the content/facts that you hear and the emotions or feelings that you believe are associated with the words. Generally, I observe that people are good at getting the content and miss the most impactful piece, the emotions/feelings behind the message. If you want to have an impact on the other person and have him or her truly feel that you are listening to him or her, then feeding back his or her emotions to him or her is very impactful. Box 10-3 gives several examples of how paraphrasing could look when connecting the content and emotions together.

Box 10-3

Examples of Paraphrases

- "Let me see if I understand what you said, 'You stayed up all night studying for a test and are disappointed that the professor did not give you the test?'"
- "What I heard you say was, 'The fullback was injured in yesterday's scrimmage, you were allowed to evaluate the athlete and came up with the same assessment as the head athletic trainer and you seem delighted that you were able to do that?'"
- "The meaning I made out of what you said was, 'John was to meet you at the library to study and he said something came up and he could not meet you and what really aggravated you was he did not call to tell you?'"

Note: See if you can determine which is the content/fact and which is the emotional or feeling part of the paraphrase.

Finally, do not worry if you are not exactly right with the content and emotions. The power in this skill is that if you are not exactly right, misinterpreted something, or left something out in your paraphrase, the sender has the opportunity to correct you so that there is a better mutual understanding. Remember, our brains can process more words/minute then we can speak and paraphrasing is one tool to help you stay connected to the other person, minimizing your "mental breaks" during a conversation. Also, if you are concentrating on paraphrasing, it is difficult to spend your mental processes on thinking about how to respond. Box 10-4 lists some of the benefits of paraphrasing.

Box 10-4

When to Use Paraphrasing

- When we are talking with someone and are not sure we completely understand what is being said to us.
- Someone who uses long, involved bursts of communication containing many issues, to slow that person down and encourage him to focus his own communication.
- Someone who seems shy, to slow you down and allow the other to bring out needed detail and affect without being steamrolled.
- Someone who seems not to be listening to him- or herself, who seems just to be filling space with sound, to help him or her stop, introspect, and focus.
- Someone it is ordinarily very difficult for you to pay attention to, forcing you to pay attention closely to find meaning in what you usually regard as unworthwhile verbiage.

Box 10-5 provides you with some lead-in examples to help you get the paraphrase started. I urge you to try out these lead-ins and see which one(s) work for you. Initially, as with all of these skills, it might seem awkward at first, but keep using them and they will become natural for you.

Perception Checking

Perception checking is the other end of the stick from paraphrasing. Here YOU (the message sender) are asking the other person(s) to paraphrase what you have been saying. You want to know if your communications are clear, if your entire message has been received, or if the person with whom you are talking has been able to absorb all that you are trying to

Box 10-5

Examples of Paraphrasing Lead-Ins

- "Did I hear you right? What you said was..."
- "Let me run that out again..."
- "Here is what I hear you say..."
- "Is this what you meant?"
- "The sense of that for me was..."
- "I hear you saying..."
- "What I got from that was... Was that the whole idea?"
- "You seem to be feeling... when you say..."
- "My feeling right now is that we do not understand each other; here is what I think you are saying..."
- "My attention wandered on the last—can you try and see if I got all you were saying..."
- "What you are saying is this...; but your face and body are saying... and what you were saying 5 minutes ago was... Can you clarify the apparent differences in those 2 statements for me?"

communicate. Box 10-6 lists some situations in which this skill is useful. The difficulty with this technique is that people believe that asking someone to basically paraphrase what they just said puts them on the spot and potentially can embarrass them if they were not listening. While this could be true in some cases, the way that the request is framed minimizes this effect. Remember, nobody is going to stay connected to what you have to say the entire time. If it is important for you to know that someone understands what you have said, use one of the lead-ins in Box 10-7.

Asking Questions

Another core listening skill is asking well-timed, appropriate questions to focus and steer a conversation. We are looking for facts when we are asking questions. There are 2 basic types of questions: 1) open-ended and 2) closed-ended. Open-ended questions call for the person to expound on the topic. Closed-ended questions usually call for a "yes" or "no" response. Uses for both open- and closed-ended questions are highlighted in Box 10-8.

Be careful of what kinds of questions you are asking. Many times you might want an open-ended answer and ask a closed-ended question. For example, if you ask the question, "Do you understand?" this calls for a closed-ended answer (ie, yes or no). If the person answers "yes," do you really know if he or she understands or what he or she understands? If you truly wanted to know what he or she understood, you would need to follow up with an open-ended question, "What did you understand?" This is also an example of a habitual (unconscious) questioning technique. We ask, "Do you understand?" and get a "yes" answer and when the results become apparent, it is evident he or she did not understand what you wanted to happen. Box 10-9 provides examples of both open- and closed-ended questions. Of the 4 listening skills presented here, I find that people are very good at this one; it is something we are unconsciously competent at (see Chapter 1).

Box 10-6

When to Use Perception Checking

- Negotiations between 2 individuals or groups where it is absolutely necessary to ensure understanding of what is being discussed.
- When you get a clue that you are misunderstood or some subtlety is escaping the person with whom you are talking.
- When you feel you may have misstated or misrepresented a position and you need to check out what has been received.
- When you feel things have moved too rapidly and some of the details are not registering.
- As a way of summarizing a discussion before moving on.

Box 10-7

Examples of Perception Checking Lead-Ins

- "I'm not sure that I was very clear. Can you read that back to me?"
- "Your last statement indicated that your idea of what I've been saying isn't quite the same as mine. Can you restate the whole idea?"
- "All right, let's review. What are the alternatives I've stated, and what are the strengths and weaknesses of each?"
- "This is a key point. I need to see that we are hearing the same thing. Would you summarize our agreement to this point?"
- "Can you paraphrase my last statement?"
- "Can you summarize what I've been saying?"
- "Where are we?"
- "What did you just hear me say?"

Box 10-8

Uses of Open- and Close-Ended Questions

Use open-ended questions when...

- You want people to participate and think
- Generating data or ideas
- Exploring options more deeply
- Improving honesty between people

Use closed-ended questions when...

- You want to find facts
- Wrapping up a discussion
- You want to obtain more specific information
- Trying to move the discussion along

Box 10-9

Open- and Close-Ended Questions

Open-Ended Questions

- "What is your reaction to that?"
- "How can this process be improved?"
- "What alternatives do we have?"
- "What suggestions do you have for ...?"
- "Why do you think there has been such a downturn in sales?"
- "How does that relate to our goal of...?"

Close-Ended Questions

- "Do you agree then that this is the best choice?"
- "Have we covered everything?"
- "Are you ready to move on?"
- "Are you willing to support this decision 100%?"
- "Is this a realistic objective for goals?"
- "Do we need more information before we can make a decision?"
- "Can you stay another 30 minutes to finish this discussion?"

Probing

Probing is a technique used to discover more information and to keep someone talking. Knowing when to probe is an important skill because probing can make a positive difference in the quality and depth of the discussion. Many people get probing confused with asking questions and actually believe they are probing when in actuality they are asking an open-ended question. A comparison of the lead-ins in Box 10-9 with 10-11 gives examples of how questioning and probing are different and may help in differentiating the two. Probing has the ability to take the conversation to a deeper level and find out the root cause(s) of a problem (Box 10-10). Examples of some probing lead-ins are listed in Box 10-11.

Box 10-10

Uses of the Skill of Probing

Probing may help:

- Find the root of an issue or problem
- Explore a concern or idea that may otherwise be overlooked
- Encourage a person to explore issues in greater depth and to value his or her own thinking process
- Open the person up to more honest sharing of information and concerns
- Increase the trust level
- Uncover key facts that have not been discussed
- Increase creativity and open-mindedness

Box 10-11

Examples of Probing Lead-Ins

- "Oh?"
- "Hmmm"
- "Why is that?"
- "What makes you think so?"
- "Tell me more about...?"
- "Does this relate to what Juan said earlier about...?"
- "Explain what you mean by...?"
- "Could you be more specific?"
- "Can you go further into that?"
- "Can you give us an example?"
- "What else happened?"
- "Can you say more about that?"

Communication between 2 or more people is a very complex process and many barriers work together to impede this process. The ability to actively listen is a core competency to minimize these barriers and improve the understanding of the spoken word. The verbal and nonverbal techniques outlined in this section can help in reducing these barriers and result in richer communication.

CONFLICT MANAGEMENT

Conflict will occur when 2 or more people are working together. Conflict will increase tension and stress, often causing work quality and morale to decrease and can ultimately result in a barrier between people if left unresolved. Some people do not care to face conflict, and if you are a leader, it is your job to work toward resolving it. This section will provide an overview of what conflict is, how it is caused, and a model that illustrates that we have 5 choices when it comes to engaging in conflict.

CONFLICT OVERVIEW

There are many definitions for conflict, but the operational definition we will use here is, "Any situation where your concerns or desires differ from another person's."[5,6] Unfortunately, in my experience of working with groups, conflict is viewed with a negative connotation, as if there should not be any conflict between people, yet on the other hand people will acknowledge that difference is important. With this difference comes conflict. Conflict left unresolved can become a destructive force and drive a wedge between people within a group. On the other hand, conflict is typically not viewed as a positive force, one in which if I choose to engage another person in difference the result could be an improved relationship.

An interesting pattern in many of these interpersonal skills is where they are obtained, since most are not taught in formal academic environments, yet are crucial in producing a productive and motivated workforce. In regards to conflict, I would suggest examining how conflict was managed in your home. Was disagreement within the household an acceptable behavior or was it something that was not dealt with? Conflict skills are generally acquired without formal education or guidance and modeled after the behavior of others.

Box 10-12 lists several sources from which conflict can stem. One of the biggest contributors to conflict is perception. Look at Figure 10-4. What do you see? If you see an old lady, you are correct. If you see a young lady, you are correct. Some people have great difficulty seeing both ladies in the picture, yet they are both there. Often we make up a story or a judgment based on what we see when in actuality there can be another story we have not considered or of which we are unaware. Most disagreements between people and in groups come from perceptions and/or inadvertently "stepping into" someone's value set, which you have no idea you have done. When this occurs, the perception is that you are rude, disrespectful, etc, when in actuality you did not have a clue about the other person's values since that is a conversation that has never occurred, yet a perception is generated just the same. As humans we have this innate ability to observe behavior and generate a story about another person, hold it as our perception and in some instances our truth, and never engage the other person about it. In most instances, we are so concentrated on the difference between us and others, particularly when they irritate us, that we never consider looking at what we may have in common. A good way to shift a situation in which conflict exists is to explore what the commonalities are or where we are in agreement versus "hanging out" in the difference.

Box 10-12

Sources of Conflict

Conflict can stem from a number of sources, including the following:

- Perception
- Aggressive or competitive nature of human beings
- Competition for limited resources
- Clashes of values and interests
- Role-based conflict
- Drives for power
- Poorly defined responsibilities
- The introduction of change
- The habits of response
- I want... versus we need...

THOMAS-KILMANN CONFLICT MODEL

The Thomas-Kilmann Conflict Model[5,6] is based on 5 approaches that people can use to engage conflict with one mode being their most preferred. The model suggests that all 5 styles have their appropriate use. The 5 conflict modes or styles are formed by 2 axes (Figure 10-5). The horizontal axis plots the amount of uncooperativeness to cooperativeness, while the vertical axis is based on the amount of assertiveness from unassertive to assertive. One engages in

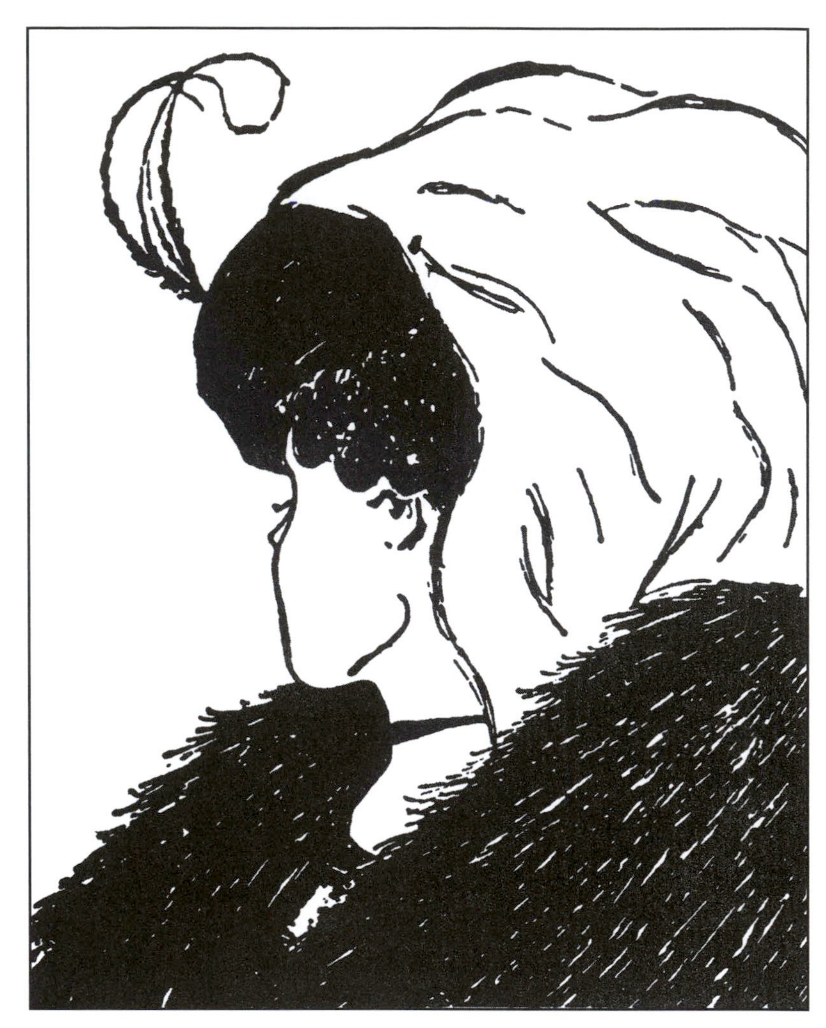

Figure 10-4. Perception exercise. Do you see an old lady? A young lady? Both?

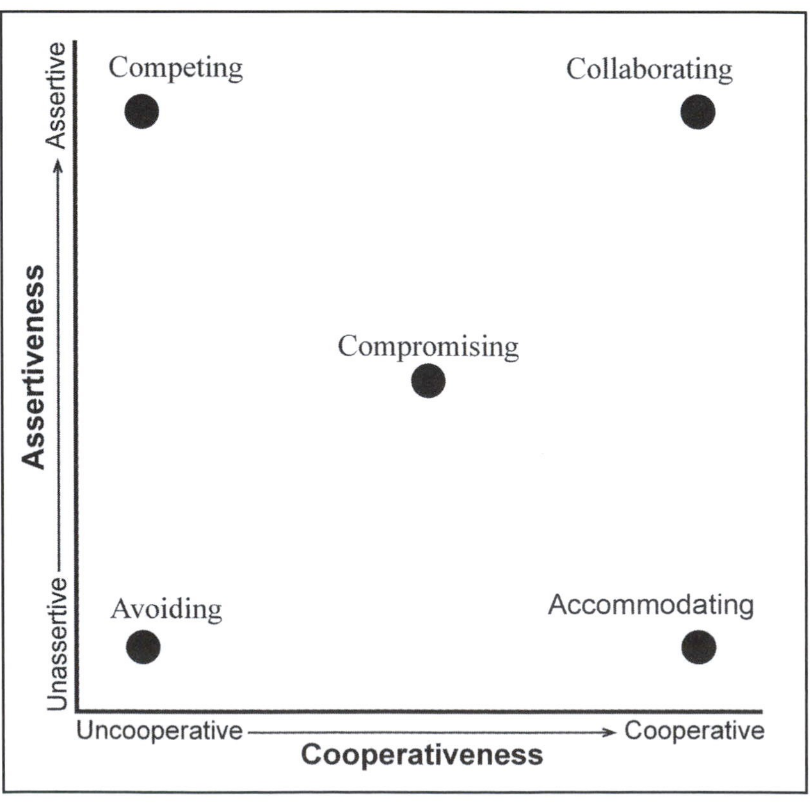

Figure 10-5. Thomas-Kilmann conflict model. (Adapted from *Conflict Workshop Facilitator's Guide*. Tuxedo, NY: Xicom, Inc; 1996.)

different conflict styles by adjusting the amount of assertive and cooperative behavior. The Thomas-Kilmann Conflict Mode Instrument[6] (CPP, Inc, Mountain View, CA, www.cpp.com) is a self-assessment that will give you an idea of which conflict style is your primary style and which one(s) you use less frequently or even at all. The learning here is that even though there are 5 styles to engage conflict, we typically fall into a primary style that is our habitual pattern to responding to conflict, leading to an overuse of one or two styles and an underuse of others. The goal is to be aware enough to know you are in conflict and make a conscious choice, instead of unconscious, about how to respond to the conflict.

All 5 conflict styles have an upside and downside (Tables 10-5 and 10-6). My experience with administering this instrument to many groups of people is that they typically place a connotation (good/bad judgment) on these labels. While avoiding generally carries with it a negative connotation, it has some wonderful uses; conversely to attempt to collaborate all the time can be very time consuming. Tables 10-5 and 10-6 give a summary of the 5 different conflict styles, eluding to their uses and the potential impact of over- and underuses.

GIVING AND RECEIVING FEEDBACK

Again, feedback is another core interpersonal skill generally not taught in formal education programs. Giving feedback is a verbal and nonverbal process through which a person lets others know his or her perceptions and feelings about the others' behavior.[7] When eliciting feedback, a person is asking for others' perceptions and feelings about his or her behavior.[7] Feedback can be a technique that helps others achieve their goals as well as a means of comparing one's own perceptions of one's behavior with others' perceptions.[7] Effective feedback should enable the receiver to walk away understanding exactly what he or she did and what impact it had. This section addresses the types of feedback we can give and receive, a model for giving effective feedback, and tips on how to frame feedback so it can be heard by another person.

FEEDBACK TYPES

There are 2 types of feedback: positive feedback and feedback for improvement (the latter might be described as negative feedback and/or constructive criticism). Words have impact and evoke emotions and feelings in people. Think about the language here. Would you rather receive negative feedback, a dose of constructive criticism, or feedback for improvement? You would probably be more open to feedback for improvement. Telling someone you have some constructive criticism for him or her tends to put him or her on the defensive, while asking someone if he or she would be open to some feedback for improvement is more acceptable.

FEEDBACK MODEL

The key to giving feedback is to be concise. The more language you use to justify the feedback or "soften the blow" only confuses the other person. If you are going to give feedback, you might as well be as impactful as possible. First, get clear on your intent for giving someone feedback (whether that be positive feedback or feedback for improvement). We often give people feedback without asking if they would like feedback. It might be possible that they are not in a place mentally to really hear what you say. What is your intent in giving this feedback? Is your intent to build this relationship even if it is feedback for improvement or is it to give someone a piece of your mind? If the latter, you might want to reconsider since given that intent the engagement with the other person will be quite different. If you are clear on your intent, you are more likely to have the impact for which you are hoping. This is referred to as intent and impact (see p. 201). We can have a pure intent and for many reasons the impact is just the opposite of what we were hoping for. Often this is based on the other person's perception and interpretation of the verbal and nonverbal communication.

There are many feedback models, and the model presented here is one I have used for many years. It works for both positive feedback and feedback for improvement. Ideally, feedback using this model is delivered in 3 statements, which makes it pithy, more likely to be heard by the other person, and have the impact you are hoping for. The model is referred to as the SBI Model.[8] SBI is an acronym that stands for situation, behavior, and impact. This model helps focus the feedback on the person's behavior, not individuals, their values, and how their behavior impacts you. Table 10-7 outlines a summary of the SBI model and gives examples of how to frame the language for each step.

Remember to keep feedback short, to the point, and timely. The closer you can connect the feedback to the situation, the greater the impact. Even feedback a day later is less powerful then feedback that occurs in the moment. The intent of the "S" part of the SBI model is to help people reconnect to the situation, and sometimes that is difficult to do days or weeks later.

Table 10-5

An Overview of Five Conflict Management Approaches

Approach	Goal	Slogans	Objective	Your Posture	Supporting Rational	Likely Outcome
Competing	To "win"	"Might makes right." "My way or the high-way"	Get your way	"I know what's right. Do not question my judgment or authority."	It is better to risk causing a few hard feelings than to abandon an issue you are com-mitted to.	You feel vin-dicated, but also defeated and possibly humiliated.
Avoiding	To "delay"	"Leave well enough alone." "I'll think about it tomorrow."	Avoid hav-ing to deal with conflict	"I'm neutral on that issue." "Let me think about it." "That is someone else's problem."	Disagreements are inherent-ly bad be-cause they create ten-sion.	Interpersonal problems do not get re-solved, causing long-term frustra-tion mani-fested in a variety of ways.
Compromising	To "find middle ground"	"Split the dif-ference." "Let's make a deal."	Reach an agree-ment quickly	"Let us search for a solution we can both live with so we can get on with our work."	Prolonged con-flicts distract people from their work and engen-der bitter feelings.	Participants become conditioned to seek expe-dient, rather than effec-tive solu-tions.
Accommodating	To "yield"	"I only live to serve." "It would be my plea-sure."	Do not upset the other person	"How can I help you feel good about this encounter?" "My position is not so important that it is worth risking bad feelings between us."	Maintaining harmonious relationships should be our top pri-ority.	Other person is likely to take advan-tage of you.
Collaborating	To find a "win/ win" solution	"Two heads are better than one."	Solve the problem together	"This is my position. What is yours?" "I'm committed to finding the best possible solution." "What do the facts suggest?"	The positions of both par-ties are equally important (though not necessarily equally valid). Equal emphasis should be placed on the quality of the outcome and the fair-ness of the decision-making process.	The problem is most likely to be resolved. Also, both parties are committed to the solu-tion and satisfied that they have been treated fairly.

Table 10-6

A Comparison of Five Conflict Management Approaches

Approach	*Description*	*Uses*	*Overuses*	*Underuses*
Competing	Competing is when you assert your position without considering opposing viewpoints. It may take the form of standing up for your rights, or throwing your weight around.	Quick action Unpopular decisions Vital issues Protection	Lack of feedback Reduced learning Low empowerment Surrounded by "yes men"	Restricted influence Indecision Slow to act Contributions withheld
Avoiding	Avoiding means that you do not satisfy your concerns or the concerns of the other person(s). You may be stalling on an issue, or ignoring it. For many people, avoiding conflict requires great discipline. You must be conscious about when and where to get involved in a situation.	Issues of low importance Reducing tensions Buying time Low power Allowing other symptomatic problems	Lack of input from you Decisions made by default Issues fester Cautious climate	Hostility/hurt feelings Too many causes Lack of prioritization/delegation
Compromising	Compromising is finding middle ground or forgoing some of your concerns in order to have others met. It can mean negotiating or splitting the difference. In order to compromise, you need to have a sense of how much each aspect of an issue means to you.	Moderate importance Equal power—strong commitment Temporary solutions Time constraints Backup for competing/collaborating	Lose big picture/long-term goals Lack of values/trust Cynical climate	Unnecessary confrontations Frequent power struggles Unable to negotiate effectively

(continued)

BUT/AND PHENOMENON

Do not sandwich a piece of feedback for improvement between 2 pieces of positive feedback. This is referred to as the good-bad-good sandwich and people will focus only on the negative piece. Another mistake people make is using the word *but*. This is generally done by taking a positive piece of feedback and connecting it to a piece of feedback for improvement by the word *but*. For example, "Carla, I observed you assessed for ligament instability but did not test for a possible meniscus lesion or fracture." The "but"

Table 10-6 (continued)

A Comparison of Five Conflict Management Approaches

Accommodating	Accommodating is forgoing your own concerns in order to satisfy the concerns of another person. It can mean an act of selfless generosity or simply obeying orders. For some people, accommodating comes very easily. However, others often do not recognize the opportunity to be accommodating until the situation has passed. You must be alert in order to seize the right opportunities, especially if you are in a leadership position.	Showing reasonableness Developing performance Creating good will Keeping "peace" Retreating Low importance	Ideas get little attention Restricted influence Loss of contribution Anarchy	Lack of support Low morale Exceptions not recognized Unable to yield
Collaborating	Collaborating is when you are concerned with fully satisfying both sides of an issue. It is working with the other person(s) to find an optimal solution. Collaborating requires time and good communication skills.	Integrating solutions Learning Merging perspectives Gaining commitment Improving relationships	Too much time on trivial matters Diffused responsibility Others may take advantage Work overload	Deprived of mutual gains Lack of commitment Low empowerment Loss of innovation

erases the positive piece and really creates an either/or situation. If both statements are true, which they are in the above example, then connect them with "and" (eg, "Carla, I observed you assess for ligament instability and I did not see you test for a possible meniscus lesion or fracture").

"I" Statements

Effective feedback must be given so that the person receiving it can hear it in the most objective and least distorted way possible in order to understand it so he or she can choose to use it or not. Being clear on your intent, framing it from an "I" point of view, and following the SBI model will allow you to give effective feedback. "I" language allows one to take responsibility for his or her words. Using words such as we, they, and them (talking in third person) circumvents ownership of the words and responsibility. For example, "We all agreed that we would study together" can be reframed as "I thought we agreed that we would study together." When using the language of the first example, you are speaking for the entire group and all group members may not share the same understanding as you, particularly in this case if you did not all meet to study. Also, the third-person language makes you wonder who they are referring to. The interesting part is that many times we do not bother to ask who "they" are or "what" is being referred to.

Table 10-7

SBI Feedback Model

Step	How/Why	Examples
Create the **S**ituation	Include: Location Time Why: Creates a context for the recipient, helping him or her remember clearly his or her thinking and behavior at the time.	"Yesterday morning, while we were discussing the posted schedule..."
Describe the **B**ehavior	Include: Actual behaviors Use verbs (avoid adjectives) What was said/done How it was said/done Why: The most critical step because behavior can be difficult to identify and describe.	"You spoke at the same time another person was speaking in the meeting." (Rude) "You leaned forward in your chair, wrote notes after other people spoke, and then said your thoughts with the group." (Engaged)
Deliver the **I**mpact	Include: Acknowledge emotional impact of the behavior on you. "When you did (Behavior), I felt (Impact)." "When you said (Behavior), I was (Impact)." Why: Relays the impact that the other person's behavior had on you.	"Jerry, this morning in the hallway you asked for my opinion about decisions for staffing the new unit. You also asked for my suggestions on which beds to purchase. That makes me feel included, part of the team."

Adapted from Weitzel S. *Feedback That Works: How to Build and Deliver Your Message*. Greensboro, NC: Center for Creative Leadership; 2000.

"You" Statements

"You" statements are accusatory statements directed at another person. They often focus on the shortcomings of the other person; are perceived as intrusive, blaming, or attacking; and/or are manipulative or coercive, which typically takes the form of either a hostile counterattack or withdrawal from the conversation. As discussed above, "I" statements are preferred to "You" statements. It is hard to argue with an "I" statement, particularly when you are disclosing your feelings, observations, or experience. Table 10-8 offers examples of "You" versus "I" statements. Starting feedback off with a "You" statement is a guaranteed way to put the receiver on the defensive and it becomes almost impossible for him or her to take the feedback as something that might be useful.

Intent and Impact

At times even if our intent is pure with feedback, the impact on the other person may not be what we hoped. In my experience, people tend to shy away from feedback for improvement because they do not want to hurt somebody's feelings or decrease their self-esteem or believe the other person will no longer like them. Unfortunately, this may happen even with the purest intentions. My experience is that if you are clear on your intent; the intent is to be helpful to someone (ie, build a relationship, or make him or her aware

Table 10-8

Examples of "You" and "I" Statements

"You" Statement	*"I" Statement*
"You make me so mad. You are not really listening to me."	"When I see you stare at the ceiling when we talk, I feel as if I am not being understood.
"Are you always so forgetful?"	"I feel not respected when you fail to return my telephone calls."
"You had better..."	"I would like it if you would..."
"You are so negative."	"My experience of you is that you tend to view things in a negative light."

of a possible "blind spot") and it is done in a kind and caring way, then the feedback comes across as such. If your intent is to give someone a piece of your mind, make him or her aware of how bad he or she messed up, and how stupid he or she is, then it will come across as such. Before giving feedback to someone, either positive or feedback for improvement, get clear on your intent. Most of the problems arise from saying words to someone before you are clear on what you want to communicate and why.

Box 10-13 lists 10 common mistakes that occur when giving feedback and Box 10-14 summarizes some dos and don'ts regarding feedback. Feedback can be a powerful tool to improve performance and mold behavior and if not used with the care it deserves, it can harm people as well. We are very competent at giving feedback for improvement and looking for what is wrong. I urge you to start looking at what is right as well. Take this challenge. Put 10 dimes in one pocket before going to work or out for the day. Every time you give someone a piece of positive feedback or encouragement during the day, move one dime to the other pocket. You might be surprised at what you find at the end of the day.

Box 10-13

Ten Common Mistakes in Giving Feedback

- The feedback does not judge the individual's actions; it judges the individual.
- The feedback is very general and vague.
- The feedback speaks for others.
- Positive messages have negative feedback sandwiched between them.
- The feedback uses many generalities.
- The feedback looks at the motives behind behavior.
- The feedback is too long.
- The feedback is threatening.
- The feedback uses humor that is inappropriate for the situation.
- The feedback is not a statement, but a question.

Adapted from Weitzel S. *Feedback That Works: How to Build and Deliver Your Message.* Greensboro, NC: Center for Creative Leadership; 2000.

DIFFICULT CONVERSATIONS

The purpose of this section is to provide an overview of what is referred to as "difficult conversations." The intent is to acknowledge that it is a part of an athletic trainer's job to have what may be considered as difficult conversations with administrators, coaches, players, players' parents, and students. There are actually several models for having a difficult conversation,[9] crucial conversation,[10] or crucial confrontation,[11] and I urge you to consult one of these resources for a model that can help you guide the conversation.

A difficult conversation is anything you find hard to talk about.[9] It can be associated with some type of physical response by yourself as a result of heightened anxiety, such as increased heart rate, nausea, "knots" in your stomach, sweating palms, dry mouth, etc. If you find yourself practicing the conversation over and over in your head and trying to figure out in advance what to say, then that can be a clue that the conversation is at the very minimum at least important to, if not difficult, for you. In my experience, simply naming a future conversation as "difficult" heightens your awareness and in some strange way can reduce the anxiety. There are multiple reasons a

Box 10-14

A Summary: The Dozen Dos and Don'ts of Effective Feedback

Do	Don't
Be specific when recalling the situation.	Assume.
Be specific when describing the behavior.	Be vague.
Acknowledge the impact of the behavior on you.	Use accusations.
Judge the behavior.	Judge the person.
Pay attention to body language.	Pass along vague feedback from others.
Use verbatim quotes.	Give advice unless asked.
Re-create the behavior, if appropriate.	Psychoanalyze.
Give feedback in a timely manner.	Qualify your feedback by backing out of the description.
Give your feedback, then stop talking.	Use examples from your own experience.
Say "I felt" or "I was" to frame your impact statement.	Generalize with words like *always* or *never.*
Focus on a single message.	Label your feedback as positive or negative.
Be sensitive to the emotional impact of your feedback.	Sandwich your feedback messages with words like *but.*

Adapted from Weitzel S. *Feedback That Works: How to Build and Deliver Your Message.* Greensboro, NC: Center for Creative Leadership; 2000.

conversation can be deemed difficult, such as the topic to be discussed, how conflictual you view the conversation to be and your preferred style of engaging conflict (see Conflict Management in this chapter), and/or having to tell someone he or she is not meeting performance standards.

A barrier to engaging someone in a difficult conversation is the "story" you make up in your mind about how it will go and the outcome. Typically, the outcome held about the conversation is not a positive one. I urge that if you are going to make up a story about a negative outcome of the conversation, then at least make up a positive one as well. The underpinnings of this are that we move toward or away from the pictures we create in our mind. It is part of the theory for use of visual imaging in athletics. The same principle applies here. If I hold a picture of a conversation in which a lot of emotions will be displayed and someone leaves mad at me, then that only heightens my anxiety about the conversation and I may choose to avoid the situation since that is something I do not care to experience. Like feedback, being clear on your intention to have the conversation and holding a positive picture of the interaction will go a long way toward success. It may not make the conversation any easier and you still might get an impact you were not expecting, but it does provide a plan for having the greatest chance of success. As a result of my job, all too often I find myself with 2 to 3 individuals or a group that is avoiding conflict and then when it does come out it is associated with a lot of emotion and does not serve the relationship or group very well moving forward. In this case, people are operating from an emotional base and, to use a metaphor, figuratively vomit all over each other with their words and emotions and obviously impact the other person in a negative way. This is a great example of when avoiding conflict should occur (ie, when it is emotionally charged). That does not mean you never engage the other person in the conflict you are having with him or her. However, the reality is that when an outburst occurs, it is really the result of unresolved conflict that has been avoided with the other person(s) building over time and then in a split second comes out because of something else the person said or did that irritated them. Try to not move from the Stimulus→Response model when there is a lot of emotion. Although the emotion may be directed at you, pausing and listening to what the other person has to say will go a long way toward resolution. Paraphrasing can go a long way here, particularly by reflecting back to the person the emotions you are experiencing from him or her (listening with empathy). Often it is the emotions that are the issue, not the topic or content. A person feels heard when you tell him or her how you are experiencing his or her emotions. When done correctly, I have seen this skill remove emotions from the equation so problem solving can begin. Finally, what one person finds difficult talking about is not difficult for another person, so do not assume that of either person. As a matter of fact, you might not label a future conversation as difficult, but when you engage the other person it could be difficult for him or her.

Having a difficult conversation is something people usually do not enjoy, yet successful assertive leaders know this is part of their job; hold a picture of a positive outcome; and engage the person in a kind, caring, and direct way. The use of the listening skills described earlier in this chapter is paramount with a difficult conversation and you will experience many of the barriers that inhibit listening. Use of the 4 listening techniques will help overcome some of these barriers. I have been told on several occasions that the reason people do not engage in difficult conversations or give feedback is that they cannot control the outcome and if there are emotions, they are not sure if they can deal with them. Even given a model and plan, you cannot predict with 100% accuracy what will happen. It is the risk you take in many instances to build a relationship.

SUMMARY

- Differentiate between assertive, aggressive, and passive behaviors.

  Assertive behavior is the ability to express one's self honestly without denying the rights of others while aggressive behavior is concerned only for the rights of one's self and passive behavior takes into account the rights of the other person at the expense of one's self. The Assertiveness Behavioral Model takes these types of behaviors into account based on the amount of consideration for others and openness of communication that are demonstrated. Sometimes assertive behavior is confused with aggressive behavior, but the key difference is the consideration for the other person's rights as well.

- Describe the communication process.

  Communication is a complex process and given the many ways people define the meaning of words for themselves, it is amazing that miscommunication does not occur more often. The process consists of transmitting a "mind picture" of what you want to say by encoding the picture with words. Another person decodes these words and based on his or her response, the transmitter determines if the original "mind picture" was decoded correctly by the receiver.

- Identify some barriers to effective communication and develop strategies to overcome these barriers.

  Barriers to effective communication can include physical, emotional, and/or intellectual barriers. Some barriers can be resolved by changing location, asking to talk at another time, or asking people to speak louder or slower or be careful of jargon usage just to name a few. One of the greatest barriers in listening to someone else is thinking about how you are going to respond to him or her. Additionally, we can mentally process 400 to 500 words/minute but can only talk at 125 words/minute, so the mind tends to wander and it is difficult to stay connected to the other person 100% of the time.

- Use verbal and nonverbal skills to actively listen.

  Since we can mentally process 400 to 500 words/minute but can only talk at 125 words/minute, we can use the verbal skills of paraphrasing, perception checking, asking questions, and probing to help us stay connected to the other person during a conversation. Additionally, body language also sends a message to people about our interest in listening to them or not. While our verbal language may be saying "yes," our body language can be saying "no," thus sending mixed messages to the other person. Unfortunately, these mixed messages are very rarely "checked out" by the person receiving these messages and confusion exists.

- Explain the Thomas-Kilmann Conflict Model.

  The Thomas-Kilmann Conflict model provides 5 different ways to engage conflict by manipulating the amount of cooperativeness or assertiveness demonstrated. While we generally have one primary style of engaging conflict, this model proposes that given the situation there are 5 possible responses to conflict that one could consciously choose to use to respond to a conflictual situation.

- Describe the SBI model for giving positive feedback and feedback for improvement and the skills necessary for this to be effective.

- The SBI model can be used to give both positive feedback and feedback for improvement. SBI stands for situation, behavior, impact (ie, when the behavior occurred, the behavior that occurred, and the impact of that behavior). Ideally, this occurs in 3 sentences. Feedback should be focused on the person's behavior and how it impacts you, not directed at the person him- or herself. The SBI model helps you meet these criteria around feedback. Avoid giving feedback in which feedback for improvement is sandwiched between 2 pieces of positive feedback. When giving feedback, frame it using the "I" point of view instead of making "you" statements, which can be accusatory in nature. It is important that you are clear on your reason (intent) for giving feedback in order to enhance the chance of having the impact you desire

- Describe what a difficult conversation is and why some conversations are considered difficult.

  A difficult conversation is anything you find hard to talk about. Several models exists that can provide you with a structure for having a difficult conversation. Generally, these types of conversations are considered difficult because of the topic to be discussed or the reactions one expects to get from the other person. Just like feedback, it is important to be clear on the intent of the conversation. Additionally, the use of active listening skills is important when having these conversations so that the conversation does not become a monologue since multiple stories generally exist around the topic at hand.

ACTIVITIES

The following activities are designed to reinforce material presented in the chapter and to allow for discussion among students and instructors.

Listening

This activity will give you practice with each of the 5 listening skills. Follow this procedure.

Step	Action
1	Find a partner. If there is an uneven number of participants, then there will have to be a triad.
2	Identify which person will be the skill user (ie, the person who uses the skill) and the skill partner.
3	Conduct the activity as instructed in each of the subsections below that are specific to each listening skill.
4	Run the activity for 3 minutes.
5	Stop the activity after 3 minutes.
6	Debrief the activity by asking what they learned as a skill user and skill partner.
7	Repeat the same activity, with the two people swapping roles.
8	Repeat steps 4 to 6.
9	Go to next listening skill.

Paraphrasing Practice

Use the following example to practice paraphrasing.

Role	Task
Skill user	Overuse the skill to become comfortable with it.
	Remember to interrupt the speaker to check your understanding.
	You are looking for both content and emotion within the message.
	Focus on a few paraphrasing lead-ins to strengthen your use of them.
Skill partner	Talk to the user about things you value deeply; specifically things you value about yourself and your work.
	Examples:
	YOURSELF. Without being humble, what do you value most about yourself as a friend, parent, citizen, etc?
	YOUR WORK. When you are feeling best about work, what do you value about it?

Perception Check Practice

Use the following example to practice perception checking.

Note: The skill user is the person telling the story.

Role	Task
Skill user	Describe/explain how to perform a technical skill. This could be something specific to your work or one of your hobbies. Try to pick a topic that your partner would not be that knowledgeable about but in which you have some expertise. Examples include how a computer works, strategies of winning at backgammon, gardening, how to bass fish, the inner workings of a trumpet, or topics specific to your work. As you tell your story, overuse perception checking.
Skill partner	Listen to what the skill user is saying.

Probing Practice

Use the following example to practice open-ended questions, close-ended questions, and probing.

Role	Task
Skill user	You are very curious as to what your partner has to say and help him or her explore the richness of this successful experience.
	For the benefit of this practice session, your goal is to overuse these skills, so that you can become familiar with them.
	Also, use your previously practiced skill of paraphrasing when appropriate.
Skill partner	Tell the skill user a story about a time when you were proud to be a member of a group/team. Why were you proud? What did you do to contribute to this? What did other team members do?

Putting It All Together Practice

Use the following example to practice paraphrasing, asking questions, probing, and perception checking.

Role	Task
Skill user	Be very curious about what your partner has to say. Help him or her explore the richness of his or her experience. Remember to use the following: Paraphrasing Asking questions Probing
Skill partner	Remember a time when you had a terrific learning experience. It might be a time when you made major strides of some sort, or developed profound understanding, achieved a significant increase in an important skill; a time when you were involved, invigorated, and excited about your learning. Tell the skill user the story of that learning experience. What made it so memorable? What did you do that contributed to this time? What did others do?
	Remember to use perception checking during the conversation.

FEEDBACK

- Think for a moment of someone to whom you would like to give a piece of feedback for improvement using the SBI feedback model (Situation-Behavior-Impact). Write down what you would say using the template below as a guide. Remember to try and keep it to a sentence. Remember to get clear on your intent first.
- Repeat the same process except using a person to whom you would like to give a piece of positive feedback.
- You could pair up in class and give your feedback to another person so you could practice actually speaking the words.

S ______________________________________

____

____

B______________________________________

____

____

I______________________________________

____

____

REFERENCES

1. Smith M. *When I Say No, I Feel Guilty.* New York, NY: Bantam Books; 1975.
2. *Interpersonal Influence Inventory.* 4th ed. King of Prussia, PA: HRDQ; 2004.
3. Fisher S. *Effective Listening.* Amherst, MA: HRD Press, Inc; 1996.
4. Covey S. *The 7 Habits of Highly Effective People.* New York, NY: Simon & Schuster; 1989.
5. *Conflict Workshop Facilitator's Guide.* Tuxedo, NY: Xicom, Inc; 1996.
6. Thomas K, Kilmann RH. *Thomas-Kilmann Conflict Mode Instrument.* Mountain View, CA: CPP, Inc; 2002.
7. Hanson P. Giving feedback: an interpersonal skill. *The Pfeiffer Library.* Vol 6. 3rd ed. San Francisco, CA: Pfeiffer; 2003:179-190.
8. Weitzel S. *Feedback That Works: How to Build and Deliver Your Message.* Greensboro, NC: Center for Creative Leadership; 2000.
9. Stone D, Patton B, Heen S. *Difficult Conversations: How to Discuss What Matters Most.* New York, NY: Penguin Books; 1999.
10. Patterson K, Grenny J, McMillan R, Switzler A. *Crucial Conversation: Tools for Talking When Stakes Are High.* New York, NY: McGraw-Hill; 2002.
11. Patterson K, Grenny J, McMillan R, Switzler A. *Crucial Confrontations: Tools for Resolving Broken Promises, Violated Expectations and Bad Behavior.* New York, NY: McGraw-Hill; 2005.

Chapter 11

IMPROVING ORGANIZATIONAL PERFORMANCE

OBJECTIVES

Upon completion of this chapter, the reader will be able to:

- Explain the benefits of strategic planning
- Discuss the pros and cons of specific evaluation and planning approaches
- Differentiate various program evaluation techniques
- Explain how systems thinking applies to athletic training health care organizations
- Draw and evaluate feedback loop diagrams as a tool to examine specific organization and administration issues
- Describe the components of a learning organization
- Identify organizational "learning disabilities" that hinder organizational progress
- Explain the relationships between organizational effectiveness (OE) and organizational trust
- Discuss how organizational structures can influence effectiveness

The literature surrounding health care administration, business administration, and educational administration is littered with catch phrases dedicated to organizational improvements. Readers can easily find themselves knee deep in the semantics of total quality management (TQM), SWOT analysis (strengths, weaknesses, opportunities, and threats), PDCA cycles (plan, do, check, act), strategic planning, outcome studies, program evaluation, etc. The list of acronyms, techniques, strategies, and philosophical approaches to organizational improvement can prove overwhelming. However, the truly effectual organizers must reach beyond techniques alone to achieve their vision. Modern athletic training health care organizations must make a paradigm shift and create learning organizations inhabited by skilled personnel trained to examine the inter-relationships, patterns, and causes that control and influence both positive and negative organizational outcomes. A broader systems thinking approach is needed. By applying a systems-based approach, an organization can be created that provides quality care to its patients and meets greater organizational demands but does not do so at the expense of the care providers.

This chapter discusses the pros and cons of traditional improvement strategies, provides a philosophical approach to learning organizations, and provides specific tools to evaluate and interpret the dynamics of ever-changing athletic training health care settings.

APPROACHING ORGANIZATIONAL EFFECTIVENESS

If athletic training educators, scientists, and clinicians were asked to define strategies to improve OE, the answers would vary in proportion to just how many people were asked. Ask 10 different people to define any one component of OE and you will get

10 different definitions. It is likely that they would stumble onto some need to have goals, to make plans, and to evaluate the effectiveness of these plans. However, it is likely they would not have a clear sense of how these fit together, nor would there be much agreement on how to best establish an overall plan for addressing these components. As varied approaches to improving the function of an organization are explored, it is imperative that organizations possess 2 key components: 1) the tools to align planning strategies with identified goals, and 2) the willingness to carry out data-driven evaluative efforts in which goals serve as a measure of progress. In the article *Why Strategies Fail*, Press[1] identifies 2 components that accurately predict the success or failure of strategies put forth in health care organizations: 1) the ability to carry out the strategy, and 2) the organization's will (or resolve) to implement it. The "doing" of organizational improvement exercises is not enough. How employees respond and participate in ongoing goal setting, planning, and evaluation strategies will largely be a reflection of the organizational culture and environment. Athletic training health care organizations must have leaders who know the key elements for improving OE and can create an organizational culture that allows employees to be genuine agents of change.

Strategic Planning

Strategic planning, sometimes referred to as strategic management, has been informally defined as "a disciplined effort to produce fundamental decisions and actions that shape and guide what an organization is, what it does, and why it does it."[2] For the purpose of this text, strategic planning for an athletic training organization is defined as a process for assessing an organization's current and anticipated environment and then identifying and implementing the best approaches for succeeding under those conditions.[3] The strategic planning process, if properly carried out, can define the organization's mission, vision, and values and translate them into tangible action by addressing its needs as follows[3]:

- Increases understanding of the organization's environment (ie, its current and anticipated opportunities and challenges).
- Stimulates innovative responses to that changing environment.
- Provides a coordinated framework for modifying the organization's desired services, processes, and capabilities to better meet future requirements.
- Identifies new capabilities that the organization and its members must obtain to succeed in the future.
- Guides daily decision making by providing a long-term context to weigh against short-term pressures.
- Provides a disciplined approach to evaluating and monitoring progress.

The strategic planning process can only meet the above outcomes if some specific underlying philosophies are accepted. The organization's existing methods of operation and current outcomes are assumed to be the baseline for the planning processes. A baseline must be established to measure performance. This is the starting point or the "where we are now" for an organization. The goals become the desired outcome or "where we want to be." A strategy to address the gap between these 2 points will be the heart of the planning document (Figure 11-1). Another fundamental assumption is that the future is assumed to be different from current operations. The extent of that difference may not be known. It is assumed that organizations must be able to adapt and change; the ability to make such adaptations is often a predictor of organizational success. In some ways, strategic planning is about designing a desired future by identifying specific goals. However, organizations must also plan in such a way as to adapt and adjust to changes that may occur along the way. The resulting process must be a guide to follow, not a specific recipe for daily activity and work. The strategic plan should be a flexible document that can be adjusted as situations change.

The outcome of a good strategic plan should yield more than just a final report. The generation of a comprehensive document is only the beginning; implementation is the key. The planning document should help employees at all levels become aligned with the direction of the plan. Alignment is an essential process that insures the organization's work processes and decisions are congruent with the broader goals. In fact, one of the most compelling reasons to undertake a strategic planning process is to develop and insure this alignment.[3] Employees guided by a well-aligned strategic plan can better evaluate all aspects of their work duties and adjust according to the strategic vision. Employees in well-aligned organizations are encouraged to evaluate their work and make changes that increase their ability to meet program goals and are recognized by their supervisors for such contributions.

The strategic planning document is not just put to use internally. Well-aligned organizations can craft a much more coherent message to both internal and external stakeholders regarding organization goals. The ability to put out a consistent message and answer the following questions (Who are we? What do we do? What are our goals? How do we serve the community?) is critical to athletic training health care

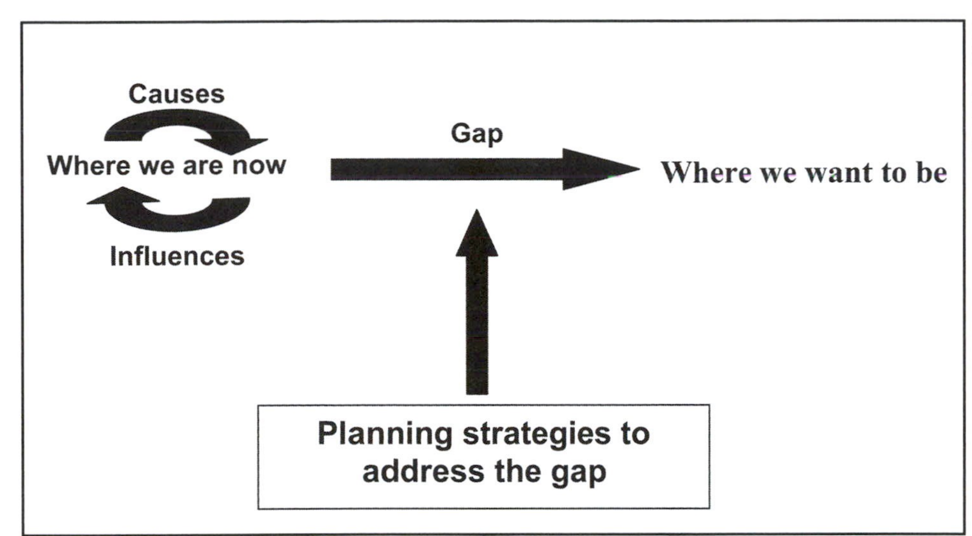

Figure 11-1. The gap diagram illustrates the need for the planning process, addressing the gap between where the organization is and where it wants to be.

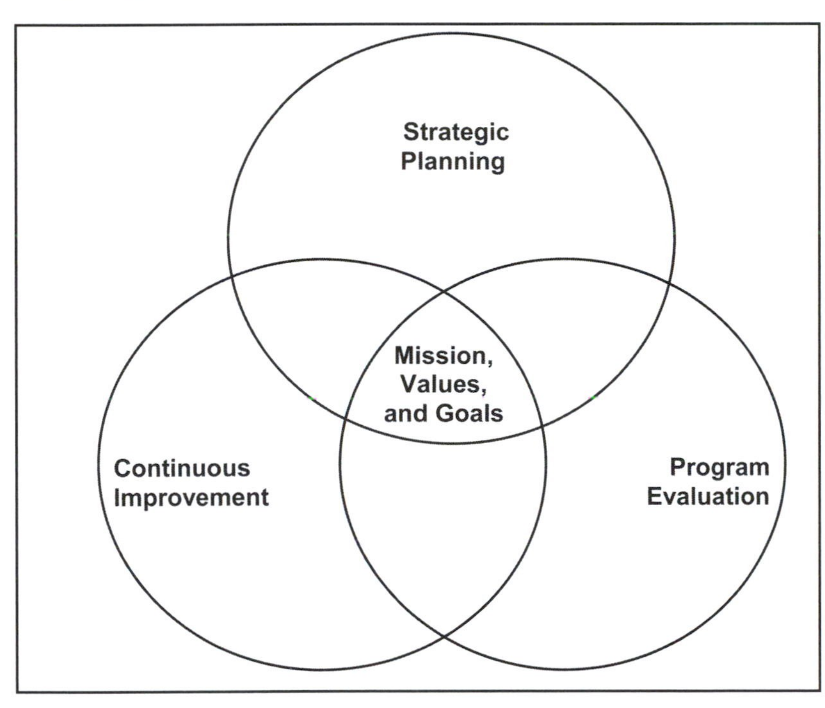

Figure 11-2. At the intersection of strategic planning, program evaluation, and continuous improvement lies the program mission, values, and goals. The broader mission, values, and goals drive the remaining processes.

organizations in both the public and private sectors. Imagine an athletic training program that is part of a private sports medicine clinic in a medium-sized city. This clinic wishes to compete for customers, develop community outreach programs, contract for services with local schools, and generally be recognized as a resource to the community. The ability to put forth a unified vision for the clinic, a set of programs and offerings that reflect this vision, and an ability to articulate that vision to the public will not happen by chance. A strategic planning process is essential when creating a well-aligned organization.

Mission

The model presented in Figure 11-2 represents how mission, values, and organizational goals lie at the intersection of planning, evaluation, and continuous improvement. Since program alignment to the broader mission is identified as an essential element for improving OE, it is worthwhile to explore the components of a mission statement and how to develop one that best fits the athletic training organization.

A mission statement should convey why an organization exists. An athletic training health care organization should have a mission statement specific to its role within the broader unit where it is housed. Even if it is part of a larger organization or institution, like a hospital or university, establishing a vision and statement of purpose is critical. Topor and Pollard[4] state that the organizational mission statement should differentiate your work from the work of others. It is the touchstone by which all offerings will be judged. It should represent your ideal state of the organization. Differentiate is the key. How is your organization unique? If you can read a mission statement from someone else, say a rival sports medicine clinic in town, and substitute your clinic name for its name, the resulting mission should sound out of place. While they may be similar, it should not read too easily. In fact, if it sounds good, chances are you have not identified the uniqueness of your organization in such a way as to differentiate your work from others. Phrases like "high quality" and "commitment to excellence" can fit any group and do not describe fundamental purposes. An organization with a clear sense of purpose that reaches beyond the everyday tasks of "work" can accomplish much more.

Sample Mission Statement

The mission of the Midwest USA Sports Medicine Clinic Athletic Training Outreach Program is to improve the health and well being of our secondary school interscholastic athletes by:

- Placing qualified dedicated staff in our local high schools committed to providing prevention, recognition, management, and rehabilitation of athletic injuries and illness.
- Establishing annual educational programming targeted to coaches and parents that promotes injury prevention and addresses sports medicine topics of interest in our community.
- Conducting research that serves to improve the health and well being of the interscholastic athlete and provides a foundation for evidence-based practice.

It Might Not Be Perfect But Let Us Get Started...

Trainer[5] states that when analytical thinkers in higher education gather to craft the perfect mission statement, it can be problematic. Planners at universities have found that there is a big difference between a model that places the central ideas of vision, values, and mission at the center of planning, assessment, and improvement and trying to write the perfect mission statement in a group setting. Such an exercise can become frustrating and serve to drain the energy from your planning before you get started. The solution is to start with broader goals and vision items in mind as opposed to the "perfect mission statement." Groups can begin the process of scanning the environment to determine the current state of the organization and determining the types of data and benchmark measures to be used in the analysis. These tasks are well suited to the analytical thinkers commonly found in our health care and higher education organizations. Allow people to participate by using their strengths. Too many attempts at planning get bogged down trying to craft the perfect vision or mission. Get started once a broader vision is decided. The things that make the organization unique and will ultimately differentiate it from others will be revealed though the process.

The Strategic Planning Process: An Overview

Strategic planning is a means for the athletic training health care organization to establish new directions. The decisions made throughout the planning process will focus resources (both fiscal and human) into these new directions to benefit the stakeholders we serve. In the athletic training setting, this may include our patients and athletes, coworkers, the organizations we serve, other care providers with which we work, and the students who participate in educational programs. These are high stakes and the process deserves our full attention to detail.

Strategic planning is sometimes, erroneously, thought of as long-range planning. This is a misnomer. A long-range plan is traditionally focused inward with little attention to the external environment in which the organization functions. Long-range planning tends to maintain the status quo over time and assumes that the future will be a linear expression of the present state of the organization.[6] The focus in long-range planning leans toward goals and objectives without consideration to the ideal vision for the organization. A strategic plan seeks to be a genuine agent for change. If done correctly, it can cause a shift in direction and a refocus of mission and result in actual changes that work toward a desired vision for the organization.

Scenarios as a Planning Tool in Athletic Training Organizations

Can we predict the future? Of course not; however, as a planning exercise, maybe it is worth our time to try. One way to explore new possibilities for your athletic training health care organization is to use scenarios as a planning tool. Bringing stakeholders together to explore possible future scenarios can help illuminate future directions and uncover areas of your organization that may be uncertain. Scenario planning allows for exploration of possibilities that have not been considered. It is an opportunity to clarify your vision of the future. Scenarios are not predictions per se. They are descriptions of a possible future. Planning scenarios should be sharp and focused possibilities of what *might* lie ahead.

An athletic training program manager or director of sports medicine may ask the following "What if" questions:

What if?

...the budget is cut by 15%

...another team is added to university sports program?

...one of my staff is on family leave for 6 months?

...our team physician has to cut back his or her time?

...the outreach program loses 2 schools?

...the hospital administration cuts my FTE load by 20% and I have to lay off someone?

Steps in Creating Scenarios

- List the driving forces that cause uncertainty for your organization.
- Rank the forces according to a) potential impact and b) degree of uncertainty.
- Select the 2 driving forces that have the highest score on both potential impact and degree of uncertainty.
- Create 4 alternatives using the "poles" of the 2 driving forces.

An Athletic Training Example

- The potential of adding a drug-testing program at your university with no increased staffing is causing uncertainty for the athletic training health care organization you supervise.
- The driving force with greatest impact centers on potentially more athletes to care for, while the greatest uncertainty is the lack of adequate funding to expand the staff.
- The resulting 2-by-2 table shows the possible extremes. While not every scenario is likely, the resulting combinations can promote plenty of "what if" thinking and allow groups to move out of their comfort zone.

(continued)

Scenarios as a Planning Tool in Athletic Training Organizations (continued)

Impact: Additional Work Load From Drug-Testing Program	High	More time on new program and less time for other athletic training duties	More time on new program and less time for other athletic training duties
		More staff available	Less staff available
	Low	Time on new program does not impact other athletic training duties	Time on new program does not impact other athletic training duties
		More staff available	Less staff available
		Low	High
Uncertainty: Staffing			

Examine each possible scenario and explore possible actions that your organization could take to capitalize on potential positive outcomes and to prevent undesired outcomes. Consider all the possibilities. While you may not think it likely that you would get additional funding or staffing, what would you do if you suddenly did have extra funds in your budget? Conversely, how would you deal with additional demands if no funding or staffing were provided?

Scenario planning is a powerful tool that allows you to explore possible outcomes on paper before you face them in a patient care setting with money, time, and good care on the line.

Bibliography

Ashley WC, Morrison JL. *Anticipatory Management: 10 Power Tools for Achieving Excellence Into the 21st Century.* Leesburg, VA: Issue Action Publications; 1995.

Planning Tools

There are countless methods that can be used to carrying out a strategic plan. Figure 11-3 outlines a complete strategic planning model. While not all plans will follow the specific path outlined in this model, a comprehensive plan must include at least 4 steps: 1) environmental scanning, 2) formulation of strategy, 3) implementation of strategy, and 4) evaluation of the change. These feedback loops, no matter what they are called, are all versions of the quality-based PDCA cycle (Figure 11-4). Actions are always followed by evaluation, and evaluation leads to more planning (scanning) to identify the needs. This constant feedback allows for continuous changes and improvements in OE. The techniques outlined below can be used at various stages in the planning process.[5] These planning tools have their own strengths and weaknesses but on balance have shown to be useful in a variety of settings.

SWOT Analysis

The SWOT analysis is one of the most familiar of all planning tools.[6] The SWOT tool is useful in the scanning portion of the planning process. It requires groups to think about the context in which organizations function. By assessing threats, groups are required to ask themselves, "Who else could perform our function?" While most strengths and weaknesses are found within the current organizational structure, opportunities and threats are more likely to sit outside of the group. Planning groups can use a range of techniques to conduct the SWOT analysis (ie, brainstorming, nominal group process, various data collection). Successful use of this tool will require a clear understanding of the competitive environment surrounding the organization, a clear vision or mission for guidance, and the ability to view the organization from both an internal and external point of view.

TOWS Analysis

A TOWS analysis can be thought of as the reciprocal of the SWOT tool. The TOWS analysis tool can only be used following a successful SWOT analysis. TOWS stands for "turning opportunities into strengths." A TOWS analysis is done using a simple 2-by-2 table (TOWS matrix). Information gathered in a SWOTS analysis is then viewed from the perspective of a TOWS matrix. This process allows planners to think about strategies that turn strengths into opportunities (SO), employ strengths to avoid threats (ST), take advantage of opportunities by overcoming

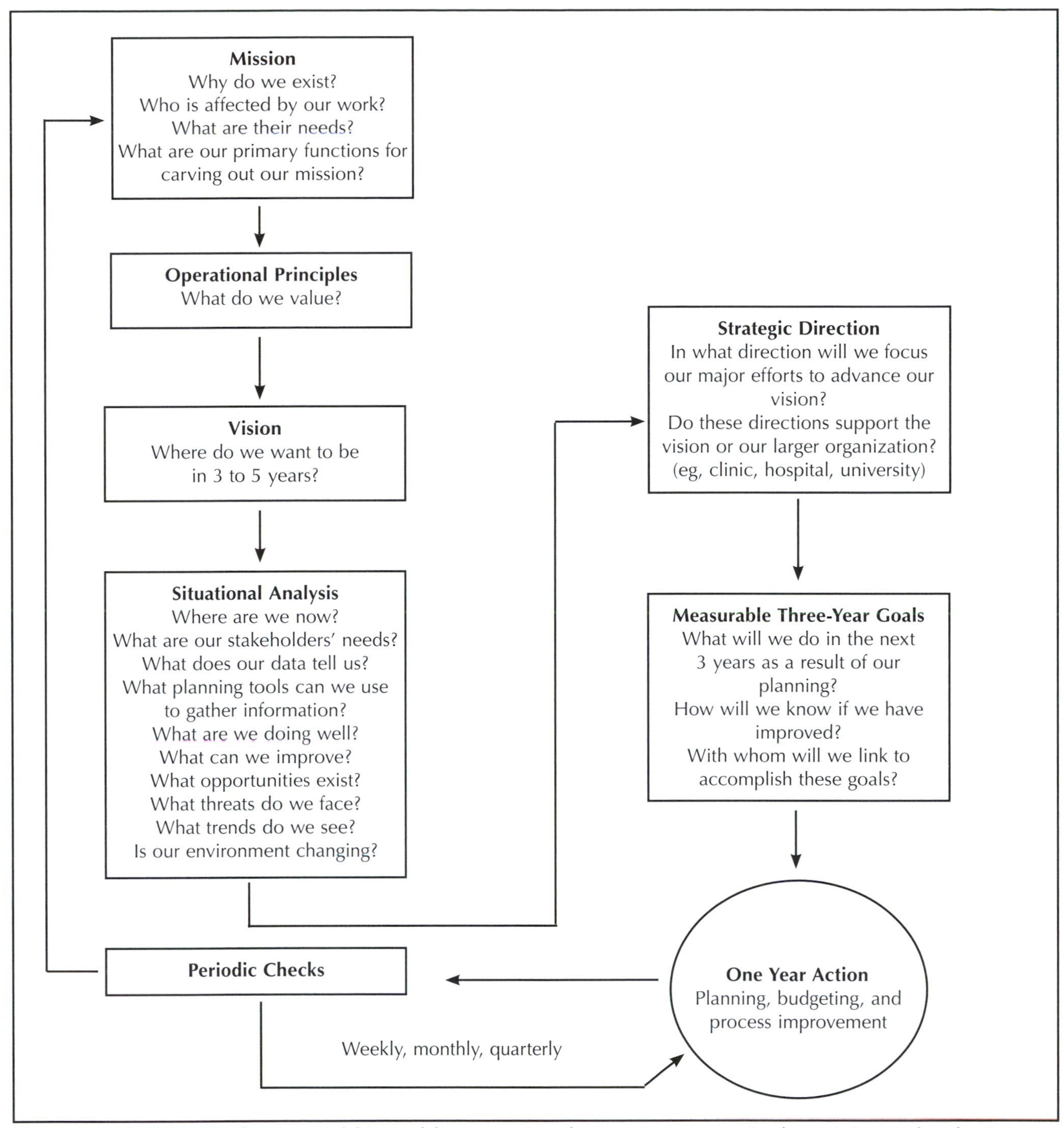

Figure 11-3. This strategic planning model is an elaborate version of a scanning, strategy, implementation, and evaluation loop. (Adapted from Office of Quality Improvement University of Wisconsin, Madison, 2000.)

weaknesses (WO), and act to minimize weaknesses and avoid threats (WT).[7] Figure 11-5 illustrates the SWOT and TOWS analysis tools.

Nominal Group Techniques

Brainstorming exercises are vital to successful planning efforts. The nominal group technique is a method that allows participants to act both in a group and alone. Participants work alone, quietly, in generating individual brainstorm lists based on a prompt (eg, develop a list of what you think are the strengths of your sports medicine staff or develop a list of the most pressing issues facing your academic program). Once everyone has developed a list, they then work again quietly to prioritize or rank their responses. A group leader or facilitator then goes around the room

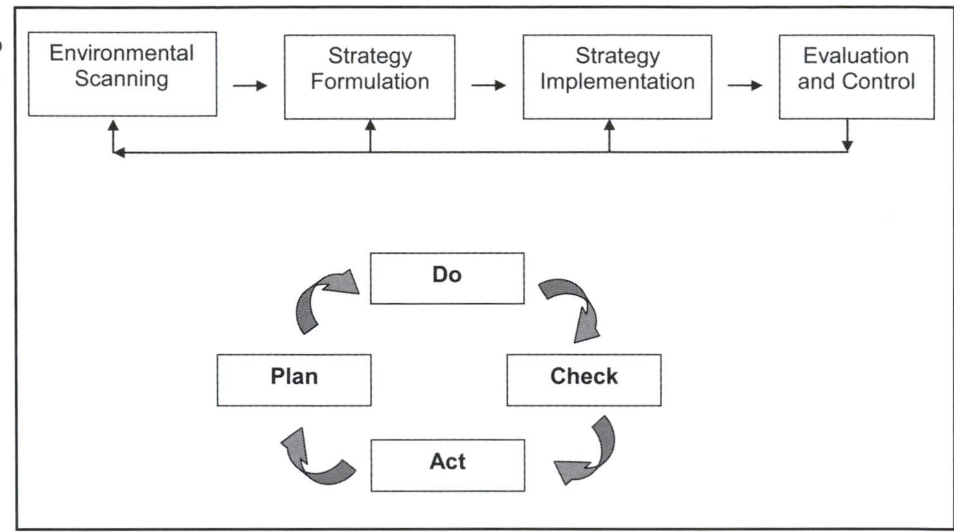

Figure 11-4. Feedback loops commonly used in planning. The 4-step scanning, strategy, implementation, and evaluation process and the PDCA cycle.

Figure 11-5. Planning data generated by brainstorming and data collection techniques is classified as strength, weakness, opportunity, or threat. The TOWS analysis uses the SWOT data to help create strategies for organizational action.

Strengths, Weaknesses, Opportunities and Threats (SWOT) Analysis

Internal to the Organization		External to the Organization	
Strengths	**Weaknesses**	**Opportunities**	**Threats**

Turning Opportunities and Weaknesses into Strengths (TOWS) Analysis

SO	ST
This cell will contain strategies that take strengths and turn them into opportunities.	This cell will contain strategies that use strengths to avoid threats.
WO	**WT**
This cell will contain strategies that attempt to take advantage of opportunities by overcoming weaknesses.	This cell will contain strategies that try to minimize weaknesses and avoid threats.

and asks participants to provide the item on the top of their list. The leader drafts a comprehensive list from all of the suggested items. If the item on the top of your list has been mentioned, then you can provide the next item. This process continues until all of the pertinent items have been placed on the common list. A variety of techniques can be used to prioritize the common list after it is developed. Giving each member a set of stickers and having him or her identify his or her top choices is a common method.

Affinity Diagrams

An affinity diagram is like a nominal group process in that the participants will work alone in silence to develop answers to specific planning prompts. In this instance, they will write their responses on a sticky note, limiting to one response per note. After all responses have been written, participants then place the notes on a table or wall. Working in silence, the group must move the notes around to cluster similar ideas together. Notes can be moved until a consensus

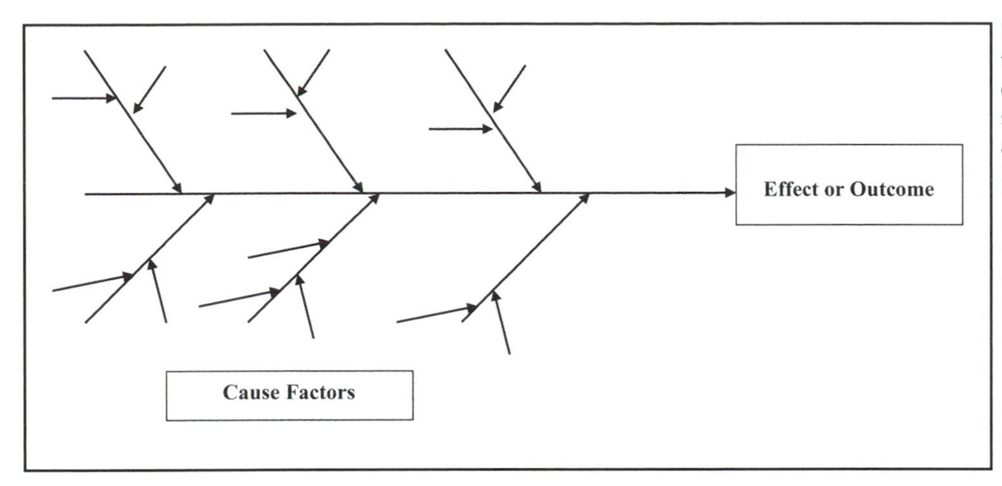

Figure 11-6. Main branches of the cause-and-effect diagram often focus on resources, personnel, policy and procedures, and environment issues that impact the effect or outcome.

is reached for which ideas belong clustered together. Once finished, the group can then discuss the themes that have emerged from the exercise.

SMART Language

SMART is an acronym for specific, measurable, achievable, results oriented, and time bound. SMART language is employed with writing goals. This can be very helpful when writing goals following the analysis of your planning data. Too often goals are too general and vague. Paying attention to SMART language can help groups write goals that are meaningful and promote genuine change.

Responsibility Matrix

The responsibility matrix is so simple, it is often overlooked. It is a method to keep track of who is taking responsibility for specific actions and steps in implementation following the planning process. Remember, plans are effective only when they yield strategies that can be put into place. It is a simple accountability and tracking process. The responsibility matrix lists in the rows the specific tasks while the columns include information on the person, group, or office responsible for taking the actions. It may also include steps in the process or target dates for completing a task. Responsibility matrices can be powerful motivational tools to see projects to completion.

Cause-and-Effect Diagrams

A cause-and-effect diagram (Figure 11-6) is sometimes called a fishbone diagram (they look like a fish skeleton when complete) or Ishikawa diagram (after the man who created them). The diagrams are graphical representations of the factors that influence a particular outcome. Recognizing the factors that influence both desired and unintended outcomes is a key element of OE (see systems thinking on p. 223). They are helpful in organizing the various causes that yield a particular effect. It could be what is contributing to the outcome of a problem, what needs to happen to obtain a desired result, or it may help determine the consequences of a decision. You need to do the following to draw cause-and-effect diagrams:

- Place the outcome or effect on the right hand side of a page.
- Draw a line across the page that connects to the effect; this is the backbone of the fish.
- Diagonal lines, or ribs, link the "cause factors" to the backbone that links to the effect.
- Additional lines can be connected to the ribs to identify "root causes" of the effect.
- The diagram is fleshed out by repeatedly asking why a certain item affects the outcome in a particular way.

Presentation of Quantitative Data

In an athletic training health care organization, gathering data will be an essential part of the planning process. There are many types of data to collect and the type will be dependent upon the nature of your organization. Some possibilities include how many initial assessments did we perform in our facility? What is the break down by sport? How many referrals to specific practitioners did we make? How many and what type of therapeutic interventions did we utilize? How did our projected budget compare to our actual costs? No matter what types of data are collected as part of the planning process, finding ways to effectively present the material is critical. The final report will need excellent tables, graphs, and charts to help clearly illustrate your points. It is imperative that the data you collect for your planning process be easily represented and explained for the audience who will read your final document.

Resources for Planning

Many readers of this text will be affiliated with institutions of higher learning. It just might be that your best resource for strategic planning is in your own backyard. Many university and college campuses have committees, offices, and full departments dedicated to strategic planning, quality improvement, and program evaluation. Take a look and chances are there is help close at hand.

Program Evaluation

The act of evaluation is a key component of the strategic planning process. Information is needed to determine if the strategic actions that grew from the planning process are having the desired effect (see Figure 11-3). Feedback loops include an evaluative component to insure that periodic adjustments can be made as plans are carried out over time (see Figure 11-4). If the strategic planning process allows organizations to look ahead, a formal program evaluation is a chance to reflect. Formal program evaluation is a systematic collection of information about the activities, characteristics, and outcomes of a program to allow for informed judgments about program improvement, program effectiveness, and decisions about future programming.[8] Priest[9] reports that programs tend go through a formal evaluation for 1 of 3 reasons: 1) accountability, 2) improvement, and 3) marketing (Table 11-1).

There are different approaches to the program evaluation based on who does the evaluation (internal or external) and the intention of the evaluation (formative or summative). The intent of the program evaluation is either formative or summative. Formative evaluations are conducted with the idea of learning how programs can be improved. Formative evaluations can be performed as part program development or on-going implementation of a program. This focus on improvement can make formative evaluations more open and less threatening. In contrast, a summative evaluation is designed to provide answers about the value of a program and the need to continue funding and carrying out the program activities. Summative evaluations are done in the interest of providing information to make major decisions on the future of a program. Who performs the evaluation can vary by setting and evaluation type. Many evaluations will utilize outside evaluators (eg, it is common practice for academic programs to have outside evaluators from like institutions). Sometimes summative evaluations will rely on neutral outside evaluators if decisions about continuation of a program could be swayed using internal evaluators. Many program evaluations will use a combination of internal and external evaluators.

Type of Program Evaluation

Program evaluation may include any or a variety of types of evaluation in order to carefully collect needed information to make decisions about a program. There are multiple models of program evaluation, but most fall under 5 categories: 1) needs assessment, 2) feasibility studies, 3) process evaluations, 4) outcome evaluations, and 5) cost analysis.[9] Table 11-2 outlines some possible athletic training applications for these evaluation types.

A needs assessment addresses the following question: What gaps in our program need to be filled? A needs assessment evaluates your current program in relation to your objectives and desired program goals. The needs assessment can help you understand the context of the program (eg, the culture, climate, and concerns of stakeholders and the communities in which the program exists). To understand this state of affairs may require surveying, interviewing, and observing staff, patients, and others who interact with the program. By establishing the gaps between the current state and the desired state of affairs, the needs assessment may also tease out underlying problems or concerns and indicated unrealized needs.

A feasibility study explores the following question: Can the program succeed given our current constraints? A feasibility study would be conducted to determine the likelihood of success for a program based on the evaluation data (resources, staff, etc). A feasibility study examines this likelihood by exploring alternative approaches and identifying the factors that may impede or assist in delivery of a program. Special attention is paid to the best use of resources such as staff, equipment, finances, space, and time. For example, if an athletic training health care organization in a collegiate setting decided to establish a mechanism to perform base line neuropsychological testing on a large number of athletes annually, a feasibility evaluation would be logical. Do we have the time? Do we have the resources? How would this program impact the other services we provide? It would be wise to determine what factors would hinder the program's attempt to provide this service, and what would facilitate their ability or provide this service. Are there alternatives to implementing the program? How could we do this in another way? These are the kinds of questions that can be addressed by examining the needs and feasibility prior to implementation. Needs assessments and feasibility studies can serve as precursors to the planning process.

A process evaluation examines the following query: How is the implementation of a program progressing?

Table 11-1

Reasons for Performing Program Evaluations

Accountability	Confirm objectives are met Make better decisions about planning and operations Authorize fiscal payments Meet grant obligations Correctly allocate resources
Improvement	Identify program strengths and weaknesses Increase educational value Enhance competence Test new ideas Decrease operating costs Establish quality benchmarks and standards
Marketing	Advertise and promote program effectiveness Indicate a track record of successful programming Promote positive public relations

Table 11-2

Program Evaluation Types: Athletic Training Examples

Evaluation Type	*Athletic Training Example*
Needs assessment	How will the addition of the women's lacrosse teams impact our sports medicine facility needs at the university?
Feasibility study	Is it feasible to build a new facility? What are the possible alternatives that have not been explored?
Process evaluation	Has our new program for referring patients to counseling services been effective? How can we evaluate it and make adjustments at this time?
Outcomes evaluation	Based on the outcome, should we continue to hold our annual educational symposium?
Cost analysis	Has the new continuing education program been worthwhile given the cost?

This type of evaluation looks at the workings of an organization. It can examine organizational offerings, staff practices, and client actions. The process evaluation measures the gap between the program plan and the actual execution of the program and determines if corrections are needed along the way, rather than waiting until the final outcome. Process evaluations contrast the information from the needs assessment with all the new needs that arise within the program. It allows you to compare what is happening with what was planned. Examining unexpected consequences is crucial to program success (see Systems Thinking on p. 223). Unexpected costs, poor estimations of staff time required, and unintended impact on other programming are all issues that would be identified in a process-oriented evaluation. To make best use of this information, staff must be willing to be flexible and make deviations from the plan if the evaluation data indicate an adjustment is needed.

An outcome evaluation places an emphasis on the program objectives or outcomes. The outcome evaluation answers the following question: Were the program goals and objectives achieved? These evaluations look at what happens to participants as a result of their participation in the program. Are the clients, customers, and community satisfied with the outcome of the program? Results of outcome evaluations are used to justify overall effectiveness and to suggest areas for program improvement. An outcome evaluation can identify levels of satisfaction, learning, or changes that were obtained by the program. They examine expected results with actual outcomes. Often, an agreed upon benchmark or standard for success will be identified a priori to program implementation and then used as a measure for the outcomes.

Many formal evaluations of health care service programs (eg, the athletic training outreach component of a private clinic, a service program housed within

Table 11-3

A Comparison of Program Evaluation Techniques

	Needs Assessment	Feasibility Study	Process Evaluation	Outcome Evaluation	Cost Analysis
Timing	Initial stages prior to program design	Precursor to formal program planning	During the delivery of the program	During and/or after the program is under way	After program completion
Measures	The gap between current and desired state or outcome	Alternate approaches, helpful and hindering factors	Gap between program plan and actual execution	Satisfaction levels and attainment of objectives	Program value and merit
Central question	What gaps in our program need to be filled?	Given our current constraints, can the program succeed?	How is the implementation of a program progressing?	Were the program goals and objectives achieved?	Was the program financially worthwhile or valuable?
Information is used to	Understand context and direct program planning	Gauge viability and best use of resources	Monitor and modify program	Improve and justify effectiveness	Decide future offerings

Adapted from Priest S. A program evaluation primer. *Journal of Experiential Education*. 2001;24(1):34-40.

an intercollegiate athletic department, or a workplace-style clinic industrial athletic training program) are hybrids of the process and outcome style, looking at both aspects of the program. Since these programs are often on going, they must look at process and outcomes at the same time.

The final evaluation type is the cost analysis. Was the program financially worthwhile or valuable? Cost analysis evaluations measure the value of a program in comparison with other alternative approaches (often these alternatives were identified in the feasibility study). Comparisons of the fiscal value of a program will determine if that program is run again, terminated, or possibly duplicated in another setting. Cost analyses identify the price, benefit, effect, utility, and efficiency of several programs and compares them. An example might be a campus-based athletic training service program that is seeking to improve its psychological counseling and referral services. The athletic training health care administrators could compare costs with a variety of options (eg, hiring staff, contracting with local services, or sharing cost with other campus entities). The cost of each option can be evaluated to determine a course of action. While a cost analysis is essential to review in association with an outcomes analysis, it can also be a part of the a priori feasibility study to explore alternatives as part of the planning process. Cost analysis and value formulas are good tools for athletic trainers to show their worth to current and potential employers. Table 11-3 provides a comparison of the previous techniques.

Methods for Collecting Evaluation Information

A variety of sources can be used to collect information for any of the described types of program evaluations. Data for the program evaluation can be gleaned from existing information or need to be collected from specific people.[10] Existing information sources include the following:

- Program documents (eg, personnel records, statistical reports, budget information, minutes of meetings, and existing strategic plans)
- Existing databases (eg, injury reporting data, treatment databases, and referral records [number and type])
- Research reports and published literature
- Data from professional organizations (eg, salary data and employment trends)

A variety of people can provide information for the program evaluation and include the following:

- Beneficiaries (ie, those individuals who benefit directly or indirectly from the program [eg, patients, student-athletes, athletic training students])

- Key informants (ie, anyone with a particular knowledge about the program and the program benefit). Coaches, administrators, other allied health professionals, and physicians would be common key informants in an athletic training setting.
- Individuals with special expertise such as site visitors, invited review teams, and hired consultants
- Program staff who directly participate in the program

Observational data may be used for some types of program evaluation. However, there are many privacy concerns that may make this technique difficult in health care settings. Videotaping is more common in controlled learning environments. This allows for later review to evaluate effectiveness. This is a viable program evaluation technique for classroom settings and under specific circumstances a tool for evaluating lab and learning environments.

Specific methods of data collection include surveys, case studies, interviews, observations, group assessments (eg, focus groups, brainstorming techniques, nominal group exercises), expert or peer review, portfolio reviews (eg, collections of materials, work samples, program data), and testimonials. Table 11-4 outlines common evaluation data collection methods and their advantages and challenges.

Generating an Evaluation Report

A comprehensive report of the program evaluation will be required to provide stakeholders with the findings of your evaluation. Boyd[11] indicates several steps that will assist in preparing a useful report.

- Consider the target audience. Keep in mind why you are performing the evaluation and what type of evaluation is being conducted. Accreditation processes and certain academic reviews have very specific formats for presentation of information.
- Include the appropriate details. The report should provide enough technical data so the reader can determine the merits of the evaluation. The basic format should address the following:
  - What—Your central question
  - Why—The purpose of the evaluation
  - Who—The sources of information (including appropriate statistical information when needed)
  - How—Full explanation of your data collection methods
  - Where—The locations from which the data were gathered
  - When—The timeline for the collection of the information.

  If the report is primarily targeted at the lay public, it may be advisable not to include as much "scientific" detail. On the other hand, if the report is designed for a professional audience, it should include specific statistical information to explain methods, sampling, and analysis.
- Exercise caution when drawing conclusions and reporting findings. Program evaluations must be careful not to overstate specific cause-and-effect relationships without appropriate evidence to support the claims regarding program outcomes. It is important to discuss results you have documented that are associated with a program and to properly describe the elements of a program, but care must be taken not to infer causation without evidence. It is also important to present results in an unbiased manner and to avoid superlatives. The report must be an objective presentation of the evaluation process and not a biased advocacy document.
- Use an evaluation team or committee to review and edit the report. Make sure all aspects of the report are readable and that tables and figures are accurate and easily understood.

Evaluation reports may determine the future of a program. A document with such power should be developed and reviewed with care. The reporting of evaluation findings may need to follow specific guidelines. In academic settings, evaluation reports will likely need to be reviewed by committees and presented to the larger department. Reports may need to be presented and accepted at various levels of an organization (eg, university, hospital administration, academic department) before they can be made public. Care should be taken to protect the content of the final report and to only release the final findings when you have followed your organizational guidelines.

The Self-Study as an Instrument of Change: Another Improvement Model

Athletic training education programs are required to develop a programmatic self-study on a regular basis. Coupled with the site visit process and subsequent administrative review by the Committee on Accreditation of Athletic Training Education (CAATE), educational programs have a clear mechanism to demonstrate their compliance with set programmatic standards. However, self-studies and accreditation reviews can reach beyond demonstrating simple compliance. They also serve as instruments of change and improvement.[12]

Table 11-4

A Comparison of Program Evaluation Data Collection Methods

Method	Overall Purpose	Advantages	Challenges
Questionnaires and surveys	Allows for the collection of lots of information from people in a nonthreatening way	Can complete anonymously Inexpensive to administer Easy to compare and analyze Administer to many people Gather lots of data Many formats already available	Might not get careful feedback Wording can bias responses Impersonal In surveys may need sampling expert Do not always get the full story
Interviews	Used when you want to understand someone's impressions or experiences or learn more about his or her answers to questionnaires	Get full range and depth of information Develops better relationship with client Allows for flexibility	Very time consuming Can be hard to analyze and compare results
Documentation review	Used to gather an impression of how a program operates without interrupting the program A review of key documentation (memos, policies, finances, etc)	Get comprehensive and historical information Information already exists Less disruption for program operation Few biases about information	Time consuming Information may be incomplete Need to be specific about what you are looking for Not flexible Data are restricted to existing information
Observation	Used to gather information about how a program actually operates, particularly about processes	View operations as they occur Can adapt to events as they occur	Can be difficult to interpret seen behaviors Can be complex to categorize observations Observation can influence the actions of the participants
Focus groups	Used to explore a topic in depth through group discussion (eg, about reactions to an experience or suggestion, understanding common concerns) Useful in evaluation.	Allows quick and reliable method to get common impressions Can be an efficient way to get much range and depth of information Can convey key information about programs	Can be hard to analyze responses Need good facilitator Can be difficult to schedule groups together
Case studies	Used to fully understand or depict a client's experiences in a program and conduct comprehensive examination through cross comparison of cases	Fully depicts client's experience in program input, processes, and results Power means to portray program to outsiders	Very time consuming to collect, organize, and describe Represents depth but little breadth about program

Adapted from McNamara C. Basic guide to program evaluation. Adapted from McNamara C. Field guide to nonprofit program design, marketing, and evaluation. Authenticity Consulting, LLC. 2006. Available at http://www.managementhelp.org/evaluatn/fnl_eval.htm#anchor1575679. Accessed February 27, 2007.

The self-study process need not be limited to our current view of its use in accreditation of athletic training educational programs. Elements of the self-study process can be applied to evaluation of athletic training health care organizations pursuing continuous improvement. At the heart of any self-study process is a program's or organization's obligation to examine itself in a critical fashion. The nature of that reflection, the questions that are deemed important for study, the types of data collected, and the participation in the process by internal and external constituents will all help determine the self-study's breadth, depth, and ultimate worth of the final report. An effective self-study can trigger change. The organizational literature sometimes refers to self-studies as potential "trigger events." A trigger event is one that may cause a perturbation or change in a loosely coupled system that can set off a pattern of new behaviors and thoughts among the members of the organization or community. Isabella[13] stated that trigger events unbalance established routines and evoke conscious thought on the part of organizational members. In short, it can be the jump-start needed to break out of old patterns and explore new thinking in an organization.

SYSTEMS THINKING

A system is a collection of parts that interact with each other to function as a more comprehensive whole. Consider this example. If we have a pile of sand in front of us and divide it in half, we are left with 2 piles of sand. The remaining piles of sand are not a functional comprehensive system; they are simply heaps of sand. A cow on the other hand is a full and functional system, but cutting the cow in half does not create 2 smaller cows.[6] Too often we look at organizations from the viewpoint of the sand (individual parts) instead of the larger whole (the cow). Systems thinking requires that we look at the "wholes" to determine how the parts influence the larger function. The concept of systems thinking relies on patterns of influence and feedback loops. Systems thinking is based on the idea that patterns of inter-related events yield specific outcomes. Systems thinking is the ability to see inter-relationships and patterns rather than snapshots or static views of events.

Feedback loops play a major role in systems thinking.[14] Loops in a system are either balancing loops or reinforcing loops. A balancing loop is feedback that provided stability to a system. These loops negate changes that have taken place (eg, if our body temperature increases, our thermoregulatory system helps cool our body and negates the change). In a reinforcing loop, any feedback is put back into the systems, thus expanding the system. Knowledge growth is a reinforcing loop. Reinforcing loops amplify disturbances or changes in a system until something changes the cycle. They need not be positive. The growth of a tumor is an unfortunate example of a reinforcing loop.

An organization is a system that is influenced by inter-related actions. The effect of decisions and actions influences other aspects of the organization and the system receives feedback, sometimes positive, sometimes negative. Understanding that the system relies on circular feedback rather than linear cause-effect thinking can influence our understanding of how organizations behave. Feedback loops help us understand causality; every action and decision can be both a cause and an effect in this circular way of thinking. Figure 11-7 shows how one decision can be both a cause and an effect.

Seeing inter-relationships will ultimately allow for a deeper understanding of how organizational problems and issues can be better addressed. Senge[14] described several archetypes or common dysfunctional patterns of organizational behavior. It is easier to interrupt dysfunctional cycles and avoid creating them in the future once they are recognized and understood. Some examples are outlined in Table 11-5. Athletic training health care organizations are not immune to these dysfunctional cycles that influence all aspects of the organization. Making the paradigm shift to systems thinking will enhance an organization's ability to participate in thoughtful planning and evaluation and ultimately improve effectiveness.

SYSTEM THINKING APPLICATIONS

Seymour[15] explains that some key points should be kept in mind when applying systems thinking to planning and decision-making organizational settings:

- Processes tend to degrade over time. A process as a "whole" needs to be monitored and continually improved. A process could refer to teaching, how patients obtain clinic appointments, patient care components, or how preparticipation exams are conducted. Without the view of the whole, the process may have many people using it but no one having a sense of responsibility for it.
- Almost any decision has both short-term and long-term consequences; these are often in opposition to one another.
- Today's problems may be yesterday's solution.[14] Every decision is both a cause and effect.
- Organizations tend to react to and try to manage "events." Systems thinking allows for better decisions because the group will have thought through the various potential effects, intended and unintended.
- Initial causes and ultimate effect may be separated by significant time and space. Learning from such delayed gaps will require conscious effort.

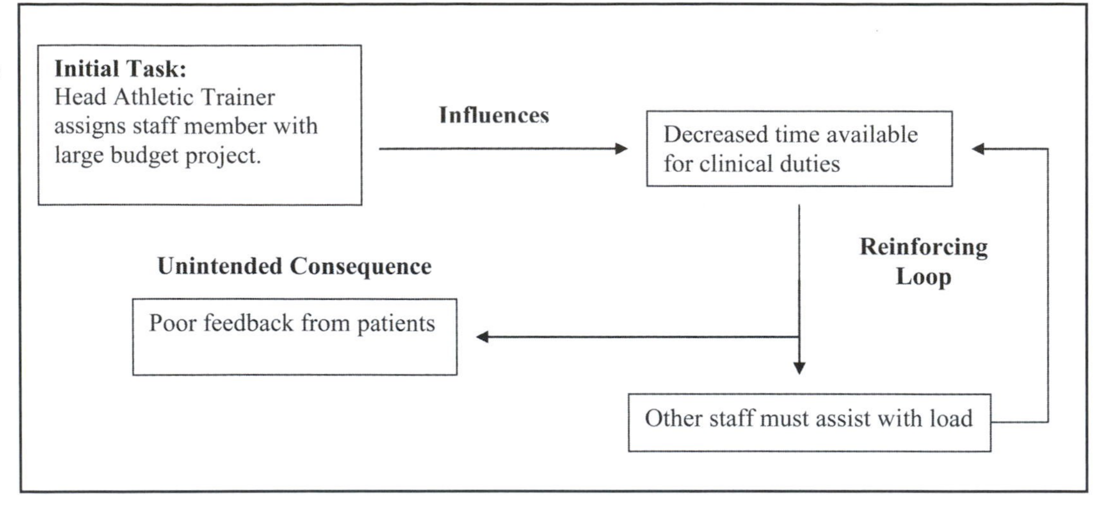

Figure 11-7. Systems thinking allows us to examine the influence and consequences (intended and unintended) of specific actions. Feedback loops are helpful as we explore cause and effect.

THE LEARNING ORGANIZATION

A learning organization is described as one that allows people to continually expand their capacity to create the results they desire.[14] Organizations that couple an individual growth with organizational performance are true learning organizations. The core "learning disciplines" of a learning organization are personal mastery, mental models, shared vision, team learning, and systems thinking.[14]

Personal mastery is learning to expand personal capacity to obtain the results that are most desired; it is creating an organizational environment that encourages all members to develop themselves toward the goals and purposes they choose. Organizations learn only through individuals who learn. Athletic training has a rich tradition of promoting personal mastery though continuing education. When properly channeled, this emphasis on personal mastery can be used to advance the effectiveness of the broader organization. To value personal mastery as a core learning organization discipline in an organization is to value the growth of the individual, an environment where employees can create their own visions, an acceptance of truth (where they are), and the willingness to see the gap between their personal vision and current state. What better resource to invest in than human resources?

Each of us carries a mental model of how we think the world works. It may be that our vision or model of how things are supposed to be gets in the way of implementing creative strategies and making good use of new insights. An organization cannot take a systems approach and see the wholes if its world view or model for how things are is impeding that progress. Mental models are really snapshots in the mind, pictures of what each person sees things to be. The business world is littered with tales of companies that could not change their mental model of how things should be done and either failed or fell behind miserably because of their world view (think American car quality in the past 20 years compared to Japanese imports). What mental models are holding us back as an athletic training profession? There are many. However, think of the creative people who changed their worldview on athletic training in such a way that we now see athletic trainers in hospitals, military bases, and industrial environments and billing third-party payers for services. That is the point. If our mental models and worldview can hold the individual or organization back and interfere with learning, why cannot the opposite be true? Why cannot a mental model be nurtured to improve learning?

The shared vision learning discipline is based on building a sense of commitment in a group by developing shared images of the future that the organization seeks to create and the principles and guiding practices that are used to get there. A shared vision is the answer to the question, "What do we want to create?" A shared vision is the commonality that gives cohesiveness to the organization's diverse activities. Employees with a strong personal vision will strengthen the opportunities for shared vision. Personal mastery is the foundation for developing such a vision. An organization that wishes to build a strong shared vision should encourage members to develop their own personal vision. If people do not have their own vision, they will latch on to someone else's. That is not commitment; it is compliance. If many individuals have a strong sense of personal direction, they can join together and create powerful shared visions.

Team learning creates results through communication and collaboration. It also centers on transforming

Table 11-5

Common Archetypes or Dysfunctional Patterns of Organizational Behavior

Pattern	*Description*
Fixes that fail	A fix, effective in the short term, has unforeseen long-term consequences that may require even more use of the same fix. Example: Adjusting a workload to meet a short-term staffing solution creates unintended consequences for other staffing area.
Tragedy of the commons	Individual uses a commonly available but limited resource solely on the basis of individual need. At first, he or she is rewarded for using it; eventually, he or she gets diminishing returns, which causes him or her to intensify his or her efforts. In time, the resource is depleted. Example: Increasing demands from 2 teams that rely on the same athletic trainer.
Balancing process with delay	An organization, acting toward a goal, adjusts its behavior in response to delayed feedback. If it is not conscious of the delay, it may overcorrect or give up because it does not see progress. Example: Making a harsh adjustment to policy prior to gathering necessary feedback.
Eroding goals	A form of burden shifting that allows short-term solutions to erode long-term fundamental goals. Example: Accepting lower academic standards for the sake of maintaining program "numbers."

Adapted from Senge PM. *The Fifth Discipline: The Art and Practice of the Learning Organization.* New York, NY: Doubleday; 1990.

Trust and Organizational Effectiveness

The relationship between organizational trust and organizational effectiveness is well established in a range of organizational studies. Employee trust has been associated with greater adaptability, responsive teamwork, effective crisis management, and overall satisfaction. Leaders in athletic training health care organizations would do well to take notice. Hidden among the complexities and challenges of managing all aspects of the organization is the road map to employee satisfaction and improved organizational effectiveness: trust. Trust is an important leadership dimension. Trustworthiness can be established through behavioral consistency, behavioral integrity, sharing, delegation of control, clear communication, and demonstration of concern. Information may hold the key. The greater the amount of information received about job and organizational issues explains the largest percentage of the variance in trust of top management and immediate supervisors. Information-receiving activities such as evaluations, decision making, organizational policies, pay and benefits, promotion and advancement opportunities, and long-term planning are all information-receiving issues. Attention to these areas and an environment of trust are a good start for any athletic training health care organization.

Bibliography

Ellis K, Shockley-Zalabak P. Trust in top management and immediate supervisor: the relationship to satisfaction, perceived organizational effectiveness and information receiving. *Communication Quarterly.* 2001;49(4):382-398.

conversational and collective thinking skills to enable groups to reliably develop intelligence and ability greater than the sum of its parts. Anyone who has seen a good basketball team play or has listened to a symphony has enjoyed the fruits of team learning. The end result yields something beyond the sum of the individual talents. Organizations that develop true team learning build on synergy, commonality of purpose, a shared vision, and an understanding of how to complement one another's efforts. Individual interests are not sacrificed for the larger vision; shared visions become an extension of personal visions. A multidisciplinary sports medicine clinic that is a learning organization with shared vision and aligned learning employees comfortable and energetic about their roles could produce remarkable results and create an amazing work environment.

Table 11-6

Examples of Organizational Learning Disabilities

Disability	*Description*
"I Am My Position"	If people in organizations focus only on "their" job or position, they have little sense of responsibility for the results of the overall group. Example: "I don't know why that happens. Things always go smoothly when my patients are seen in clinic." Reality: Any clinic that does not run smoothly reflects on the entire organization.
"The Enemy Is Out There"	Anything that may go wrong in an organization must be because of something outside of the group. No one will take ownership. Example: "The administration just doesn't give us enough support. No wonder we are having troubles." Reality: Issues that are internal to the group are as likely to blame for problems.
"The Fixation on Events"	Too often we only fixate on short-term events. Therefore, we only have short-term explanations. Example: "It always seems like one difficult case puts my clinic schedule behind for the whole day." Reality: If the schedule is always behind, the true influences and causes have not been explored.
"The Illusion of Taking Charge"	Too often proactive action is just reaction in disguise. It is a combination of the enemy out there and a fixation on events. True proactiveness comes from seeing how we contribute to our own problems. Problems require broader systems thinking. Example: "I am going to see to it that the clinic staff stays on schedule." Reality: Without understanding the true underlying causes of the schedule falling behind, this is just being reactive disguised as being proactive.

Adapted from Senge PM. *The Fifth Discipline: The Art and Practice of the Learning Organization.* New York, NY: Doubleday; 1990.

Systems thinking has been discussed previously. It is the fifth of the learning disciplines. In fact, Senge[14] titled his book *The Fifth Discipline* as recognition of how important systems thinking was to the practice of the 5 learning disciplines for a learning organization. It is an integration of the preceding 4 disciplines into a complete practice. It is a way of thinking about and a language for describing and understanding the forces and inter-relationships that shape the behavior of systems. The 5 disciplines for a learning organization are designed as a group. For example, vision without systems thinking paints a nice image of the future without any understanding of the forces at work that influence how to get there. Without personal mastery, people tend to be reactive and threatened by the idea of systems thinking. In turn, systems thinking is dependent upon personal mastery, mental models, shared vision, and team learning to reach its full potential for an organization.

Does Your Organization Have a Learning Disability?

Senge[14] describes various types of organizational learning disabilities (Table 11-6). Most organizations do not learn well. The way they are designed and managed, the way people think about their jobs, and how they interact all contribute to this low level of learning. Smart people with good ideas working very hard often try to fix organizational problems and the results are even worse. Understanding the root causes of organizational problems, and the learning disabilities that prevent the organization from being a true learning organization is the key to correcting this problem. Before they can be fixed, they must be identified.

Leadership and the Learning Organization

It is worth noting that in a learning organization, the role of leaders may vary from our traditional views of leadership. In learning organizations, the roles of the leaders are thought of as a designer, teacher, and steward. Leaders help build a shared vision, help challenge prevailing mental models, and foster a greater understanding of systems thinking.[16] In the role of designer, leaders help construct the social architecture in which others operate within the organization. The leader helps shape a vision, purpose and mission, and operating structure to support the learning disciplines within the organization. The leader as teacher develops the individual and group capacity to gain insight from the current reality. In learning organizations, leaders teach through facilitation, foster strategic thinking, and foster in their employees the ability to achieve insight into the complexity of their worldview and mental models and coping with them in a constructive manner. Stewardship is the third type of leadership role in a learning organization. The leader as steward serves as a guardian for both the people he or she leads and the larger purpose of the organization. The leader as steward role is heightened in a learning organization since participants are encouraged to promote a shared vision and sense of ownership for the organizational mission. If the leaders fail in this setting, there is the potential for greater impact on the employees who have developed a stake in the outcomes.

PROFESSIONAL DEVELOPMENT: IMPROVING THE ORGANIZATION ONE EMPLOYEE AT A TIME

The strategic planning and evaluation techniques discussed in this chapter focus on organization-wide approaches to improving organizational performance. However, athletic training health care administrators should never lose sight of the people who must be the agents of change. If planning is really planning, then something has to happen. That something is change, and change requires people to carry the plans forward. Investing in the staff around you will only make them better suited to carry forward the vision of the organization. Allowing ways for individuals to invest in their own improvement so that they may give back to the broader organization is a fundamental goal of professional development.

Most views of professional development seem to center on attending meetings and conferences, but these may not be the most cost effective or learning-centered mechanisms for improvement. What else could you do to learn something new that would assist you in your athletic training duties? You might observe someone else, read a book, research a project, subscribe to a new journal, undertake a literature review, take a class, participate in a list serve, join a teaching circle, visit another organization, or seek out a mentor. These are just a handful of ideas. Keep in mind, professional development is not unlike the other processes we have discussed in this chapter. It too requires planning, a link to broader organizational goals, and specific attention to cost and detail.

Administrators should encourage employees to develop annual professional development plans (Figure 11-8). This planning tool allows for the development activities to be linked to the broader goals of the department or work unit. This can ensure that the group meets its capacity to fulfill its stated purpose. The plans can also be shared. Looking at common themes among employees can shed light on broader needs.

Athletic training health care administrators should develop plans for themselves as well. While his or her staff may rightfully focus on more patient care goals, the athletic training administrator may wish to expand his or her organizational or management skills.

Organizational Structure and Effectiveness

How an organization is formally structured can make a difference in the effectiveness of the program services. Many questions can guide a discussion of the physical structure of the organization:

- Is your organization too vertical?
- Does it have many layers of management?
- Do individuals have the authority to make decisions on their own?
- Is the organization too flat with everyone on the same level?
- How do people communicate across the organization?
- How have responsibilities been divided?
- How are activities coordinated?

Asking such questions allows consultants on organizational structure to uncover many common organizational problems. Bolman and Deal[17] identified some examples of structurally related organizational problems:

Annual Professional Development Plan for:

____

Professional Learning Goal	Related Department/Office Goal	Proposed Activity (what, when, where?)	Cost (including travel)
Learn how to use database software program.	Better organization of medical record information.	Take workshop at campus computer center.	$125.00
Learn more about university strategies for improving diversity.	Develop a candidate pool for job openings that is more representative.	Contact campus Office of Human Resources for information on available resources.	$ 0.00
Improve manual therapy skills.	Provide a broader range of treatments to our clients.	Identify a regional workshop on myofascial release.	$1200.00
Think "outside the box" and develop more information about organizational improvement.	Stay in step with our commitment to quality.	Read *Good to Great* Share thoughts with staff and consider purchase for them.	$ 30.00

Chair / Supervisor Comments:

Chair / Supervisor Signature:___________________________ Date: ____________

Figure 11-8. The development of an individual professional development plan can allow employees and supervisors to work together to select activities that are well aligned with the broader program goals. (Adapted from Office of Quality Improvement University of Wisconsin-Madison, 2000.)

- Overlap. This occurs when 2 or more individuals are doing the same thing. Unnecessary duplication of activities wastes effort and can lead to turf battles.
- Gaps. Important tasks and responsibilities are not assigned and fall through the cracks.
- Under use. Some individuals or units have too little work.
- Overload. Some individuals are so overloaded that their work suffers in many areas.
- Excessive autonomy. Individuals or groups that are too loosely coupled the feel isolated and unsupported, and their efforts become uncoordinated with others in the program. This easily happens when many people of the same unit are in multiple locations.
- Too many meetings. It is common to hold a meeting or form a committee for every new issue that arises. With too many meetings and committees, little else gets done. Lack of accountability and no shared ownership become a problem.
- Diffuse authority. No one knows or is in agreement about who is in charge of specific important program tasks. Confusion will limit initiative and stifle creativity.
- Structure/technology mismatch. Does the organization have the proper technology in place that is appropriate for the structure, or vice versa? How do members communicate? Is the group overly dependent upon technology and not meeting face to face enough?

No one structure will fit an organization. Athletic training health care organizations may take many shapes and forms. The problems identified above are common to any organization from the smallest of athletic training staffs at a college to the large multidisciplinary groups found at large sports medicine clinics.

Asking questions about organizational structure and recognizing specific problems is another tool that can aid in improving OE.

SUMMARY

- Explain the benefits of strategic planning.

  Successful strategic planning can increase the understanding of the organization's current and anticipated opportunities and challenges; stimulate innovative responses to a changing environment; and provide a coordinated framework for modifying the organization's services, processes, and capabilities to meet future requirements. Strategic planning helps identify new capabilities that the organization and its members must obtain to succeed in the future and can guide daily decision making.

- Discuss the pros and cons of specific evaluation and planning approaches.

  This chapter has addressed a range of strategic planning and program evaluation tools, techniques, and applications for athletic training health care organizations. The efficacy of any planning or evaluation tool lies in a clear understanding of the purpose of the evaluation or planning process. Formative evaluations are conducted with the idea of learning how programs can be improved. A summative evaluation is designed to provide answers about the value of a program and the need to continue funding and carrying out the program activities.

- Differentiate various program evaluation techniques.

  Program evaluation may include a variety of types of evaluation in order to carefully collect needed information to make decisions about a program. There are multiple models of program evaluation. The most common types are needs assessment, feasibility studies, process evaluations, outcome evaluations, and cost analysis.

- Explain how systems thinking applies to athletic training health care organizations.

  Systems thinking requires looking at the "wholes" to determine how the parts influence the larger function. The concept of systems thinking relies on patterns of influence and feedback loops. Systems thinking is based on the idea that patterns of inter-related events yield specific outcomes. Systems thinking is the ability to see inter-relationships and patterns rather than snapshots or static views of events.

- Draw and evaluate feedback loop diagrams as a tool to examine specific organization and administration issues.

  Feedback loops are common tools used in planning and evaluation processes. The PDCA cycle is an example of such a feedback loop. Any process that provides continuous feedback and allows for adjustments can be considered a feedback loop. The ability to make adjustments based on evaluative feedback is essential.

- Describe the components of a learning organization.

  A learning organization is described as one that allows people to continually expand their capacity to create the results they desire. Organizations that couple an individual growth with organizational performance are true learning organizations. The core "learning disciplines" of a learning organization are personal mastery, mental models, shared vision, team learning, and systems thinking.[14]

- Identify organizational "learning disabilities" that hinder organizational progress.

  Various types of organizational learning disabilities have been identified. Most organizations do not learn well. Understanding the root causes of organizational problems and the learning disabilities that prevent the organization from being a true learning organization is the key to correcting this problem.

- Explain the relationships between OE and organizational trust.

  The relationship between organizational trust and OE is well established in a range of organizational studies. Employee trust has been associated with greater adaptability, responsive teamwork, effective crisis management, and overall satisfaction.

- Discuss how organizational structures can influence effectiveness.

  How an organization is formally structured can make a difference in the effectiveness of the program services. Many questions can guide a discussion of the physical structure of the organization. Examining organizational structure can uncover many common organizational problems.

ACTIVITIES

The following activities are designed to reinforce material presented in the chapter and to allow for discussion among students and instructors.

Scenario Planning

Review the Chapter 11 box on scenario planning (p. 213) and consider the following case.

The sports medicine program at Anytown Tech (a small Division III program) is thinking of adding another sport. The athletic director has asked you, the head athletic trainer, to develop a scenario planning document to examine the impact on adding men's and women's lacrosse in the next year.

You will recall that Anytown Tech currently offers 12 sports (men's and women's soccer, softball, baseball, men's and women's indoor track and field, men's and women's outdoor track and field, volleyball, wrestling, and men's and women's basketball) and has 2 athletic trainers (including yourself) on staff.

Consider the following:

- How will this impact current staffing?
- What is the fiscal impact on your supplies and services budget?
- What steps could Anytown Tech take to assist the athletic training staff in absorbing these additional demands?

Program Evaluation

The athletic training outreach program at the local sports medicine clinic in your community provides high school outreach services to 3 local schools in your community. The clinic has 2 sports medicine physicians (one family medicine specialist and one orthopedic surgeon), one physician assistant, and 3 athletic trainers who provide outreach services. In addition, the clinic also provides rehabilitation services provided by one physical therapist and one athletic trainer. You have been asked to develop a plan to assess the effectiveness of the athletic training outreach program for the purpose of providing a formative evaluation to improve the outreach services.

Consider the following:

- What additional information do you need before you can begin your evaluation?
- What type of information would you want to gather to perform this evaluation?
- What methods would you employ?
- Beyond input from people, what data would you collect?
- How would you organize your report on such an evaluation?

REFERENCES

1. Press C. Why strategies fail. *Health Forum Journal.* 2001;March/April:26-31.
2. Bryson JM. *Strategic Planning for Public and Nonprofit Organizations: A Guide to Strengthening and Sustaining Organizational Achievement.* San Francisco, CA: Jossey-Bass; 1995.
3. American Society for Quality. The art and process of strategy development and deployment. *The Journal of Quality and Participation.* 2005:10-17.
4. Topor R, Pollard, E. The Toper-Pollard test for evaluating your mission statement. Marketing Higher Education Newsletter. Available at http://www.marketinged.com/library/newsltr/1202mhe.txt. Accessed February 26, 2007.
5. Trainer JF. Models and tools for strategic planning. *New Directions for Institutional Research.* 2004;123:129-138.
6. Paris K. A collection of planning corner articles. University of Wisconsin Board of Regents. Available at http://www.wisc.edu/oqitest/strplan/collection.pdf. Accessed February 27, 2007.
7. Hunger JD, Wheelen TL. *Essentials of Strategic Management.* 3rd ed. Upper Saddle River, NJ: Prentice Hall; 2003.
8. McNamara C. Basic guide to program evaluations. In: McNamara C, ed. Field Guide to Nonprofit Program Design, Marketing and Evaluations: Authenticity Consulting, 2006. Available at http://www.managementhelp.org/evaluatn/fnl_eval.htm#anchor1575679. Accessed February 27, 2007.
9. Priest S. A program evaluation primer. *The Journal of Experiential Education.* 2001;24(1):34-40.
10. Taylor-Powell E. *Sources of Evaluation Information, Quick Tips #11.* Madison, WI: University of Wisconsin-Extension; 2002.
11. Boyd HH. *Basics of Evaluating Reporting, Quick Tips #14.* Madison, WI: University of Wisconsin-Extension; 2002.
12. Martin RR, Manning K, Ramaley JA. The self-study as a chariot of strategic change. *New Directions for Higher Education.* 2001;113:95-115.
13. Isabella LA. Managing the challenges of trigger events: the mindsets of governing adaptation to change. *Business Horizons.* 1992;35:59-66.
14. Senge PM. *The Fifth Discipline: The Art and Practice of the Learning Organization.* New York, NY: Doubleday; 1990.
15. Seymour D. *Once Upon a Campus: Lessons for Improving Quality and Productivity in Higher Education.* Phoenix, AZ: American Council on Education and the Oryx Press; 1995.
16. Knutson KA, Miranda AO. Leadership characteristics, social interest, and learning organizations. *The Journal of Individual Psychology.* 2000;56(2):205-213.
17. Bolman LG, Deal TE. *Modern Approach to Understanding and Managing Organizations.* San Francisco, CA: Jossey-Bass; 1984.

Chapter 12

EMPLOYMENT ISSUES IN ATHLETIC TRAINING
ORGANIZATIONAL INFLUENCES AND SOCIALIZATION FOR PROFESSIONAL ROLES

William A. Pitney, EdD, ATC

OBJECTIVES

At the conclusion of this chapter, the reader will be able to:

- Define professional socialization and identify its phases
- Explain the importance of professional and organizational socialization in preparing for specific professional roles
- Identify various organizational socialization tactics and provide examples of each
- List the components of role strain and explain their potential negative impact on athletic trainers
- Identify the fundamental organizational structures and describe the characteristics of each
- Appraise the practical implications of employment issues as they relate to the field of athletic training

Once credentialed and licensed, an athletic trainer will enter an employment organization such as a hospital, sports medicine clinic, college, or high school and embark on what is hoped to be a long and successful career. As an athletic trainer is immersed in an organizational context, however, he or she will encounter many experiences and a complex blend of factors that influence his or her perceptions as well as how he or she performs and functions in the professional role.[1]

Socialization into professional roles offers a framework for examining how professionals are influenced within organizations as they attempt to perform their responsibilities. Socialization for roles contends how one performs a given role, such as providing health care, and is influenced by the social context, structure, and the individuals within that context.[1,2] As health care professionals such as athletic trainers work within an organization, they will interact with other professionals in the organization's structure to provide the delivery of health care. We must recognize that organizations are social systems and individuals function within the system and interact with others to accomplish the varied role expectations or responsibilities associated with their employment.[3]

While each organization is different, there are fundamental aspects of organizations' structures that are predictable; these create rather predictable influences on individuals within the organization as well. An understanding of various aspects of socialization as it relates to organization and employment issues is critical; therefore, in order to positively influence this process, an organization can facilitate individuals' attainment of goals and objectives and be successful in their roles. This chapter will first provide an overview of the professional socialization process, with an emphasis on organizational socialization and the various socialization tactics organizations may utilize. Second, role strain and its components that result during the socialization process will be discussed. Third, organizational structure will be examined and specific strategies for use by employers and employees to facilitate successful organizational socialization will be explicated.

PROFESSIONAL SOCIALIZATION

Professional socialization is the process of learning specific values and attitudes as well as a particular knowledge and skill set associated with a specific discipline.[4,5] Professional socialization can influence the success one may experience in the work environment.[6] The professional socialization process has many aspects, including the recruitment, pre-service (formal education in an athletic training education program), and organizational socialization experiences. The recruitment and pre-service aspects are likely the most familiar to individuals because they relate to the experiences prior to and during a formal academic program. Collectively, the recruitment and pre-service aspects are known as the anticipatory socialization experiences. As the name implies, these experiences allow an individual to anticipate the expected professional responsibilities for a specific professional role.

Professional socialization is the process by which an individual learns the knowledge, skills, values, attitudes, and dispositions associated with a professional role.

> Scholars have used different terminology to organize and present the phases of socialization for professional roles. While the terminology may differ, common elements amongst the socialization process are anticipatory experiences, a period of transition into a formal role, and organizational experiences.

ANTICIPATORY SOCIALIZATION

The anticipatory socialization process has been scarcely investigated in athletic training. Mensch and Mitchell[7] have found that many potential athletic training students, or athletic training recruits, identify the sport culture as an appealing aspect of the athletic training profession. This corroborates with Pitney, Ilsley, and Rintala,[8] who found that a love of sports was a major draw to the profession for athletic trainers working in the collegiate setting.

> The identification with the sport culture during anticipatory socialization is related to what has been called a "team" orientation, which refers to being a part of the sports team. This runs in contrast to the more traditional health care model of anticipatory socialization in which a preprofessional is more likely to identify with the "patient" orientation.

ORGANIZATIONAL SOCIALIZATION

While the anticipatory socialization experiences are critical for preparing individuals for their professional roles, it is the beginning of a long process of professional development across the course of a career. Following the anticipatory socialization phase, individuals will select an employment setting, transition into a professional role, and enter an organization. The process of learning one's professional role within a specific job setting is termed *organizational socialization*. The experiences encountered in the employment setting, or organization, will be either consistent with or different from the anticipatory socialization experiences prior to taking a job, and an individual will reflect on and consider all of these experiences to formulate his or her perceptions of the new professional role.

> The induction phase of organizational socialization is often identified as the first year or 1.5 years of a job. Following the induction phase, a professional will continue his or her role (role continuance) and become an "insider" or veteran in the organization.

Figure 12-1 provides a model of the professional socialization process and captures the relationship between the anticipatory socialization experiences and the organizational socialization experiences.

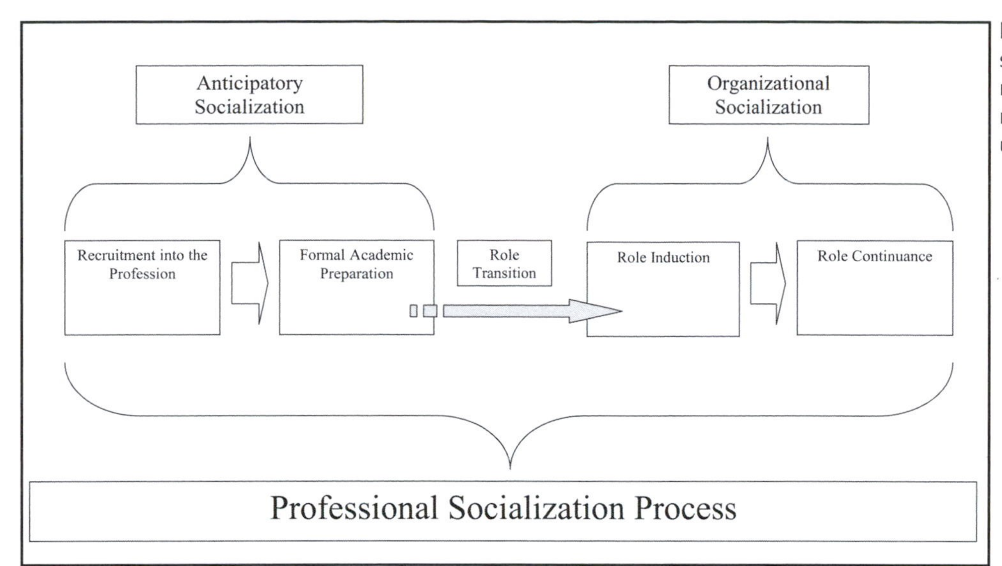

Figure 12-1. The professional socialization process consists of recruitment, formal education, role transition, induction, and ultimately role continuance.

Organizational socialization relates to how individuals learn their roles within an organization and how to deal with the various job demands.[6] The organizational socialization process is a key factor that contributes to whether a professional is satisfied with his or her job and prospers in the workplace or is dissatisfied and experiences a level of strain in his or her role. Although each organization operates and functions differently, they also have many aspects in common.[9] For example, as individuals are socialized into their organizational roles, they are likely to experience any number of socialization tactics. Understanding these tactics can help both employers and employees gain a better appreciation of how one's experiences can affect his or her role performance.

ORGANIZATIONAL SOCIALIZATION TACTICS

Many scholars refer to the organizational socialization process as "learning the ropes" of a job or "learning to fit in" with the organization. Ideally, the transition from school to an employment setting should be an easy one, although this is rarely the case. Indeed, many individuals will experience a degree of difficulty adjusting to the demands of a specific work organization and these difficulties will be discussed later. There are, however, strategies that can be employed to help improve the transition into a new organization and facilitate a professional's success in his or her work role.

The classic work of Van Maanen and Schein[10] identifies several dimensions of socialization tactics that are utilized, whether purposefully or not, within an organizational context. These tactics are basically ranges of experience that can influence how an individual responds to his or her employment setting, learns the ropes, fits in, and functions within the organization. The relevant tactical dimensions of socialization experiences are formal or informal, collective or individual, sequential or random, investiture or divestiture, and serial or disjunctive. Each of these are further explained next and summarized in Table 12-1.

FORMAL AND INFORMAL TACTICAL DIMENSIONS

Formal socialization experiences refer to extremely structured and tailored events that explicitly orient an individual to his or her role. Such experiences, as Van Maanen and Schein[10] state, leave no doubt as to what tasks should be performed and how they should be performed within an organization. A clear example of such a tactic is with medical documentation and processing of medical forms. Because many sports medicine clinics employ multiple personnel to treat patients yet process the reimbursement for services through a single office, it is often imperative that the medical notations, treatments, and services rendered conform to the same structure and function so information can be accessed, shared, and processed in an efficient manner. Thus, many clinics will provide very structured tutorials on the medical documentation process after an individual is hired. Such experiences make an individual's role extremely clear and leave little, if any, room for deviation.

Informal socialization experiences, on the other hand, do not structure experiences or make an attempt to provide an explicit level of orientation to a new role. These experiences are described as loose and relaxed; the employee is left to figure out how best to complete

Table 12-1

Summary of the Tactical Dimensions of Socialization Experiences

Socialization Experience	*Definition*
Formal	Refers to extremely structured and tailored events that explicitly orient an individual to his or her role
Informal	Does not structure experiences or make an attempt to provide an explicit level of orientation to a new role
Collective	Refers to having several individuals and placing them in a group so they encounter the same experiences together as they learn their professional role within an organization
Individual	Refers to having a unique set of experiences for a single person to encounter so he or she can learn a specific and tailored role within an organization.
Sequential	Relates to a specific sequence of events being necessary to complete prior to an employee being able to move into a determined organizational role
Random	The sequence of experiences necessary to take on an organizational role is unclear or ambiguous
Investiture	Occurs when an individual's attributes, characteristics, values, and attitudes are affirmed and valued by the organization and the organization does not wish to change them
Divestiture	Attempt to change an individual's attitude, values, skills, and patient interaction techniques to match the organization
Serial	Refers to the presence of a role model or mentor to orient and instruct individuals who are entering an organization
Disjunctive	Refers to a lack of role models or mentors to orient a new employee

his or her new role. In a study of the socialization of athletic trainers in the high school setting, Pitney[6] found that informal learning processes were common and many participants stated they learned their role by trial and error.

Collective and Individual Tactical Dimensions

Collective socialization refers to having several individuals and placing them in a group so they encounter the same experiences together as they learn their professional role within an organization. An example of this tactic is having approved clinical instructors for an athletic training education program complete a training program as a group. In this example, the collective socialization experiences often promote the requirements and expectations of the athletic training program and build consensus on how to address shared problems that the group may encounter in their roles.

Individual tactics refer to having a unique set of experiences for a single person to encounter so he or she can learn a specific and tailored role within an organization.[11] Individual socialization experiences are often used to differentiate an individual's responsibility apart from others and facilitate more innovation.[10]

Sequential and Random Tactical Dimensions

Sequential socialization tactics relate to a specific sequence of events being necessary to complete prior to an employee being able to move into a determined organizational role. A typical example of sequential socialization is found with mid and upper management positions. If, for example, an athletic trainer wished to manage a sports medicine center and oversee both the clinical and outreach components, the organization's upper management may make it clear that the prerequisite is having at least 1 year of full-time clinical experience and at least 2 years of clinical high school experience. In this instance, an employee can perhaps negotiate his or her role to obtain the necessary experience to move on to his or her desired management position.

With random socialization, the sequence of experiences necessary to take on an organizational role is unclear or ambiguous. As such, an employee wishing to obtain a new role within an organization or climb the organizational ladder will likely experience anxiety and stress.[10]

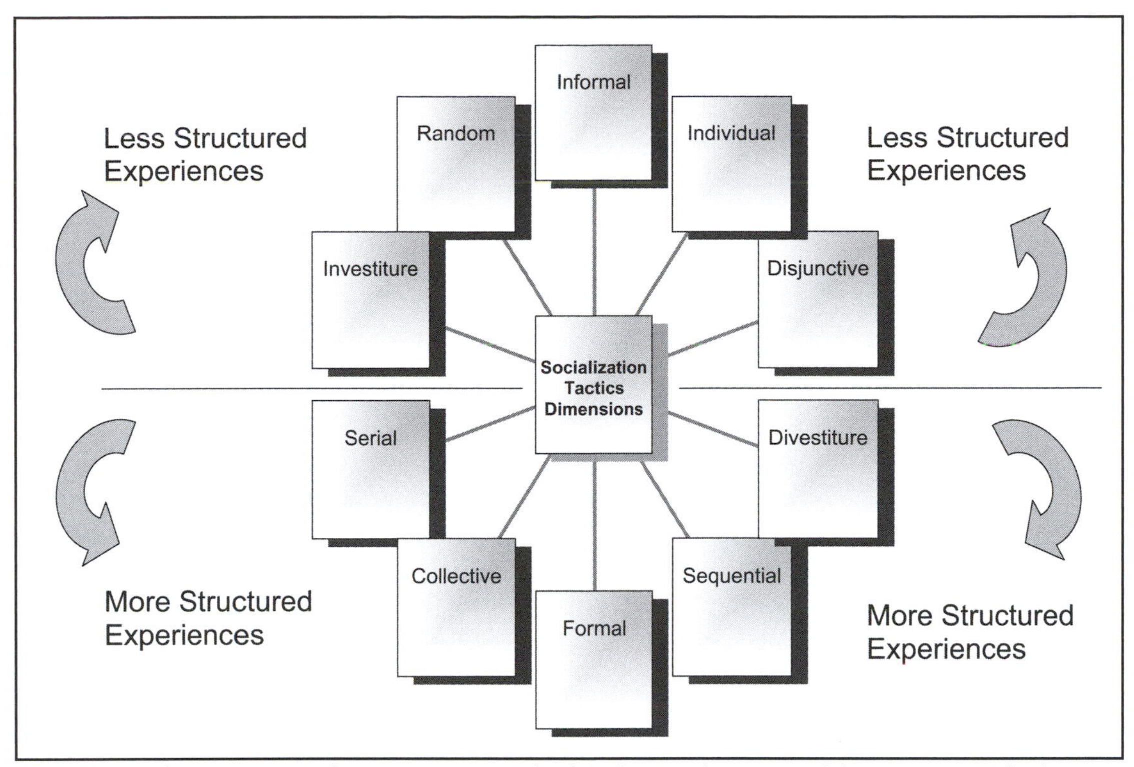

Figure 12-2. The various socialization tactics are displayed. Note the nature of the tactics (ie, whether or not they are structured) is identified.

Investiture and Divestiture Tactical Dimensions

Investiture socialization occurs when an individual's attributes, characteristics, values, and attitudes are affirmed and valued by the organization and the organization does not wish to change them. In such instances, the organization will support individuals in many different ways in hopes of facilitating a smooth transition into the work setting.

Divestiture socialization experiences, on the other hand, attempt to change an individual's attitude, values, skills, and patient interaction techniques to match the organization. To illustrate this tactic, consider an athletic training student who just completed an internship at a clinical setting where she was able to give 45 to 60 minutes of personal attention to each patient. Upon taking a position at a different clinic with higher case loads, the new athletic trainer will be socialized to an environment that requires more concise communication with the patients and the ability to multitask and instruct 2 patients simultaneously.

Serial and Disjunctive Tactical Dimensions

Serial socialization refers to the presence of a role model or mentor to orient and instruct individuals who are entering an organization. In many instances, serial tactics are used to facilitate the attainment of consistent set of values, skills, and attitudes within an organization.[10]

Disjunctive socialization simply refers to a lack of role models or mentors to orient a new employee. Such a tactic can allow the development of fresh perspectives and innovation, leading to new ways of performing within the organization.

Figure 12-2 displays the various tactics and identifies whether they are more or less structured. The type of socialization tactics used in an organizational setting facilitates the social structure and relationships that develop; as such, the tactics contribute to how a professional is influenced and how he or she perceives his or her professional role.

Conceptualizing the Relationships of the Organizational Socialization Tactics

It is important to understand that the various socialization tactics will not occur in isolation; rather they will occur in an integrated fashion within an organization. The types of tactics used in combination can have a substantial influence on how an employee responds and fits within the organization.

Less structured and more casual socialization tactics such as individual, informal, random, disjunctive, and investiture procedures will tend to facilitate innovation as an employee takes on a new role. Such an orientation can allow newcomers to an organization to challenge the status quo[10-13] and facilitate needed changes within an organization. The problem with an absence of structure, however, is it can also create ambiguity for employees,[14] leading to stress and conflict in one's job.

Socialization tactics that are more structured and less casual such as sequential, serial, and involve divestiture tend to promote an organization's status quo and a passive receipt of an organization's values and operational procedures.[14] The systematic and planned nature of these organizational tactics, though, tends to reduce ambiguity and conflict[14] so employees are clear on their roles and responsibilities within an organization. Some scholars[15] have linked these socialization tactics with the development of good compatibility between individuals and the organizations in which they work, often referred to as person-organization fit.

If an organization desires good person-organization fit and wishes to foster a clear role and easy transition for an employee, the use of more structured socialization tactics is warranted. If an organization desires to change its way of functioning and seeks different ways to obtain its objectives, then a less structured series of tactics is appropriate to foster employee innovation.

ORGANIZATIONAL INFLUENCES AND SOCIALIZATION OUTCOMES

Despite the best intentions to hire individuals who are distinctly qualified for an employment position and will fit well within an organization, the reality is that an athletic trainer's work environment is very complex and demanding. In many instances, athletic trainers will experience a number of perceptions related to work within an organization, including reality shock,[16] role stress/strain,[17] job dissatisfaction,[18] and concern about one's quality of life.[19] The next several paragraphs further explain these organizational influences that are framed as outcomes to organizational socialization.

REALITY SHOCK

Individuals who transition into a professional role within an organization are likely to experience a period of realization that work life differs from the educational experiences incurred during the anticipatory socialization phase.[20] This experience is termed *reality shock* and is derived from the work of Kramer[21] and Schmalenberg and Kramer.[22]

In discussing the work of Minkler and Biller,[23] Hardy and Hardy[17,24] explain that reality shock exists when there is a discrepancy between the professional role one anticipates and the actual role one is expected to perform within an organization.

The discrepancies in the anticipated and actual role have led to the thought that reality shock is the result of inappropriate anticipatory socialization processes. That is, the recruitment and formal educational experiences failed to adequately prepare an individual for a specific role.

In a study on the professional socialization of athletic trainers working in the intercollegiate setting, Pitney, Ilsley, and Rintala[8] found that there was a period of uncertainty and adjustment upon taking a job and entering the college setting for most participants, despite individuals having had 1 or 2 years' experience as a graduate assistant in a similar setting. Results from this study suggested that even with formal academic preparation in athletic training and having experienced a graduate assistantship, entering a formal work setting often resulted in increased levels of responsibility, longer work hours, higher volume of patients, and exposure to previously unseen aspects of the work environment. In total, these aspects of reality shock are stressful for the new employee.

These findings are consistent with athletic trainers beginning a position in the high school setting. Pitney[6] found that athletic trainers went through an adjustment period when entering the high school setting from a previous position, including transitioning from a bachelor's or master's degree program or a previous employment setting.

Both the Pitney et al[8] and Pitney[6] studies corroborate with Schwertner, Pinkston, O'Sullivan, and Denton[25] that physical therapists continue to be socialized into their roles after transitioning into employment settings.

The good news is reality shock will eventually lessen and professionals will soon recover from the intensity of the shock. The bad news is the shock is bound to happen to some extent. Organizations, however, can take proactive steps to help new employees through this transitional process. Formalized mentor programs can help during this process as they tend to offer a level of support. Moreover, orientation activities and collegial networking can also be of help. Pitney[6] found that athletic trainers working in the high school setting relied on networking with other professionals to adjust to their new roles in the organizations.

Activity 12-1

List experiences required of you as a student that may be designed to fully prepare you for your role as a professional and minimize the shock that is often experienced in a real work setting.

Role Related Problems: Components of Role Strain

As Hardy and Hardy[17,24] suggest, if an organization creates instances where an individual's professional roles are perceived as complex, conflicting, difficult, or simply too demanding, role strain will result. Role strain "...is a subjective state of emotional arousal in response to the external conditions of social stress" (p. 165)[17] while performing or attempting to perform a professional role. Role stress is "...a social structural condition in which role obligations are vague, irritating, difficult, conflicting, or impossible to meet" (p. 165).[17] There are many aspects or contributing factors of role strain that can make a professional role extremely complex in nature.

The relevant components of role strain, or role complexity, for most allied health professions include role conflict, role ambiguity, role incompetence, role incongruity, and role overload. Each of these components will be further explained and are summarized in Table 12-2.

Role Conflict

Role conflict relates to a professional feeling as though his or her expected role(s) is/are contradictory. That is, an athletic trainer feels as though addressing one expectation of the job interferes with completing another. If, for example, an individual was dual credentialed (as a BOC certified athletic trainer and an NSCA Strength and Conditioning Specialist) and was hired by a high school to be both the athletic trainer and strength and conditioning coach, a potential exists for a great deal of role conflict. A majority of the role conflict in this example is likely to occur during the after school hours when the need to facilitate the off-season conditioning of athletes interferes with the simultaneous need to prepare in-season athletes for practice and games. With this example, the conflict is the result of performing 2 distinct roles simultaneously and is referred to as inter-role conflict.

An individual need not have 2 positions to experience role conflict. An athletic trainer, for instance, may find it difficult to attend to the medical documentation required by the sports medicine center because of the need to closely supervise his or her current patient load. Intrarole conflict is when conflict exists because an individual is trying to achieve the responsibilities required of one role.

Role Ambiguity

The term *role ambiguity* is used to denote a set of professional responsibilities or expectations within an organization that are unclear, vague, or substantially lacking information to complete a role.[17,24,26] Imagine being hired to function as an athletic trainer in a college setting with the responsibility to work with volleyball and softball, only to learn later that you are also responsible for clinical instruction of athletic training students, yet this aspect of your role has not been explained. You might lack clarity about how the students are to be evaluated, what specific competencies you are to teach and evaluate, or how much direct supervision you must provide each of them. Producing even more ambiguity, you may not yet have learned the courses the students have completed, making it nearly impossible to expect them to integrate their knowledge and skill into the clinical setting.

As aforementioned, job settings that use less structured socialization tactics are likely to create situations that are ambiguous. This can lead to anxiety, job dissatisfaction, and lack of commitment to the organization,[26] all of which can contribute to attrition or an employee leaving his or her position, which is costly for an organization.

Role Incompetence

Role incompetence simply relates to a lack of knowledge and/or skill to adequately and acceptably perform a set of job expectations. Competence in one's professional role is related to adequate knowledge, skills, ability, and motivation to perform at an acceptable and successful level.[17] Provided an individual continues to engage in continuing professional education, he or she is likely to maintain a minimal level of competence to perform his or her role. Organizations can mitigate role incompetence by encouraging and promoting continued learning via financial support for educational conferences, in-services, workshops, and aggressive human resource development activity.

Role Incongruity

Role incongruity relates to an employee having incompatible abilities, attitudes, values, and/or

Table 12-2

Summary of the Components of Role Strain

Component	Definition
Role conflict	The presence of contradictory professional roles and expectations.
Role ambiguity	Having professional responsibilities that are vague or unclear.
Role incongruity	An instance where an employee has incompatible skills, values, or attitudes in relation to the professional role.
Role incompetence	A lack of knowledge and/or skill to perform a specific professional role.
Role overload	Having professional responsibilities that are too voluminous, leaving inadequate time to complete them.

dispositions for a required employment position or professional role in an organization. Role incongruity may occur, for example, when an assistant athletic trainer is promoted to a head athletic trainer position. Only after assuming the position does he or she realize that the heavy administrative responsibilities leave little time to deliver patient care, which he or she genuinely values. In this instance, the individual's "fit" with the role is not optimal.

To help prevent role incongruity, individuals need to reflect on and consider their values, skills, and abilities prior to taking a position. Moreover, they need to weigh and consider their values, skills, and abilities with what the organization expects from them to help with creating situations where there are role congruity and a good person-organization fit.

Organizations can prevent incongruity by making job descriptions clear and thoroughly interviewing individuals to ensure they recognize the expectations and responsibilities prior to taking a position. Moreover, a thorough interview can help employers determine that an employee's abilities, disposition, values, and attitudes are a good match for a given job.

Role Overload

Perhaps the most commonly experienced aspect of the athletic trainer's complex role is overload. Role overload is having more job responsibilities and obligations than time to complete them. An employee may, in order to fulfill his or her role, utilize personal time, resulting in a perceived imbalance in the time allotted for work and personal life. In a recent study by Pitney, Stuart, and Parker,[27] athletic trainers who were also teachers in the high school setting identified role overload as the most prevalent component of role strain (see Table 12-2).

Role Strain—Relationships Amongst the Components

As identified in the previous citations, a fair amount of research has investigated the various components of role strain experienced by athletic trainers and other health care providers. Additionally, recent socialization research in athletic training has exposed the prevalence of some of these components with evidence to suggest they critically influence an athletic trainer's roles. Role strain has been linked to a variety of negative organizational outcomes, including job dissatisfaction, depreciated commitment, attrition, or leaving a position, and lowered productivity.[28] This section will examine other research findings that have examined the relationship among and between these components of role strain.

Role conflict and role ambiguity have perhaps been more widely researched than the other components. Traditional research examined by Klenke-Hamel and Mathieu[29] revealed that both role ambiguity and role conflict lead to depreciated job satisfaction and an inclination to leave a position within an organization. More recently, this literature base has been verified and, indeed, role conflict and role ambiguity are directly related to overall job satisfaction, stress, and organizational commitment.[30]

Johnson, LaFrance, Meyer, Speyer, and Cox[26] studied the relationship between formalization, role conflict, and role ambiguity. Formalization was conceptualized as the extent to which occupational roles were explicit and supported with such things as job descriptions, rules, regulations, and policy manuals. Their findings showed that formalization was negatively related to both role ambiguity and role conflict; formalization predicted role ambiguity and role conflict. More formalized organizational procedures such as written policies, clear job descriptions, and explicit procedures lead to less role conflict and less role ambiguity.

In one of the earliest studies on organizational factors related to burnout in athletic trainers, Capel[31] examined the relationship of role conflict, role ambiguity, and role overload with dimensions of burnout, including emotional exhaustion, depersonalization, and personal accomplishment. The findings of her study revealed that high levels of role ambiguity and role conflict as well as higher numbers of athletes to treat and longer work hours (aspects of role overload) resulted in a higher intensity and frequency of burnout amongst athletic trainers, though the level of burnout found with athletic trainers was generally low.[31]

> There is no single definition of burnout, although burnout is often related to stress and results in emotional exhaustion, detachment from a job (lack of motivation to perform a role), and low levels of personal accomplishment.

In a more recent study of burnout in athletic training, Clapper and Harris,[32] like Capel,[31] found that burnout was not necessarily problematic. The authors did find, however, that time commitment, as an aspect of role overload, tended to be high among the athletic trainers.[32]

A key point is that the expectations an organization has for employees can lead to role-related problems, including, but not limited to, role conflict, role ambiguity, role incongruity, role overload, and role incompetence. Further, the incidence of these components of role strain can lead to substantial issues for the organization and the individuals working within it. These issues include depreciated job commitment, propensity to leave (attrition), symptoms of burnout, and job dissatisfaction (Figure 12-3). If not remedied, these issues can lead to costly problems such as lack of productivity and termination of employment.

Activity 12-2

With a partner, discuss why job dissatisfaction is costly for an organization. Make a list of the problems job dissatisfaction can cause.

STRUCTURAL ASPECTS OF ORGANIZATIONS AND THEIR POTENTIAL INFLUENCE ON ATHLETIC TRAINERS

Organizations exist to provide services and achieve specific social goals, such as delivering rehabilitation services, preventing injuries, and increasing patients' quality of life. To that end, all organizations will have an identifiable hierarchy, specific individuals to perform specific roles (termed *division of labor*), and established procedures for making informed decisions.[9] The goal for organizations is to deliver a service or product as efficiently and effectively as possible.[3]

Beyond these commonalities, an organization may have 1 of 2 orientations: 1) bureaucratic or 2) professional.[3] A bureaucratic orientation involves substantial hierarchy of authority, top-down decision making, division of labor, and formal rules and regulations.[9,10,26] A professional orientation differs in that the hierarchy of authority is not as substantial (often referred to as a flat organizational structure), which gives employees more autonomy to make decisions. Employees in this structure tend to have collegial relationships[3] rather than using control and authority to attain goals.

Bureaucratic orientations seem to offer substantial challenges for employees. In a recent study, athletic trainers working in the intercollegiate setting indicated that they often dealt with the bureaucratic tendencies of their organizations.[19] Though the athletic trainers were able to make decisions related to the health care of their athletes and function somewhat autonomously, the work environment was found to be political in nature and some of the participants in the study felt as though they were low in the organization's hierarchy and unable to influence how their job was structured (ie, when practices might be conducted). Many individuals in this study were surprised by the bureaucratic influences; this suggests that their anticipatory socialization did not expose them to such work environments.

As Pitney[19] identified, bureaucratic influences can lead to increased work volume and lack of administrative support and appreciation. Both high work volume and low support can lead to increased stress and negative perceptions of the organization's environment or climate. In fact, another key finding in the Pitney[19] study was that the organizational influences of high

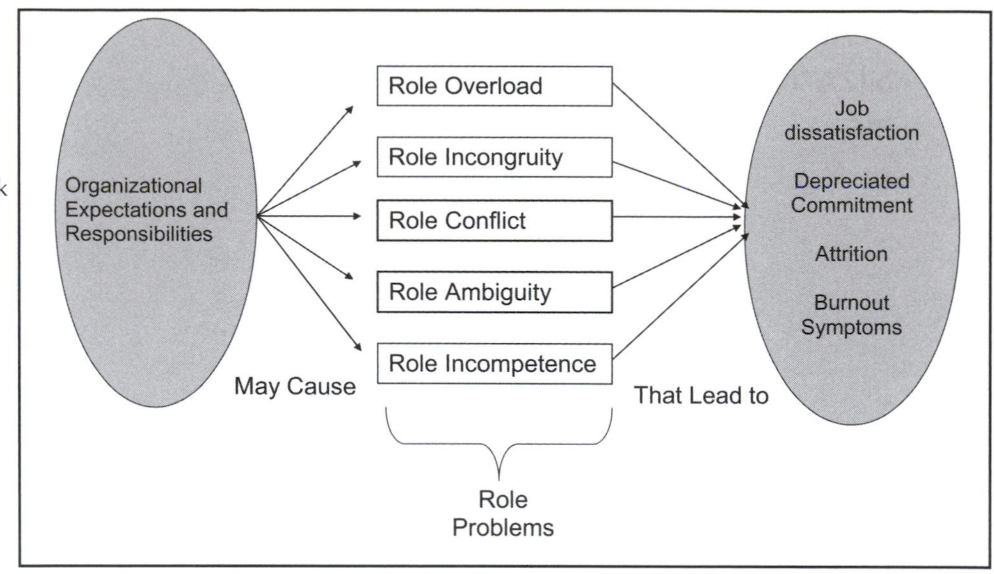

Figure 12-3. The expectations an organization presents to employee can result in role-related problems that are components of role strain. If not attended to, many consequences can result that produce a lack of productivity and turnover.

work demands such as long hours and high volume of patients, as well as lack of administrative support, led to a fear of burnout and inability to maintain a balance between work and personal life.

Activity 12-3

Role play a conversation with a mock employer with the goal of negotiating some strategies to establish more of a balance between your work life and personal life.

Concluding Thoughts Related to Organizational Structure

There exists an interesting paradox in considering the literature related to professional socialization, role strain, and organizational influences. An employment situation that is ill defined, ambiguous, and leads an athletic trainer to perform conflicting responsibilities can result in various negative consequences such as role ambiguity, role conflict, and role incongruity. To combat these negative consequences, an organization may utilize clearly delineated job descriptions, clear lines of authority, and formalized procedures for completing job-related responsibilities—all of which have bureaucratic characteristics. The paradox exists in that on one hand less structured and formalized procedures can result in stressful situations and so too can more formalized, bureaucratic tendencies.

The solution to this paradox likely rests with a balance in the dimensions of an organization's structure. That is to say, it is likely for organizational leaders to create and utilize clearly defined roles, responsibilities, and formalized procedures, yet still include professionals in the organization's decision-making process. Moreover, it is likely possible, with effort, for a bureaucratically oriented organization to periodically examine the work volume of employees and make adjustments as necessary.

Practical Applications for Encouraging Successful Organizational Socialization

For some readers, the previous paragraphs may paint a bleak picture of employment within an organization, but rest assured many organizations take great measures to facilitate the success of their employees while still accomplishing the goals of the organization. Moreover, professionals themselves can also take action to ensure successful role performance in a healthy and productive manner. The following sections provide practical strategies for both organizational leaders and athletic trainers to facilitate successful role transition and minimize the possibility of role-related problems such as role conflict, ambiguity, overload, incongruity, and incompetence.

Practical Suggestions for Organizational Leaders—What the Organization Can Do to Facilitate Successful Socialization

Although in the preceding sections I have eluded to what organizations can do to facilitate employee success and limit role strain, additional suggestions are offered. These suggestions are written in terms of what organizational leaders can do and summarized in Box 12-1.

- Consider the anticipatory socialization experiences of potential employees to determine the extent to which they are prepared for their role and to lessen the possibility of role incongruity.

  While graduates of athletic training education programs will have demonstrated clinical proficiency and achieved very specific educational competencies, not all programs emphasize the same clinical rotations. For example, some programs may provide students with a large amount of clinical education in the high school and college setting while minimizing exposure to sports medicine centers or hospitals. Certainly the opposite could also be true. In either event, employers must understand that a student's anticipatory socialization experiences set the stage for his or her career and the more one's anticipatory experiences differ from an employment setting, the more reality shock and role incongruity are likely to occur.

- Utilize formal orientation sessions and chances for employees to network with others in the organization to facilitate a successful adjustment to a new role.

  Despite carefully screening employees to determine a good fit to an organization, there is still a lot for employees to learn. To avoid role ambiguity and role conflict, orientation sessions should be utilized to provide instruction, discussion, and elaboration on an expected role.[8] Moreover, providing a chance to network with veteran employees can help new employees learn to adjust to their new role.[6] In fact, involving existing employees in the orientation of new hires provides an opportunity for them to meet one another, share ideas and experiences, and perhaps to connect with one another and develop a mentoring relationship.

- Understand that reality shock may occur during the role transition phase of socialization. Consider using planned mentoring activities to facilitate learning the professional role. Mentors can give practical advice to new employees and help them adjust to the employment demands.

  Mentoring relationships are key to learning about the structure and function of an organization and has been identified as a key factor to the development of expert athletic trainers.[36] The benefits of a mentoring relationship cannot only be obtained by newly inducted employees but also more veteran employees as well. Veteran

Box 12-1

What Organizational Leaders Can Do to Facilitate Successful Socialization Into Professional Roles

- Consider the anticipatory socialization experiences of potential employees to determine the extent to which they are prepared for their role and to lessen the possibility of role incongruity.
- Utilize formal orientation sessions and chances for employees to network with others in the organization to facilitate a successful adjustment to a new role.
- Understand that reality shock may occur during the role transition phase of socialization. Consider using planned mentoring activities to facilitate learning the professional role. Mentors can give practical advice to new employees and help them adjust to the employment demands.
- Create clear and explicit descriptions of job responsibilities to mitigate role ambiguity and role conflict.
- Provide in-service learning opportunities and support for continuing education activities to avoid professional obsolescence and role incompetence.
- Conduct periodic examinations of the responsibilities given to employees to see whether they are in conflict with one another or whether the responsibilities are too voluminous.
- Implement conflict and stress management training to help deal with role stress and strain.
- Consider using less structured socialization tactics when organizational change is needed, but be sure to communicate this to employees so they are aware of why there is a lack of structure.
- Include employees in the organization's decision-making process.

employees can become reinvested in their roles and facilitate their professional development.

- Create clear and explicit descriptions of job responsibilities to mitigate role ambiguity and role conflict.

  A great deal of role ambiguity and conflict stems from vague expectations and conflicting role responsibilities. Putting the organization's expectations for professionals in writing makes expectations explicit and clear.

- Provide in-service learning opportunities and support for continuing education activities to avoid professional obsolescence and role incompetence.

  Although learning is a two-way street, organizational leaders should expect professionals to stay current in their discipline. To this end, organizations should contribute to professional learning. Structuring learning experiences such as in-services is an excellent way to share knowledge between and among employees and send a message that learning is valued. Organizations should also contribute to continuing education financially to support employee learning. Keep in mind that one aspect of a bureaucracy is a lack of administrative support. Financial support and release time to learn new knowledge and skills related to the job reveals the existence of support. Many organizations expect employees who have attended a formal continuing education program to provide instruction (usually in the form of an in-service) to other employees. Such events help reinforce learning.

- Periodically examine the responsibilities given to employees to see whether they are in conflict with one another or whether the responsibilities are too voluminous.

  Change is inevitable and in many instances an employee's job becomes more complex. Periodic examinations of an employee's roles can allow the employer to update the job description to mitigate role ambiguity. Moreover, it allows an employer to get a sense of the work volume with which an employee is dealing. Only then can workloads be adjusted to prevent work overload.

- Implement conflict and stress management training to help deal with role stress and strain.

  We have discussed the negative consequences of role conflict and role ambiguity and identified that these can result in job dissatisfaction and symptoms of burnout. In many instances, helping employees deal with the stress and conflict is essential, especially since we do not work in isolation. Indeed, we interact with others constantly, and any dissatisfaction and burnout can strain our inter-relationships. Organizations should be proactive and utilize training to help employees through these issues.

- When organizational change is needed, consider using less structured socialization tactics, but communicate this to employees so they are aware of why there is a lack of structure.

  Vague expectations and unclear responsibilities can lead to role ambiguity. Organizations may see a need, however, to let a professional role unfold or develop over time, and thus wish to maintain less formalization so an employee can determine how best to function as a professional and accomplish a role. An example here can help to clarify. Let us take a scenario such as a sports medicine center that has decided to offer an athletic training outreach program to a local school district. The district has 2 high schools but can only afford to hire one athletic trainer to work for the district. When an individual is hired to fulfill the role, there will be several dynamics occurring: 1) one professional to serve 2 athletic programs at 2 different sites, 2) clinical responsibilities during the morning hours, 3) multiple levels of communication—the employee will likely need to communicate with the athletic director, clinical director, coaches, principals, and others. In this instance, it would be very difficult to hammer out a clear and unwavering job description until the needs of each high school and clinic are known. Indeed, the clinic may not want to overload the new athletic trainer and will want to "wait and see" what the volume of hours are like at the district prior to determining which mornings and at what times the athletic trainer will perform clinical duties. With this example, having this information can help an employee understand the socialization tactics and be more tolerant of the ambiguity. In fact, such tactics would allow the employee to negotiate or bargain what the job expectations should be as the role becomes clearer with time. This could possibly be very empowering for the employee.

- Include employees in the organization's decision-making process.

  Recall that bureaucracies often limit the input and decision-making ability of employees and that bureaucratic influences are challenging for professionals working within organizations. Despite having a definitive hierarchy and chain of command, organizations can borrow from the professional dimensions of an organization structure and seek input from employees to inform the decision-making process. This sends a message that employees are valued members of the organization and their input is respected, thus establishing a positive organizational climate.[3]

Practical Suggestions for the Professional—What the Employee Can Do to Facilitate Successful Socialization

Just as organizations can implement practical strategies to facilitate successful role socialization, professionals themselves can act in this process as well. These suggestions are written in terms of what a professional working within organizations can do and are summarized in Box 12-2.

- Prior to taking a job, ask for a clear job description and be sure to explore the organization's values, expectations, and interactions with employees to facilitate having a good fit with your values, knowledge, and skills.

  As an employee, you have a right to know your responsibilities within an organization. Understanding role expectations prior to accepting a job is one facet of gaining an understanding of the job and whether you will be a good fit in the organization. This can help alleviate role incongruity and ambiguity.

- Connect and network with colleagues in the same or similar work settings to help navigate the organizational context and various influences to which you will be exposed.

  Interacting with others who have become veterans within an organization can aid in understanding how the organization functions and facilitate a successful transition into one's role.[8] If this is not possible within the organization itself, individuals can seek to interact with colleagues in similar work environments. Pitney[6] learned that athletic trainers in the high school setting purposefully took opportunities to travel with teams so they could meet other athletic trainers in high school settings and discuss how best to deal with their work environments. These actions helped them adjust to their professional role.

- Understand that with less structured organizational socialization tactics, informal learning will likely be required of you to learn about the various facets of a job and how the organization works.

Box 12-2

What Professionals Can Do to Facilitate Successful Socialization Into Their Professional Roles

- Prior to taking a job, ask for a clear job description and be sure to explore the organization's values, expectations, and interactions with employees to facilitate having a good fit with your values, knowledge, and skills.
- Connect and network with colleagues in the same or similar work settings to help navigate the organizational context and various influences to which you will be exposed.
- Understand that with less structured organizational socialization tactics, informal learning will likely be required of you to learn about the various facets of a job and how the organization works.
- Understand that socialization is an interactive process and you can be proactive in how you respond to your role requirements.
- Engage in continuing education to prevent role incompetence.
- Communicate with others openly and honestly in a respectable manner and explore conflict management training opportunities.
- Prevent burnout by exploring psychological skills and techniques.
- Engage in a healthy lifestyle, including individually appropriate physical activity and proper nutrition in order to maintain wellness.

It appears that a great deal of learning amongst athletic trainers working in organizations relies heavily on informal processes or learning experiences with little if any structure.[8] This form of learning is common within organizations and is often related directly to problems that arise in the workplace. Understanding that not all information will be formally provided is helpful when taking a job so the extent of reality shock is lessened.

- Understand that socialization is an interactive process and you can be proactive in how you respond to your role requirements.

  Though you will experience many influences that will shape you as a professional within an organization, you have the capacity to reflect on your experiences and decide how to act and perform your role. For example, in instances where one role seems in conflict with another or you feel overloaded with a number of responsibilities, you may need to negotiate or participate in role bargaining.[17,24] Role negotiation relates to a professional communication with others within the organization, usually a supervisor, to figure out how best to work through a conflict. In a study on role strain among dual position teachers and athletic trainers in the high school setting, Pitney, Stuart, and Parker[27] found that those experiencing less role strain often used role negotiation to remedy their conflicts and overload.

- Engage in continuing education to prevent role incompetence.

  Not having appropriate knowledge or skill to fulfill your role obligations is a component of role strain and, as described previously, has many negative consequences. As a professional, you are obligated to stay current in the field and engage in continued, lifelong learning. Engage in purposeful continuing education to prevent professional obsolescence and maintain role competence.

- Communicate with others openly and honestly in a respectable manner and explore conflict management training opportunities.

  Collegial relationships are a characteristic of organizations with a professional orientation, as opposed to a bureaucratic orientation. Collegiality is based on respect for one another and can facilitate a positive organizational climate.[3] This, however, does not mean that conflicts will not occur because in fact they will. Seek conflict management training opportunities to learn how best to deal with conflict in a positive and constructive manner and maintain a good working environment.

- Prevent burnout by exploring psychological skills such as relaxation techniques and self-talk.

  Capel[31] suggests that in addition to good communication and other organizational strategies, professionals take an active role in preventing burnout. She recommends learning and incorporating psychological skills such as self-talk and relaxation techniques. Seek opportunities related to these psychological skills and others to take a proactive role in minimizing your risk for symptoms of burnout.

- Engage in a healthy lifestyle, including individually appropriate physical activity and proper nutrition, in order to maintain wellness.

  Research findings reveal that bureaucratic organizations can lead to depreciated employee wellness and actions should be taken to attend to one's health.[37] As health professionals, we know the benefits of proper exercise and diet; we must remember to heed our own advice and remember that despite the problematic aspects of the organizations in which we work we must take care of ourselves.

SUMMARY

- Define professional socialization and identify its phases.

  Professional socialization is the process of an individual or group learning various knowledge, skills, values, and attitudes related to a particular professional role. The phases of professional socialization include recruitment, pre-service (formal education), and organizational experiences. The recruitment and pre-service phases are often collectively referred to as the anticipatory phase.

- Explain the importance of professional and organizational socialization in preparing for specific professional roles.

  The anticipatory socialization phase allows individuals to foresee what will be expected of them in their professional role. If successful, the anticipatory socialization process will allow individuals to select a profession that is appropriate for them and gain a rich learning experience that prepares them for a specific work context. Each organization is different, however, and the organizational socialization process allows individuals to understand how the work setting operates and learn the organizational values, acceptable attitudes, and any specialized skills that are required. The organizational socialization process is a key factor that contributes to whether a professional is satisfied with his or her job and prospers in the workplace or is dissatisfied and experiences a level of strain in his or her role.

- Identify various organizational socialization tactics and provide examples of each.

  There are many tactics involved with organizational socialization. These tactics include formal or informal, collective or individual, sequential or random, investiture or divestiture, and serial or disjunctive.

  Formal socialization experiences refer to extremely structured and tailored events that explicitly orient an individual to his or her role. An example of this is a formal orientation session for processing patients as they enter a clinic. Conversely, informal processes lack a specific structure and an employee must eventually figure out how to process a patient. Collective socialization refers group experiences whereby a set of new employees would learn the patient processing procedures together. This contrasts with an individual tactic in which a single individual is taught a set of procedures. Sequential socialization tactics involve an explicit sequence of experience prior to moving into an organizational role. An example is when an organization articulates that an individual needs to have experience as an associate athletic trainer before becoming a head athletic trainer. Random tactics are ambiguous and an organization makes any requirements unclear. Investiture tactics involve an organization supporting and affirming an individual's characteristics. An example is having an employee with a strong customer service orientation and the work setting values that in the employee and does not wish to change it. Divestiture tactics, on the other hand, lead to the organization hoping to change an individual's characteristics, values, or ways of acting. If an employee, for example, did not speak politely to clients and yet the organization values customer service, then the organization would likely work to change the employee's attitude. Serial socialization refers to a new employee having a former mentor to assist him or her to learn a role. Disjunctive socialization simply refers to a lack of role models or mentors to orient a new employee.

- List the components of role strain and explain their potential negative impact on athletic trainers.

  The components of role strain include role conflict, role ambiguity, role incompetence, role incongruity, and role overload. When any of these components are experienced or perceived, individuals can experience lowered productivity, stress and anxiety, job dissatisfaction, lack of professional commitment, inclination to leave a position, and even burnout.

- Identify the fundamental organizational structures and describe the characteristics of each.

  An organization will have either a bureaucratic or professional structure. A bureaucratic orientation involves an explicit hierarchy of authority, top-down decision making, division of labor, and formal rules and regulations.[33-35] A professional orientation differs in that the hierarchy of authority is not as substantial (often referred to as a flat organizational structure), which gives employees more autonomy to make decisions. Employees in this structure tend to have collegial relationships[8] rather than using control and authority to attain goals.

- Appraise the practical implications of employment issues as they relate to the field of athletic training.

  The socialization process is complex and has the potential to positively or negatively influence new employees. Those who are socializing agents within an organization and the new employees themselves have roles to facilitate the successful transition into the workplace.

ACTIVITIES

The following activities are designed to reinforce material presented in the chapter and to allow for discussion among students and instructors.

Case Study 1: Professional Socialization

Jennifer Dillman is a recently certified athletic trainer who has just accepted a position at Anytown Sports Medicine Center (ASMC). Her job description states that she will work in the clinical setting from 8:00 am to 12:00 pm, performing rehabilitation and then service 2 local high schools from approximately 2:00 to 6:00 pm, covering practices. She was excited about her new job, especially the outreach services for which she felt very well prepared. She was a bit nervous about her clinical responsibilities, however.

She received a letter from her supervisor, John Earlman, identifying her specific start date and instructing her to meet with human resource services to select insurance coverage and benefits in the next 2 weeks. The only other information Jennifer received was the ASMC dress code.

Jennifer arrived at work early on her start date and was shocked to enter the lobby where 6 patients were waiting. Only one other staff member, Bobby Durango, was available and he was setting up the rehabilitation center area in order to initiate treatments. Bobby was not expecting Jennifer, but he graciously introduced himself and said she could go ahead and pick a patient and get started. Jennifer's anxiety level escalated and she was in shock that she was to begin treating patients, yet she was not familiar with how patients were processed and she noticed that much of the equipment was different from that which she was used to.

Debriefing Questions

- What do you see as the primary problem in this case?
- How could Jennifer be better socialized into her new role? What strategies would you suggest?
- Whose responsibility is it to help an employee become accustomed to his or her role? Explain.
- What form of role strain is Jennifer likely suffering from and what suggestions would you give to prevent similar instances from happening at ASMC in the future?

Case Study 2: Professional Socialization

Marty Cool had just changed jobs after working in the clinical setting for 10 years. He believed his clinical experience allowed him to become an expert at orthopaedic injury rehabilitation, but he missed working in the exciting world of college athletics.

When Marty started his job as one of three assistant athletic trainers at Anywhere University, the most senior assistant, Ken Maybury, was assigned as his mentor. Marty was pleased that Ken took the time to teach him about such things as the injury tracking system, the referral procedures, and general interworkings of the department.

As Marty's first year unfolded and he settled into his role working with the men's basketball team, Ken was sure to answer all of Marty's questions and help him understand the various job responsibilities. Marty was starting to become concerned, however, about 2 aspects of his job.

Though Marty was hesitant to express dissatisfaction, he decided to talk to Ken about how his work day was structured. He articulated that having to attend staff meetings at 7:00 am, perform morning treatments from 8:30 am to 1:00 pm, prep for practice from 1:30 to 3:00, cover practice from 3:00 to 6:00, and then clean the facilities after practice, was getting him home at 7:00 pm and he hardly saw his kids. He assured Ken that he was committed to his job, but the days were very long. Ken assured Marty that he was not alone and that they all worked long, hard hours and that was to be expected. Marty also confided in Ken that he was also uncomfortable with his lack of autonomy. It seemed that the head athletic trainer, Joe Oversight, seemed to be micromanaging Marty's treatment and rehabilitation procedures and insinuating that "this isn't how we do it at Anywhere University!" Marty expressed his concern with this because his treatments were based on the latest research and evidence published in the literature. Ken again assured Marty that he was not alone in his thoughts and that all of the other staff often felt that way about Joe. Ken stated, "Sometimes you just have to let your concerns go."

Marty left the conversation feeling anxious about how he would deal with this aspect of his role. While he appreciated Ken's willingness to "show him the ropes," Marty felt these concerns would be difficult to manage.

Debriefing Questions

- How would you describe the socialization tactics used in this case?
- What forms of role strain have resulted for Marty?
- How do you think Marty could have prevented these types of role strain, if at all?
- As you think about Marty's situation, what questions might you ask when interviewing for a job to get a sense of how the roles are structured? Explain what information or insights these questions would provide you.

References

1. Mensch J, Crews C, Mitchell M. Competing perspectives during organizational socialization on the role of certified athletic trainers in high school settings. *Journal of Athletic Training.* 2005;40:333-340.
2. McGarvey BD, Chambers MGA, Boore JRP. The influence of context on role behaviors of perioperative nurses. *Association of Operating Room Nurses Journal.* 2004;80(6):1103-1120.
3. Grigsby KA. Perceptions of the organization's climate: influenced by the organization's structure? *J Nurs Educ.* 1991;30(2):81-88.
4. Clark PG. Values in health care professional socialization: implications for geriatric education in interdisciplinary teamwork. *Gerontologist.* 1997;37:441-451.
5. McPherson BD. Socialization into and through sport involvement. In: Luschen GRF, Sage GH, eds. *Handbook for Social Science of Sport.* Champaign, IL: Stipes; 1981.
6. Pitney WA. The professional socialization of certified athletic trainers in high school settings: a grounded theory investigation. *Journal of Athletic Training.* 2002;37:286-292.
7. Mensch, J, Mitchell M. Choosing a career in athletic training: exploring the perceptions of potential recruits. *Journal of Athletic Training.* 2008;43:70-79.
8. Pitney WA, Ilseley P, Rintala J. The professional socialization of certified athletic trainers in the National Collegiate Athletic Association Division I Context. *Journal of Athletic Training.* 2002;37:63-70.
9. Conway ME. Organizations, professional autonomy and roles. In: Hardy ME, Conway ME, eds. *Role Theory: Perspective for Health Care Professionals.* 2nd ed. Norwalk, CT: Appleton and Lange; 1988:111-132.
10. Van Maanen J, Schein E. Toward a theory of organizational socialization. In: Staw B, ed. *Research in Organizational Behavior.* Greenwich, CT: JAI; 1979:209-261.
11. Ashforth BE, Saks AM, Lee RT. Socialization and newcomer adjustment: the role of organizational context. *Human Relations.* 1998;51(7):897.

12. Lawson HA. From rookie to veteran: workplace conditions in physical education and induction into the profession. In: Templin TJ, Schempp PG, eds. *Socialization Into Physical Education: Learning to Teach*. Indianapolis, IN: Benchmark; 1989.
13. Siegel PH, Agrawal S, Rigsby JT. Organizational and professional socialization: institutional isomorphism in an accounting context. *Mid-Atlantic Journal of Business*. 1997;33(1):49-68.
14. Kim T, Cable DM, Kim, S. Socialization tactics, employee proactivity, and person-organization fit. *J Appl Psychol*. 2005;90:232-241.
15. Cable DM, Parson CK. Socialization tactics and person-organization fit. *Personnel Psychology*. 2001;54:1-22.
16. Wilson A, Startup R. Nurse socialization: issues and problems. *J Adv Nurs*. 1991;16:1478-1486.
17. Hardy ME, Hardy WL. Role stress and role strain. In: Hardy ME, Conway ME, eds. *Role Therapy: Perspective for Health Care Professionals*. 2nd ed. Norwalk, CT: Appleton and Lange; 1988:159-239.
18. Ostroff C, Kozlowski SWJ. Organizational socialization as a learning process: the role of information acquisition. *Personnel Psychology*. 1992;5:849-874.
19. Pitney WA. Organizational influences and quality-of-life issues during the professional socialization of certified athletic trainers working in the National Collegiate Athletic Association Division I setting. *Journal of Athletic Training*. 2006;41:189-195.
20. Flynn SP, Hekelman FP. Reality shock: a case study in the socialization of new residents. *Fam Med*. 1993;25(10):633-636.
21. Kramer M. *Reality Shock: Why Nurses Leave Nursing*. St. Louis, MO: Mosby; 1974.
22. Schmalenberg C, Kramer M. *Coping With Reality Shock: The Voices of Experience*. Wakefield, MA: Nursing Resources; 1979.
23. Minkler M, Biller R. Role shock: a tool for conceptualizing stresses accompanying disruptive role transitions. *Human Relations*. 1979;32:125.
24. Hardy ME, Hardy,WL. Managing role strain. In: Hardy ME, Conway ME, eds. *Role Therapy: Perspective for Health Care Professionals*. 2nd ed. Norwalk, CT: Appleton and Lange; 1988:241-255.
25. Schwertner RM, Pinkston D, O'Sullivan P, Denton B. Transition from student to physical therapist: changes in perceptions of professional role and relationship between perceptions and job satisfaction. *Phys Ther*. 1987;67:695-701.
26. Johnson DJ, LaFrance BH, Meyer M, Speyer JB, Cox D. The impact of formalization, role conflict, role ambiguity, and communication quality of perceived organizational innovativeness in the cancer information service. *Evaluation and the Health Profession*. 1998;21(1):27-51.
27. Pitney WA, Stuart ME, Parker J. Role strain among dual position physical educators and athletic trainers working in the high school setting. *The Physical Educator*. 2008;65:157-168.
28. Mobily PR. An examination of role strain for university nurse faculty and its relation to socialization experiences and personal characteristics. *J Nurs Educ*. 1991;30(2):73-80.
29. Klenke-Hamel KE, Mathieu JE. Role strains, tension, and job satisfaction influences on employee's propensity to leave: a multiple-sample replication and extension. *Human Relations*. 1990;43(8):791-807.
30. Wolverton M, Wolverton ML, Gmelch WH. The impact of role conflict and ambiguity on academic deans. *Journal of Higher Education*. 1999;70(1):80.
31. Capel SA. Psychological and organizational factors related to burnout in athletic trainers. *Res Q Exerc Sport*. 1986;57(4):321-328.
32. Clapper D, Harris LL. Determining professional burnout of certified athletic trainers employed in the big ten athletic conference. Presented at: Great Lakes Athletic Trainers' Association Winter Meeting and Clinical Symposium; Madison, WI; March 18, 2006.
33. Hall RH. The concept of bureaucracy: an empirical assessment. *American Journal of Sociology*. 1963;69:32-40.
34. Hall RH. Professionalization and bureaucratization. *American Sociological Review*. 1968;33:92-104.
35. Nixon HL, Frey JH. *A Sociology of Sport*. Belmont, CA: Wadsworth; 1996.
36. Malasarn R, Bloom GA, Crumpton R. The development of expert male National Collegiate Athletic Association Division I certified athletic trainers. *Journal of Athletic Training*. 2002;37:55-62.
37. Hamil M. Wellness for professionals. In: Young WH, ed. *Professional Education in Transition: Visions for the Professions and New Strategies for Lifelong Learning*. Malabar, FL: Krieger; 1998:21-42.

Appendix A

EXAMPLES OF TYPES OF INTERVIEW QUESTIONS

GENERAL INTERVIEW QUESTIONS

- What were your major responsibilities?
- What were some of the toughest parts of that job?
- Describe the most significant project you have worked on so far.
- Have you held other positions like the one for which you are applying? Tell me about them.
- What did you like most about your last or most recent job?
- How have you benefited from your work with your last company?
- What could your past employers count on you for without fail?
- What kind of career progress did you make in your last job?
- In your last job, what problems did you identify that had previously been overlooked?
- Tell me about the most boring job you ever had.
- What did you do in your last job that made you more effective?
- If you were to hire someone to replace you in your last job, what kind of person would that be?
- How do you start a project when you get no direction from your supervisor?
- When is it OK to break the rules?
- What did you do to make your last job more interesting?
- Have you ever felt as if you had outgrown a job? Tell me about it.
- What did you do in your last job that made you feel proud?
- What kinds of rewards are most satisfying to you?
- What motivates you to put forth your best effort?
- Why do you think initiative is important?
- In your opinion, what does it take to be a "success?"
- What does it take to challenge you?
- If you saw a coworker doing something dishonest, would you tell your boss? What would you do about it?
- If you took out a full-page ad in a newspaper and had to describe yourself in only 3 words, what would those words be?
- How would you describe your personality?
- If I call your references, what will they say about you?
- What kind of people "bug" you?
- Describe the appropriate relationship between a supervisor and subordinates.
- What kind of relationship do you have with your associates, both at the same level and above and below?
- What is your management style? How do you think your subordinates perceive you?
- What do you think you owe your employer?
- What are your short-term or long-term career goals?

- What do you think it takes to be successful in a company like this one?
- Is there anything you wanted me to know about you that we have not discussed?
- Do you have any questions for me?
- Tell me how your patients would describe you and give examples.
- Why do you want to leave your current position?
- What do you expect to find in our organization that you have not found with your current employer?

BEHAVIORAL INTERVIEWING

- Describe your activities during a typical day on your last or current job.
- Tell me about a project that you were responsible for initiating.
- Tell me about your efforts to "sell" a new idea to your boss.
- How do you reward and encourage others?
- What have you done about your own professional development in the last 5 years?
- In what business situations do you feel dishonesty would be appropriate?
- Do you consider yourself a risk taker? Describe a situation in which you had to take a risk.
- What are 2 or 3 examples of tasks that you do not particularly enjoy doing? Indicate how you remain motivated to complete those tasks.
- As a manager, have you ever had to fire anyone? If so, what were the circumstances, and how did you handle it?
- Have you ever been in a situation where a project was returned for errors? What effect did this have on you?
- Think about a time when you had a patient of the opposite sex feel uncomfortable with rendering care to him or her. How did you handle that situation?
- Describe how you have responded when you have entered a patient's room and the patient did not want you in there.
- How have you responded in the past when you were given instructions by your manager that you did not agree with?
- Give me an example of a stressful situation that you found yourself in and how did you handle it?
- How do you respond when you have been given several assignments to do at one time?
- Since you are applying for a ________ position, tell me some qualities that make you the right person for this job.
- Tell me about a time when you had several important tasks to complete and how you accomplished them.
- Give me a specific example of how you made a project more effective in your last job.
- Give me an example of a task that you particularly do not enjoy and indicate how you have remained motivated to complete the task.

QUESTIONS THAT TARGET SPECIFIC JOB-SKILL REQUIREMENTS

- Give an example of a time when you could not participate in a discussion or could not finish a task because you did not have enough information. How did you move forward?
- Give an example of a time when you had to be relatively quick in coming to a decision.
- Give me an example of when you felt you were able to build motivation in your coworkers or subordinates.
- Tell me about a specific occasion when you conformed to a policy even though you did not agree with it.
- Describe the most significant written document, report, or presentation that you have completed.
- Give me an example of an important goal you set and tell me about your progress in reaching that goal.
- Give me an example of a time when you were able to communicate successfully with another person, even when that individual may not have personally liked you.
- Describe the most creative work-related project you have completed.
- Describe a time when you felt it was necessary to modify or change your actions in order to respond to the needs of another person.
- What did you do in your last job to contribute to a teamwork environment? Be specific.

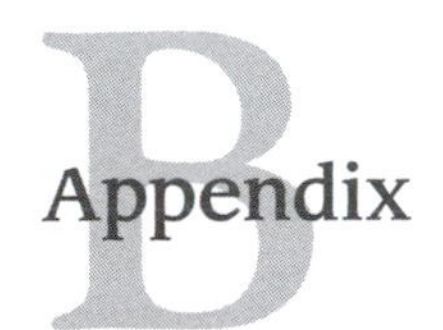

Appendix

SAMPLE ATHLETIC TRAINING OUTREACH CONTRACTS

ATHLETIC TRAINING EVENT COVERAGE: SAMPLE MEMO OF UNDERSTANDING

MEMORANDUM OF UNDERSTANDING BETWEEN
The (School/Institution/Organization) and Anytown Sports Medicine Clinic

The (Anytown Sports Medicine Clinic) has established an athletic training outreach program to provide athletic training services to high schools, small colleges, and other organizations/institutions. Under this program, a licensed athletic trainer from the (Anytown Sports Medicine Clinic) may provide athletic training services to a contracted institution or organization under the direction of a consulting Anytown Sports Medicine Clinic Sports Medicine Physician.

The (School/Institution/Organization) wishes to obtain the athletic training services of a (Anytown Sports Medicine Clinic) certified athletic trainer. Therefore, the (School/Institution/Organization) and the (Anytown Sports Medicine Clinic) agree to the following:

Athletic training services will be provided at (School/Institution/Organization) sponsored events by (Anytown Sports Medicine Clinic) athletic trainers as determined by the leadership of (School/Institution/Organization) and the supervisor of athletic training services for the (Anytown Sports Medicine Clinic).

Duties of the (Anytown Sports Medicine Clinic) athletic trainer include:

- Provision of first aid services on site.
- Provision of medical supplies customarily used by and supplied by athletic trainers in the course of on-site first aid.
- Initial injury evaluations and treatment.
- Record all time loss injuries and all other necessary record keeping.
- Advise athletes on the rehabilitation of athletic injuries.
- Precompetition set up.

The scope of these services will be limited to those services that an athletic trainer may provide on site with only off-site supervision by a consulting physician.

A (Anytown Sports Medicine Clinic) athletic trainer will assist in facilitating referral to a physician for care of any identified injury or emergency medical condition of an athlete.

The (Anytown Sports Medicine Clinic) and the Institution understand that (Anytown Sports Medicine Clinic) athletic trainers are considered "health care providers" under the Health Insurance Portability and Accountability Act of 1996 ("HIPAA") and are subject to HIPAA's rules and regulations. The (Anytown Sports Medicine Clinic) and the Institution agree that coaching staff, officials, and the executive director of the (School/Institution/Organization) are "involved in the care" of the student-athlete. This allows the coaches, officials, and the Executive Director of the (School/Institution/Organization) to receive information necessary to address injuries and to receive information concerning involvement in practice or competition to protect the health and safety of the athlete. If HIPAA is interpreted in a different manner in the future, the parties agree that the flow of information will need to be adjusted to comply.

All services would be provided under the off-site direction, supervision, and review of the licensed athletic trainer's consulting physician of the (Anytown Sports Medicine Clinic) and clinics sports medicine program. The athletic training services provided would in no way substitute for those of a physician.

The (Anytown Sports Medicine Clinic) will include the (Anytown Sports Medicine Clinic) athletic trainer providing services under this agreement within the professional liability coverage provided for (Anytown Sports Medicine Clinic) employees. The liability coverage applies solely to actions of the (Anytown Sports Medicine Clinic) athletic trainer as an employee of the (Anytown Sports Medicine Clinic) within the scope of his/her own duties and responsibilities. Claims against the athletic trainer or (Anytown Sports Medicine Clinic) are subject to section 893.80, (Your State) Stat. (Anytown Sports Medicine Clinic) does not provide liability coverage for the supervising physician(s). The supervising physician(s) are employed by (Anytown Sports Medicine Clinic) and are covered by the insurance program in accordance with and subject to section 893.82, (Your State) Stat.

The terms of this agreement shall be from 1/01/2007 through 12/31/2007. The agreement shall automatically renew for an additional year on each January 1 unless by the prior November 1 one party sends the other party written notice terminating the agreement.

The fee for this service will be $25.00/hour.

Both parties will review the agreement on an as-needed basis to determine if it is continuing to meet the needs and expectations of both parties. Either party may terminate this agreement at any time without cause by providing the other party with sixty (60) days written notice of termination.

For (Anytown Sports Medicine Clinic)	For the (School/Institution/ Club)
______________________________	______________________________
Chief Operating Officer	Chief Executive Officer
Date: ____________	Date: ________________

ATHLETIC TRAINING SCHOOL COVERAGE TWICE A WEEK: SAMPLE CONTRACT

(Anytown Sports Medicine Clinic) has established an athletic training outreach program to provide athletic training services to high school and small college athletic departments. Under this program, a licensed athletic trainer from the (Anytown Sports Medicine Clinic) may provide athletic training services to a contracted institution or organization under the direction of a consulting Anytown Sports Medicine Clinic Sports Medicine Physician.

(Name of School or Athletic Organization) wishes to provide the athletic training services of a (Anytown Sports Medicine Clinic) certified athletic trainer for the student-athletes at Institution. Therefore, the Institution and the (Anytown Sports Medicine Clinic) agree to the following terms :

Bi-weekly athletic training coverage will be provided at times determined by the athletic director from the Institution and assigned (Anytown Sports Medicine Clinic) athletic trainer. Sessions will last as long as needed to address the sports medicine needs of 7th through 12th grade athletes. In general, the sessions will last approximately 1 hour.

- Duties of the (Anytown Sports Medicine Clinic) athletic trainer include:
  - Initial injury evaluations and treatments
  - Physician referrals when appropriate
  - Record all time loss injuries
  - Direct the rehabilitation of athletic injuries
  - Implement injury prevention programs when necessary

Additional athletic training coverage of athletic events will be provided by a (Anytown Sports Medicine Clinic) athletic trainer as requested by the Institution's athletic director at a rate of $22.00/hour. This coverage is beyond the contracted 3 hours. The Institution will be billed for 15 minutes of set-up time prior to the event in addition to the actual athletic event time.

- Duties of the (Anytown Sports Medicine Clinic) athletic trainer include:
  - Precompetition set-up
  - Meeting with opposing coaches
  - Evaluating and treating athletic injuries within the scope of athletic training practice
  - Provide visiting teams with athletic training services as needed

Funding for necessary sports medicine supplies and equipment will be provided by the Institution.

A (Anytown Sports Medicine Clinic) athletic trainer will advise Institution officials on topics relevant to the health, safety, and performance enhancement for athletes at all levels on a continuing basis.

A (Anytown Sports Medicine Clinic) athletic trainer will facilitate referral to appropriate physicians in the timeliest manner possible for any injury or medical condition of an athlete.

A (Anytown Sports Medicine Clinic) athletic trainer will provide free skinfold testing for all of the Institution's wrestlers.

The (Anytown Sports Medicine Clinic) and the Institution understand that (Anytown Sports Medicine Clinic) athletic trainers are considered "health care providers" under the Health Insurance Portability and Accountability Act of 1996 ("HIPAA") and are subject to HIPAA's rules and regulations. The (Anytown Sports Medicine Clinic) and the Institution agree that school coaching staff are "involved in the care" of the student-athlete. This allows the coach to receive information necessary to address injuries and to receive information concerning involvement in practice or competition to protect the health and safety of the student-athlete.

The Institution agrees that starting in the fall of 2003, it will distribute information and collect documents supplied by (Anytown Sports Medicine Clinic) that are necessary for the (Anytown Sports Medicine Clinic) to comply with HIPAA. This information will be distributed as part of the agreement that the student-athlete and parents must sign at the beginning of each school year.

All services would be provided under the direction, supervision, and review of the licensed athletic trainer's consulting physician of the Anytown Sports Medicine Clinic Hospital and Clinics sports medicine program. The athletic training services provided would in no way substitute for those of a physician.

The (Anytown Sports Medicine Clinic) will provide professional liability coverage for the (Anytown Sports Medicine Clinic) athletic trainer providing services under this agreement. The liability coverage applies solely to actions of the (Anytown Sports Medicine Clinic) athletic trainer as an employee of the (Anytown Sports Medicine Clinic) within the scope of his or her own duties and responsibilities.

The period of agreement would be for:

The 2003/2004 and 2004/2005 school years @ a rate of $1800.00 annually.

The 2005/2006 and 2006/2007 school years @ a rate of $1975.00 annually.

The Institution will be invoiced each September for the amount indicated above.

Both parties will review the agreement on an as-needed basis to determine if it is continuing to meet the needs and expectations of both parties. Either party may terminate this agreement at any time without cause by providing the other party with sixty (60) days written notice of termination.

Additional event coverage as determined jointly by the Institution and the respective (Anytown Sports Medicine Clinic) athletic trainer will be billed separately to the athletic director at the Institution. These additional invoices will be sent in early November, March, and June of each school year to coincide with the end of the fall, winter, and spring sport seasons.

_______________________________	_______________________________
Date: _______________	Date: ______________________
For the (Anytown Sports Medicine Clinic)	For the School/Institution

DAILY ATHLETIC TRAINING COVERAGE: SAMPLE CONTRACT

The (Anytown Sports Medicine Clinic)) has established an athletic training outreach program to provide athletic training services to high school and small college athletic departments. Under this program, a licensed athletic trainer from the (Anytown Sports Medicine Clinic) may provide athletic training services to a contracted institution or organization under the direction of a consulting Anytown Sports Medicine Clinic sports medicine physician.

(Name of School or Athletic Organization) wishes to provide the athletic training services of a (Anytown Sports Medicine Clinic) certified athletic Trainer for the student-athletes at Institution. Therefore, the Institution and the (Anytown Sports Medicine Clinic) agree to the following terms:

Athletic training coverage will be provided by a (Anytown Sports Medicine Clinic) athletic trainer on Monday through Friday. This coverage will be 3 hours in duration each day. The athletic director from the Institution and the assigned (Anytown Sports Medicine Clinic) athletic trainer will determine the 3-hour time slot. The athletic training services will address the sports medicine needs of 7th through 12th grade athletes as well as staff.

- Duties of the (Anytown Sports Medicine Clinic) athletic trainer include:
    - Initial injury evaluations and treatments
    - Physician referrals when appropriate
    - Record all time loss injuries
    - Direct the rehabilitation of athletic injuries
    - Implement injury prevention programs when necessary

Additional athletic training coverage of athletic events will be provided by a (Anytown Sports Medicine Clinic) athletic trainer as requested by the Institution's athletic director at a rate of $20.00/hour. This coverage is beyond the contracted 3 hours. The Institution will be billed for 15 minutes of set-up time prior to the event in addition to the actual athletic event time.

- Duties of the (Anytown Sports Medicine Clinic) athletic trainer include:
    - Precompetition set up
    - Meeting with opposing coaches
    - Evaluating and treating athletic injuries within the scope of athletic training practice
    - Provide visiting teams with athletic training services as needed

Funding for necessary sports medicine supplies and equipment will be provided by the Institution.

A (Anytown Sports Medicine Clinic) athletic trainer will advise institution officials on topics relevant to the health, safety, and performance enhancement for athletes at all levels on a continuing basis.

A (Anytown Sports Medicine Clinic) athletic trainer will facilitate referral to appropriate physicians in the timeliest manner possible for any injury or medical condition of an athlete.

A (Anytown Sports Medicine Clinic) athletic trainer will provide free skinfold testing for all of the Institution's wrestlers.

The (Anytown Sports Medicine Clinic) and the Institution understand that (Anytown Sports Medicine Clinic) athletic trainers are considered "health care providers" under the Health Insurance Portability and Accountability Act of 1996 ("HIPAA") and are subject to HIPAA's rules and regulations. The (Anytown Sports Medicine Clinic) and the Institution agree that school coaching staff are "involved in the care" of the student-athlete. This allows the coach to receive information necessary to address injuries and to receive information concerning involvement in practice or competition to protect the health and safety of the student-athlete.

The Institution agrees that starting in the fall of 2003, it will distribute information and collect documents supplied by (Anytown Sports Medicine Clinic) that are necessary for the (Anytown Sports Medicine Clinic) to comply with HIPAA. This information will be distributed as part of the agreement that the student-athlete and parents must sign at the beginning of each school year.

All services would be provided under the direction, supervision, and review of the licensed athletic trainer's consulting physician of the Anytown Sports Medicine Clinic Hospital and Clinics sports medicine program. The athletic training services provided would in no way substitute for those of a physician.

The (Anytown Sports Medicine Clinic) will provide professional liability coverage for the (Anytown Sports Medicine Clinic) athletic trainer providing services under this agreement. The liability coverage applies solely to actions of the (Anytown Sports Medicine Clinic) athletic trainer as an employee of the (Anytown Sports Medicine Clinic) within the scope of his/her own duties and responsibilities.

The period of agreement would be for :

The 2003/2004 and 2004/2005 school years @ a rate of $6800.00 annually.

The 2005/2006 and 2006/2007 school years @ a rate of $7200.00 annually.

The Institution will be invoiced each September for the amount indicated above.

Both parties will review the agreement on an as-needed basis to determine if it is continuing to meet the needs and expectations of both parties. Either party may terminate this agreement at any time without cause by providing the other party with sixty (60) days written notice of termination.

Additional event coverage as determined jointly by the Institution and the respective (Anytown Sports Medicine Clinic) athletic trainer will be billed separately to the athletic director at the Institution. These additional invoices will be sent in early November, March, and June of each school year to coincide with the end of the fall, winter, and spring sport seasons.

______________________________	______________________________
Date: ______________	Date: ____________________
For the (Anytown Sports Medicine Clinic)	For the School/Institution

POSITION DESCRIPTION: PHYSICIAN EXTENDER/OUTREACH ATHLETIC TRAINER

The primary responsibilities of the clinic/outreach athletic trainer are to assist with clinic operations, work alongside other health care providers to provide injury evaluation and treatments, provide rehabilitative care to injured patients and athletes, to educate patients, school personnel and the public on injury prevention and other health-related issues.

Degree and area of specialization:

- Bachelor's degree required in athletic training or related field. Master's degree preferred. NATA-BOC certification and state licensure.

Minimum number of years and type of relevant work experience:

- One to 3 years of clinical experience working as a physician extender and outreach provider.

HOURS OF OPERATION

The normal time frame that an athletic trainer works within is from approximately 8:30 am to 5:30 pm. They work alongside other health care providers in the morning and are contracted with daily schools to be present for 3 hours daily in the afternoon. They are contracted with bi-weekly schools to be present twice per week at a predetermined time. However, the athletic trainers will cover up to 75 athletic contests per year per staff member on weekends and evenings at the schools that they are assigned.

General description of types of patients cared for, including age range:

- The patients that we primarily care for are adolescent and young adult athletes within the schools in our athletic training outreach program. In addition, we care for youth and an adult population when covering recreational events in the area. The age range would be from approximately 8 to 70 with most patients being between the ages of 12 and 19 years of age.

Major conditions/most frequent diagnoses treated:

- The primary conditions that are treated are sports-related musculoskeletal disorders and sports-related medical conditions. The injuries most commonly seen and treated involve the ankle, knee, and shoulder, but all sports injuries are treated by our athletic training staff in a field and clinical setting.

SPECIFIC DUTIES

Clinic

Athletic trainers work alongside the other health care professionals on a daily basis. The purpose of this is to enhance the quality of the clinic visit by improving services provided to the patient by the physician staff. Duties include but are not limited to:

- Triage the patient to make sure this is an appropriate referral
- Update medical records for current medication list and drug allergies
- Obtain the medical history
- Perform the initial injury evaluation
- Order diagnostic tests such as x-rays that will facilitate the physician evaluation
- Document the findings and dictate the clinic note for the physician examination
- Preparation for administration of injections
- Write referrals for rehabilitative services and provide initial rehabilitation guidelines
- Fit appropriate, noncustom orthotics, braces, or casts as ordered by the physician
- Assist in scheduling follow-up appointments for further physician visits or other diagnostic tests such as magnetic resonance or electromyography

Outreach

The outreach athletic trainer has the added responsibility of working daily in the athletic training room of a local school with which the clinic has a current contract for medical coverage. Coverage may be given at high schools, elementary/middle schools, or community colleges. As in any athletic training room, the certified athletic trainer is the primary and often sole caregiver and works under the supervision of a team physician. Specific duties include but are not limited to:

- Prevention, recognition, evaluation, and immediate care, rehabilitation, and reconditioning of athletic injuries
- Maintaining appropriate medical records and relevant paperwork
- Communicating with athletes, parents, athletic director(s), coaches, and physicians regarding athletes' playing status and ability to return to competition
- Referring athletes for appropriate physician care, diagnostic, and follow-up procedures and subsequent injury tracking
- All outreach and clinical athletic trainers will occasionally be asked to provide medical coverage at outside games, practices, and/or tournaments

Appendix C

ATHLETIC TRAINING INITIAL EVALUATION

Patient:______________________________ MD:______________________________
DX:______________________________
MD precautions:______________________________
W/C:______________________________
Today's date:______________________________ Date of surgery:______________________________

Subjective:
Date of onset/mechanism of injury/previous Rx:______________________________
____
____
Social Hx:______________________________
Chief complaint/functional limitations:______________________________
____
____
____
____
Medical/surgical Hx:______________________________
____
Medications:______________________________
____
Work/school/recreational tasks/activities:______________________________
____
____
____
MD work/school/recreational restrictions:______________________________
____

Objective:
Pain scale:______________________________
Skin integrity:______________________________
Posture:______________________________
____
Edema:______________________________
____
Proximal joint screen:______________________________
Distal joint screen:______________________________
Pt tenderness:______________________________

ROM: Joint motion	R	L	Strength: Muscle	R	L

Joint mobility:____________________

Muscle length:____________________

Neurological system:____________________

Special tests:____________________

Proprioception:____________________

Functional tests:____________________

Assessment:

Athletic training Dx/impairments and related functional limitations:

Prognosis:____________________

Plan of Care:

Goals:____________________

Frequency and duration:____________________

Athletic training interventions:____________________

Licensed Athletic Trainer:____________________ Date:__________

MD comments:____________________

MD:____________________ Date:__________

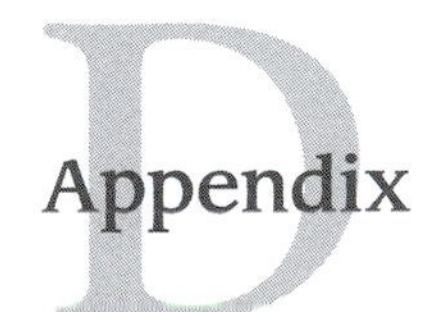

Appendix D

EXAMPLES OF FUNCTION AND IMPAIRMENT-BASED GOALS

ELBOW/HAND

1. Impairment based: Increase R elbow AROM = to L so Pt can reach into the back seat of the car for his or her briefcase without pain (4 wks).
2. Function based: Increase R UE grip strength, so Pt can carry his briefcase and luggage x 300 ft across the airport in his R UE without pain (6 wks).

SHOULDER

1. Function based: Increase R shoulder AROM so Pt can return to washing and combing hair 3 consecutive days independently (6 wks).
2. Impairment based: Increase R shoulder PROM = to L so Pt can don/doff T-shirt without pain (6 wks).

LOW BACK

1. Function based: Increase segmental spine mobility, so Pt can tolerate 45 min of sitting with $\leq$2/10 pain (4 wks).
2. Function based: Pt will demonstrate safe body mechanics with squatting and lifting 20# from floor to waist ht 3x without verbal cues from athletic trainer for return to safe lifting of grocery bags at home (6 wks).

HIP/KNEE

1. Function based: Increased L knee (hip) AROM so Pt can return to don/doff socks and tying shoes independently without modification (2 wks).
2. Function based: Increase L LE strength, so Pt can perform 5 L unilat mini-squats without UE support with good eccentric quad control and no hip IR for safe return to reciprocal stair amb (10 wks).

ANKLE

1. Impairment based: Increase R ankle PROM = to L so Pt can walk and accommodate to uneven surfaces to collect wood in the backyard safely (4 wks).
2. Function based: Increase R ankle strength so Pt can perform squat to kneel with R LE leading 3x without pain or loss of balance so Pt can perform safe floor transfers to play with her toddler at home (6 wks).

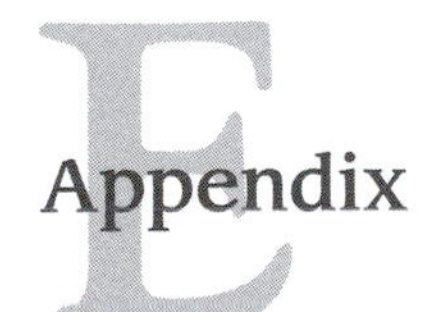

GOAL WRITING TIPS

The following are examples of functional activities included in goals in order of progressing function.

TEMPOROMANDIBULAR JOINT

- Chewing all foods, including hard and chewy foods
- Talking loudly without pain
- Yawning without pain or painful clicking
- Able to undergo a dental cleaning without pain

CERVICAL-THORACIC SPINE

- Uninterrupted sleep (hours or consecutive nights)
- Looking down to read a book (number of minutes)
- Typing at a computer and using a mouse (number of minutes)
- Putting on jacket/hooking bra behind back
- Turning to check for blind spots while driving
- Driving/holding/turning the steering wheel
- Time without tension headaches
- Looking up to change a light bulb
- Getting hair shampooed in salon shampoo chair without pain

LUMBOSACRAL SPINE

- Uninterrupted sleep (hours or consecutive nights)
- Bed mobility and transfers (speed and ease)
- Sitting, standing, walking endurance (minutes or hours) tied to community function
- Tolerance to home and work activities (hours or minutes)
- Floor transfers, picking up objects off floor
- Demonstrate safe lifting and pivoting without cues from licensed athletic trainer (pounds and pounds with number of repetitions)
- Return to exercise for cardiac fitness without pain (number of minutes of activity)

HAND/ELBOW

- Using eating utensils I
- Gripping pen/pencil, using mouse, holding keys, using pinch grip
- Holding full glass, drinking coffee, carrying dishes without dropping
- Uninterrupted sleep (hours or consecutive nights)
- Putting on and taking off jewelry (manipulation with clasps, etc)
- Driving (gripping and turning key to start car, stick shift, turning, putting seatbelt on, closing car door, etc) (number of min)

- Dressing independently (ie, tucking shirt, don/doff T-shirt, don/doff pants, hooking bra, zipping zipper)
- Grooming/washing/combing hair (number of minutes)
- Activity tolerance for office, home, computer work (minutes or hours)
- Reaching above head (number of inches) for putting dishes into overhead cupboards, hang up a jacket, change a light bulb, placing books into locker, etc
- Using garden tools, pruners, trimmers
- Lifting gallon of milk (7#) (or other object) in and out of fridge
- Lifting and carrying full grocery bags, briefcase, suitcase, laptop
- Other lifting (pounds lifted and sets/reps and over what distance or to what height)

SHOULDER

- Using eating utensils I
- Uninterrupted sleep (hours or consecutive nights)
- Driving (stick shift, turning, putting seatbelt on, closing car door, etc) (number of minutes)
- Dressing independently (ie, tucking shirt behind back, don/doff T-shirt, hooking bra behind back)
- Grooming/washing/combing hair (number of minutes)
- Activity tolerance below 90 degrees for office, home, computer work (minutes or hours)
- Returning to household activities (ie, vacuuming, dusting high surfaces, scrubbing shower/tub, washing car or other vehicle, washing windows, raking lawn, shoveling snow, fertilizing lawn, pushing a lawn mower, starting a lawn mower)
- Reaching above head (number of inches) for putting dishes into overhead cupboards, hanging up a jacket, changing a light bulb, placing books into locker, etc
- Lifting gallon of milk (7#) (or other object) in and out of fridge
- Lifting garbage bags, full grocery bags, briefcase, suitcase, laptop, 12- or 24-pack of soda, lifting children (into car seat) and/or carrying children
- Other lifting (pounds lifted and sets/reps and over what distance or to what height)

LOWER EXTREMITY

- Uninterrupted sleep (hours or consecutive nights)
- Ambulation (without antalgic gait, without assist device, altering speed, to cross street)
- Ability to rise from toilet I (knee flexion 95 degrees), basic and advanced transfers
- Tie and don/doff shoes I
- Kneeling to wash floor (number of minutes), pick up groceries off floor (number of reps), to get up from floor (number of reps), etc
- Stair ambulation (reciprocal pattern, without UE support on railing, safe, efficient, can carry objects)
- Stepping up to heights (curbs, stairs, step-stool or ladder, chair seat, climbing ladders, stepping up on playground equipment, etc)
- Single limb stance—reaching overhead without loss of balance (LOB) (number of times), don/doff pants, bend/squat without LOB
- Return to exercise for cardiac fitness without pain (number of minutes of activity)
- Ability to participate in physical education class (number of minutes) without limitation
- Landing appropriately/safely without mis-stepping (from number of inches/ft height); ex: step down from curb, stairs, step-stool or ladder, chair seat, treatment table, playground equipment

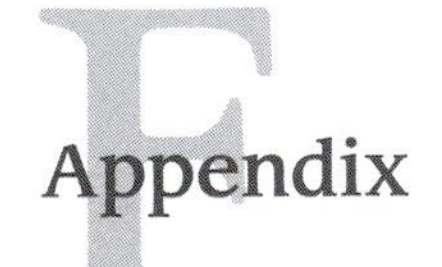

Appendix F

DAILY NOTES

Patient:______________________ MD:______________________

DX:____

MD Precautions:______________________ Date of surgery:______________________

Visits approved:______________________

Date: Visit #:___/___ Units billed/time:	Date: Visit #:___/___ Units billed/time:	Date: Visit #:___/___ Units billed/time:
S:	S:	S:
O: Modalities: HEP/Pt/family education: Education format: Pt/family response:	O: Modalities: HEP/Pt/family education: Education format: Pt/family response:	O: Modalities: HEP/Pt/family education: Education format: Pt/family response:
A:	A:	A:
P: LAT:	P: LAT:	P: LAT:

Cancelled appts: ______________________ No Shows: ______________________

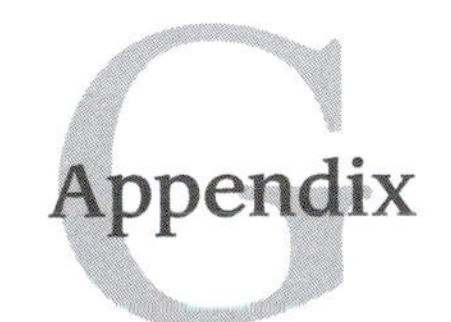

ATHLETIC TRAINING PROGRESS/DISCHARGE NOTE

____ Progress Note ____ Discharge Note

Patient:_______________________ MD:_______________________

DX:____

Today's date:_______________________ Date of surgery:_______________________

Date of 1st visit:_______________________ Date of last visit:_______________________

Patient compliance: Visits attended:__________ Visits scheduled:__________

Athletic Training Interventions:

Subjective (chief complaint; functional limitations):

Objective:

Assessment:

Plan of Care:

Goals (met, modified, continued):

Frequency and duration of additional rehab:

Athletic Training Interventions:

Certified Athletic Trainer:_______________________ Date:_______________

Cont athletic training:_______ D/C:_________

MD comments:____

____

____

MD signature:_______________________ Date:_______________

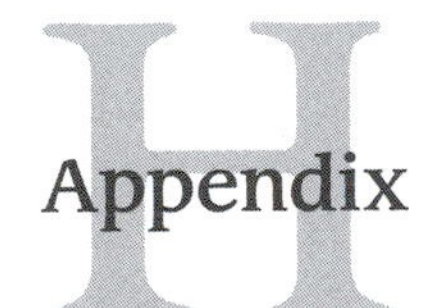

ATHLETIC TRAINING CHART REVIEW

	YES or N/A	NO
INITIAL EVALUATION		
Intake Paperwork/Subjective		
1. MD order with specific diagnosis, signed and dated (timeframe for script expiration dependent on individual state laws)	______	______
2. Medical history form	______	______
3. Medications listed	______	______
4. Date of injury onset listed	______	______
5. Patient's specific functional limitations noted	______	______
6. Patient's previous level of function listed	______	______
7. Patient's societal role listed	______	______
8. Patient's goal(s) listed	______	______
9. MD/work restrictions indicated	______	______
10. MD precautions listed, if applicable	______	______
Objective		
11. Functional limitations measured (numbers)	______	______
12. Work/task requirements described quantitatively	______	______
Assessment		
13. Athletic training diagnosis	______	______
14. Impairments related to functional limitations	______	______
15. Prognosis	______	______
16. Patient barriers listed, if applicable	______	______
17. Assessment clearly demonstrates Pt's need for rehab	______	______
Plan		
18. Duration of visits	______	______
19. Frequency of visits	______	______
20. Intervention list	______	______
21. Goals for every 2 to 3 wks of rehab	______	______
22. Goals are quantifiable/measurable	______	______
23. Goals create clear criteria for discharge	______	______
24. Specific, functional task listed in every goal	______	______
25. Time deadline for every goal	______	______
26. Impairment addressed in every goal	______	______
27. Goals relate specifically to plan of care/interventions	______	______

Comments:

DAILY NOTES	YES or N/A	NO
1. All SOAP sections filled in	______	______
2. One item reassessed every visit	______	______
3. Reason why modality was performed is listed, if applicable	______	______
4. Specific modality info listed, if applicable	______	______
5. Interventions selected clearly demonstrate need for LAT skills	______	______
6. Interventions are nonroutine and nonrepetitive	______	______
7. Evidence of skilled feedback with exercises presented	______	______
8. Exercises that can be performed at home are given in home exercise program	______	______
9. Assessment states patient's response to Rx specifically	______	______
10. Goals are reassessed every 2 to 3 visits	______	______
11. Plan lists specific ideas for next treatment	______	______
12. Modifications to treatment plan are listed	______	______
13. Communication with patient, MD, case managers documented	______	______
14. Changes in work status/restrictions noted	______	______
15. Pt/family education noted at least every 2 visits	______	______
16. Cancelled and no show appointments listed with dates	______	______
17. Visit number (actually attended) listed	______	______
18. Date of visit listed	______	______
19. Treatment time listed in minutes	______	______
20. All entries signed and dated	______	______
21. Total of billed treatment does not exceed treatment time	______	______
22. All treatment time billed required skilled intervention	______	______
23. Correct use of group therapy charges	______	______

Comments:

PROGRESS AND DISCHARGE NOTES	YES or N/A	NO
1. Functional abilities regained noted	______	______
2. Functional limitations remaining noted	______	______
3. Quantified objective data	______	______
4. Functional tests performed	______	______
5. Assessments address changes in impairments and function	______	______
6. Note refers back to previous notes, if applicable	______	______
7. Goals reassessed	______	______
8. Modified goals and reason why modified, if applicable	______	______
9. Timeline for all new goals	______	______
10. Frequency and duration for continued treatment listed	______	______
11. Modified intervention list	______	______
12. Comment on interventions eliminated and why	______	______
13. Statement on new focus of treatment for this bout of care	______	______
14. Demonstrate clinical decision-making skills if continuing or discontinuing rehab	______	______
15. Reasons for unmet goals on discharge notes	______	______
16. Further treatment recommendations on discharge notes (if applicable)	______	______
17. Re-certification obtained for additional visits (beyond those requested in initial evaluation)	______	______
18. MD signed initial evaluation and progress/discharge notes	______	______

Comments:

Appendix I

SAMPLE INSURANCE APPEAL LETTER

February 17, 2009

To Whom It May Concern:

I am the treating athletic trainer for Mr. T (DOB: 3/3/45), who is a member of your ABC insurance company plan. Mr. T underwent a right rotator cuff repair on 11/23/08 and has been seen in rehabilitation for 17 visits to date. A concern Mr. T and I shared at the start of his rehabilitation was whether the 20 visits Mr. T had been authorized for by ABC insurance company was a maximum number of visits, or whether additional visits might be available with additional authorization. Due to this concern, Jane, Sports Medicine Clinic patient financial counselor, contacted ABC. Per Jane's notes of the telephone conversation on 1/9/09, Mr. T's visits are 100% covered with a $20 co-pay, with 20 visits per calendar year allowed, then authorization would be needed (please see Jane's computer records). Jane passed this information along to me, and then I shared this information with Mr. T. On 2/1/09, it was clear that Mr. T would need additional visits, so Jane faxed over a Progress Note to request additional visits. On 2/16/09, Danelle from ABC called back and told Jane that this is a new ABC plan and that the 20 visits is a maximum number of visits available. Danelle also stated that ABC is sending out an alert to their customer service people to make sure they know it is a 20-visit limit. On 2/17/09, I called ABC and spoke with Tara, who recommended that I file an appeal on Mr. T's behalf.

I believe the reasons why this appeal should be granted are quite clear. Had Jane or myself been told that the 20 visits was a maximum number of visits, I would have further rationed Mr T's visits over that time period to somehow make this inadequate number of visits work. Receiving the wrong information guided my decision to give Mr. T the best start possible in rehabilitation utilizing the 20 visits, assuming that more would be available if medically necessary. After 17 visits have been used, now ABC says there are no more visits available. I understand that this patient and his employer selected this particular health plan, and that 20 visits is the maximum number of physical therapy visits available under this plan. However, we double checked the particulars with ABC and were misled. Now Mr. T is in definite need of the additional visits requested in the last progress note, but now they are not available unless he self-pays. This puts the patient in a very unfortunate situation that was not his fault and will likely lead to future shoulder and cervical dysfunction in the near future if additional visits are not granted. Please do not punish this extremely compliant patient due to a miscommunication from and among ABC customer service representatives. If you have any questions, please do not hesitate to contact me at 920-444-4444.

Sincerely,

Jill Murphy, MPT, LAT, CSCS
Sports Medicine Clinic

Appendix J

STANDARD MEDICAL ABBREVIATIONS

These abbreviations are the language of medicine. At the same time, it must be noted that acceptable abbreviations can vary by practice setting and institution, so only the most standard abbreviations are listed here. Also of note is the medical community's current emphasis on writing out full words instead of using abbreviations to help eliminate medical errors.

$\bar{a}$	before
A	assessment
AC	acromioclavicular
ACL	anterior collateral ligament
Amb	ambulation
AAROM	active assistive range of motion
AROM	active range of motion
ATC	athletic trainer, certified
B	bilateral
BPM	beats per minute
BBS	Berg Balance Scale
BID	twice per day
$\bar{c}$	with
C-spine	cervical spine
Ca	cancer
CHF	congestive heart failure
cm	centimeters
CMS	Center for Medicare and Medicaid Services
COG	center of gravity
contralat	contralateral
CPT	common procedural terminology
CSCS	certified strength and conditioning specialist
CT	computed tomography
CVA	cardiovascular accident
DDS	dentist
df	dorsiflexion
DIP	distal interphalangeal
DVT	deep venous thrombosis
Dx (s)	diagnosis (-es)
ER	emergency room
ERS	extended, rotated, and side bent (in reference to spinal segment)
ever	eversion
FCE	functional capacity evaluation
FHP	forward head posture
FRS	flexed, rotated, and side bent (in reference to spinal segment)
Fx	fracture
GH	glenohumeral
HEP	home exercise program
ht	height
Htn	hypertension
Hx	history
I	independently
ICD-9	*The International Classification of Diseases, Ninth Revision*
ICU	intensive care unit
ILA	inferior lateral angle (of sacrum)
inf	inferior
inv	inversion
Jt	joint
L	left
L-spine	lumbar spine
lat	lateral
LAT	licensed athletic trainer
LCL	lateral collateral ligament
LE	lower extremity
LOB	loss of balance
MCL	medial collateral ligament
MD	physician
med	medial
MFR	myofascial release
MI	myocardial infarction
mL	milliliters

MMT	manual muscle test
Mob(s)	mobilization (s)
MRI	magnetic resonance imaging
MVA	motor vehicle accident
NP	nurse practitioner
NSAIDS	nonsteroidal anti-inflammatory drugs
QID	four times per day
O	objective
OA	osteoarthritis
OT	occupational therapy
$\overline{p}$	after
P	plan
PCL	posterior collateral ligament
PE	pulmonary embolism
pf	plantarflexion
PIP	proximal interphalangeal
PNF	proprioceptive neuromuscular facilitation
POC	plan of care
PPT	physical performance test
PROM	passive range of motion
Pt	patient
PT	physical therapy
PTG	patellar tendon graft
R	right
RA	rheumatoid arthritis
RCL	radial collateral ligament
RD	registered dietician
R/O	rule out
ROM	range of motion
RTC	rotator cuff
Rx	treatment
$\overline{s}$	without
S	subjective
SAD	subacromial decompression
Scap	scapular
sec	seconds
SLS	single limb stance
SNF	skilled nursing facility
SOB	short of breath
s/p	status post
stab	stabilization
STM	soft tissue mobilization
sup	superior
Sx(s)	symptom (s)
T-spine	thoracic spine
THA	total hip arthroplasty
TID	three times per day
TKA	total knee arthroplasty
TMJ	temporomandibular joint
TSA	total shoulder arthroplasty
Tx	traction
UCL	ulnar collateral ligament
UE	upper extremity
unilat	unilateral
US	ultrasound
W/C	workman's compensation
WFL	within functional limits
y. o.	year old

Appendix K

BOARD OF CERTIFICATION STANDARDS OF PROFESSIONAL PRACTICE

INTRODUCTION

The mission of the Board of Certification Inc. (BOC) is to certify Athletic Trainers and to identify, for the public, quality healthcare professionals through a system of certification, adjudication, standards of practice and continuing competency programs. The BOC has been responsible for the certification of Athletic Trainers since 1969. Upon its inception, the BOC was a division of the professional membership organization the National Athletic Trainers' Association. However, in 1989, the BOC became an independent non-profit corporation.

Accordingly, the BOC provides a certification program for the entry-level Athletic Trainer that confers the ATC® credential and establishes requirements for maintaining status as a Certified Athletic Trainer (to be referred to as "Athletic Trainer" from this point forward). A nine member Board of Directors governs the BOC. There are six Athletic Trainer Directors, one Physician Director, one Public Director and one Corporate/Educational Director.

The BOC is the only accredited certification program for Athletic Trainers in the United States. Every five years, the BOC must undergo review and re-accreditation by the National Commission for Certifying Agencies (NCCA). The NCCA is the accreditation body of the National Organization for Competency Assurance.

The BOC Standards of Professional Practice consists of two sections:

- I. Practice Standards
- II. Code of Professional Responsibility

I. PRACTICE STANDARDS

Preamble

The Practice Standards (Standards) establish essential practice expectations for all Athletic Trainers. Compliance with the Standards is mandatory.

The Standards are intended to:

- Assist the public in understanding what to expect from an Athletic Trainer
- Assist the Athletic Trainer in evaluating the quality of patient care
- Assist the Athletic Trainer in understanding the duties and obligations imposed by virtue of holding the ATC® credential

The Standards are NOT intended to:

- Prescribe services
- Provide step-by-step procedures
- Ensure specific patient outcomes

The BOC does not express an opinion on the competence or warrant job performance of credential holders; however, every Athletic Trainer and applicant must agree to comply with the Standards at all times.

Standard 1: Direction

The Athletic Trainer renders service or treatment under the direction of a physician.

Standard 2: Prevention

The Athletic Trainer understands and uses preventive measures to ensure the highest quality of care for every patient.

Standard 3: Immediate Care

The Athletic Trainer provides standard immediate care procedures used in emergency situations, independent of setting.

Standard 4: Clinical Evaluation and Diagnosis

Prior to treatment, the Athletic Trainer assesses the patient's level of function. The patient's input is considered an integral part of the initial assessment. The Athletic Trainer follows standardized clinical practice in the area of diagnostic reasoning and medical decision making.

Standard 5: Treatment, Rehabilitation and Reconditioning

In development of a treatment program, the Athletic Trainer determines appropriate treatment, rehabilitation and/or reconditioning strategies. Treatment program objectives include long and short-term goals and an appraisal of those which the patient can realistically be expected to achieve from the program. Assessment measures to determine effectiveness of the program are incorporated into the program.

Standard 6: Program Discontinuation

The Athletic Trainer, with collaboration of the physician, recommends discontinuation of the athletic training service when the patient has received optimal benefit of the program. The Athletic Trainer, at the time of discontinuation, notes the final assessment of the patient's status.

Standard 7: Organization and Administration

All services are documented in writing by the Athletic Trainer and are part of the patient's permanent records. The Athletic Trainer accepts responsibility for recording details of the patient's health status.

II. CODE OF PROFESSIONAL RESPONSIBILITY

Preamble

The Code of Professional Responsibility (Code) mandates that BOC credential holders and applicants act in a professionally responsible manner in all athletic training services and activities. The BOC requires all Athletic Trainers and applicants to comply with the Code. The BOC may discipline, revoke or take other action with regard to the application or certification of an individual that does not adhere to the Code.

The Professional Practice and Discipline Guidelines and Procedures may be accessed via the BOC website, www.bocatc.org.

Code 1: Patient Responsibility

The Athletic Trainer or applicant:

- 1.1 Renders quality patient care regardless of the patient's race, religion, age, sex, nationality, disability, social/economic status or any other characteristic protected by law
- 1.2 Protects the patient from harm, acts always in the patient's best interests and is an advocate for the patient's welfare
- 1.3 Takes appropriate action to protect patients from Athletic Trainers, other healthcare providers or athletic training students who are incompetent, impaired or engaged in illegal or unethical practice
- 1.4 Maintains the confidentiality of patient information in accordance with applicable law
- 1.5 Communicates clearly and truthfully with patients and other persons involved in the patient's program, including, but not limited to, appropriate discussion of assessment results, program plans and progress
- 1.6 Respects and safeguards his or her relationship of trust and confidence with the patient and does not exploit his or her relationship with the patient for personal or financial gain
- 1.7 Exercises reasonable care, skill and judgment in all professional work

Code 2: Competency

The Athletic Trainer or applicant:

- 2.1 Engages in lifelong, professional and continuing educational activities
- 2.2 Participates in continuous quality improvement activities
- 2.3 Complies with the most current BOC recertification policies and requirements

Code 3: Professional Responsibility

The Athletic Trainer or applicant:

- 3.1 Practices in accordance with the most current BOC Practice Standards

3.2 Knows and complies with applicable local, state and/or federal rules, requirements, regulations and/or laws related to the practice of athletic training

3.3 Collaborates and cooperates with other healthcare providers involved in a patient's care

3.4 Respects the expertise and responsibility of all healthcare providers involved in a patient's care

3.5 Reports any suspected or known violation of a rule, requirement, regulation or law by him/herself and/or by another Athletic Trainer that is related to the practice of athletic training, public health, patient care or education

3.6 Reports any criminal convictions (with the exception of misdemeanor traffic offenses or traffic ordinance violations that do not involve the use of alcohol or drugs) and/or professional suspension, discipline or sanction received by him/herself or by another Athletic Trainer that is related to athletic training, public health, patient care or education

3.7 Complies with all BOC exam eligibility requirements and ensures that any information provided to the BOC in connection with any certification application is accurate and truthful

3.8 Does not, without proper authority, possess, use, copy, access, distribute or discuss certification exams, score reports, answer sheets, certificates, certificant or applicant files, documents or other materials

3.9 Is candid, responsible and truthful in making any statement to the BOC, and in making any statement in connection with athletic training to the public

3.10 Complies with all confidentiality and disclosure requirements of the BOC

3.11 Does not take any action that leads, or may lead, to the conviction, plea of guilty or plea of nolo contendere (no contest) to any felony or to a misdemeanor related to public health, patient care, athletics or education;, this includes, but is not limited to: rape; sexual abuse of a child or patient; actual or threatened use of a weapon of violence; the prohibited sale or distribution of controlled substance, or its possession with the intent to distribute; or the use of the position of an Athletic Trainer to improperly influence the outcome or score of an athletic contest or event or in connection with any gambling activity

3.12 Cooperates with BOC investigations into alleged illegal or unethical activities; this includes but is not limited to, providing factual and non-misleading information and responding to requests for information in a timely fashion

3.13 Does not endorse or advertise products or services with the use of, or by reference to, the BOC name without proper authorization

Code 4: Research

The Athletic Trainer or applicant who engages in research:

4.1 Conducts research according to accepted ethical research and reporting standards established by public law, institutional procedures and/or the health professions

4.2 Protects the rights and well being of research subjects

4.3 Conducts research activities with the goal of improving practice, education and public policy relative to the health needs of diverse populations, the health workforce, the organization and administration of health systems and healthcare delivery

Code 5: Social Responsibility

The Athletic Trainer or applicant:

5.1 Uses professional skills and knowledge to positively impact the community

Code 6: Business Practices

The Athletic Trainer or applicant:

6.1 Refrains from deceptive or fraudulent business practices

6.2 Maintains adequate and customary professional liability insurance

INDEX